BEYOND RESULTS

The Practitioner's Guide to Functional Lab Analysis in Pregnancy

SARAH THOMPSON

Author of *Functional Maternity: Using Functional Medicine and Nutrition to Improve Pregnancy and Childbirth Outcomes*

modern wisdom
PRESS

modern wisdom
PRESS

Modern Wisdom Press
Crestone, Colorado, USA
www.ModernWisdomPress.com

Hardcover ISBN: 978-1-951692-50-6

Cover design: Raúl Peña

Visit the author's website at www.FunctionalMaternity.com.

Table of Contents

Introduction

As practitioners, it is our job to provide the most comprehensive care for our patients. This begins with understanding how to read lab work, not just in diagnosing and managing overt disease but also in analyzing function to prevent disease and maximize physiology. Whether you are a midwife, physician, nutritionist, or other medical professional who treats pregnant women, this guide will help you better understand how blood chemistry can help you improve your patient care.

Pregnancy presents a unique challenge in lab work interpretation. Many parameters used outside of pregnancy and reference ranges in lab work are inaccurate during this period. This can make lab work analysis a complex task for healthcare providers who are not well versed in these changes. It's time to equip ourselves with the necessary knowledge to overcome these challenges!

My goal is to increase knowledge about the unique physiology of maternity care, and to help reduce pregnancy and childbirth complications by focusing on supporting the functional health of the mother through nutrition and lifestyle.

This is a comprehensive guide to laboratory testing, but it is not complete. For various reasons, some indices may not be included.

This guidebook divides the information into groups based on the standard blood-work analysis run during pregnancy. For ease of understanding, I've grouped panels and individual labs that are best run together or used to assess specific conditions.

The nutrition guidelines, supplements, and other preparations suggested in this book should be considered adjunctive to standard medical treatments. They should only be prescribed under the direct supervision of a trained medical provider. This guide is not a substitute for medical care.

Each section will summarize the individual indices or analytes and physiological changes associated with pregnancy, and describe how these changes affect values. You will be provided with evidence to support the various changes in standard reference ranges and possible causes of abnormal values. In addition, there may be evidence-based suggestions for dietary, lifestyle, and supplemental treatments. There may also be suggestions for additional labs. Because this list is incomplete, other indices may help you with differential diagnosis.

This is a guide and not a protocol list. It is your job to use this information to differentiate the correct diagnosis and use your excellent critical-thinking skills to create a specific protocol for your patient.

Reference ranges are variable. Each lab has its own range based on guidelines from organizations and their research. Science is never static; it is constantly changing. The ranges set forth in the book are also variable. Use them as a guide. No single value should be taken on its own. A good practitioner looks for patterns in the blood work in conjunction with patient health history, symptomology, and other lab analyses. The reference ranges in this book have been taken from various sources (see the reference lists at the end of each section), research, and other providers. Nothing is set in stone. As more studies are done, these ranges and guidelines may change. The information in this guidebook should not be considered a claim or a representation of absolute fact.

Standard ranges have been taken from LabCorp 2024. Pregnancy-specific standard reference ranges are taken from the American College of Obstetricians and Gynecologists (ACOG). Ranges are for six weeks postpartum unless otherwise specified. Functional ranges are based on studies that associate specific values with risk; they may vary and are not exact. As research databases continue to grow, these values and ranges may change.

White Blood Cell (WBC) Count

The total white blood cell (WBC) count measures the total amount of WBC found in a blood sample. It is found in the complete blood count (CBC) panel.

WBCs are also known as leukocytes. These cells are part of the immune system and help to fight infections and inflammation. They are further divided into categories based on function. (See the following differential analysis sections.) The WBC count is a valuable tool in assessing maternal health. Levels that are too high or too low may indicate dysfunction and may be a predictive factor for complications. Note that any stressful situation can increase WBC production, including both physical stress and emotional stress.

Based on their progenitor cells, leukopoiesis can be divided into two categories: myelopoiesis and lymphopoiesis.

Myelo- is Greek for "marrow." Myelopoiesis is the production of white blood cells from myeloid progenitors, such as agranulocyte monocytes and granulocytes. Interleukin-3 (IL-3), interleukin-5 (IL-5), macrophage colony-stimulating factor (M-CSF), and granulocyte-macrophage colony-stimulating factor (GM-CSF) stimulate the formation of monocytes. IL-3, IL-5, and granulocyte colony-stimulating factor (G-CSF) stimulate the formation of granulocyte white blood cells.

The major types of white blood cells include:

Basophils are involved in the inflammatory response and the release of histamines, which are important in allergic reactions and inflammation.

Eosinophils are primarily involved in defending against parasitic infections and allergic reactions. They release toxic substances to destroy parasites.

Lymphocytes are a critical component of the adaptive immune system. They include β cells, which produce antibodies, and T cells, which play a role in cell-mediated immunity.

Monocytes are another type of phagocyte that circulates in the bloodstream before differentiating into macrophages when they migrate into tissues. Macrophages are essential for clearing away cellular debris and pathogens.

Neutrophils are the most abundant type of white blood cell in circulation. They are phagocytes, meaning they engulf and digest bacteria and other microorganisms.

White blood cells serve several critical functions in the body's immune response. They constantly patrol the bloodstream and tissues to identify and eliminate foreign invaders, such as bacteria, viruses, fungi, and parasites. Neutrophils and monocytes are adept at engulfing and destroying pathogens. They ingest and digest microorganisms and cellular debris to prevent infection. Lymphocytes, particularly β cells, play a significant role in the adaptive immune response. They produce antibodies specific to a particular pathogen, and these antibodies can provide long-lasting immunity to that pathogen. Basophils and eosinophils are involved in the inflammatory response and reactions to allergens. They release chemicals like histamine, which can trigger inflammation, vasodilation, and increased blood flow to infected or damaged areas. Macrophages are crucial in the process of tissue repair and healing. They help remove damaged tissue and promote the regeneration of healthy tissue.

Pregnancy

In pregnancy, the upper reference limit for WBC is elevated by 36%, which is primarily driven by the rise in neutrophils. The WBC count may be 1.5 to 2 times higher than the nonpregnant baseline. The upper limit for neutrophils is 55% higher in pregnancy. The upper limit for lymphocytes is 36% lower in pregnancy. Monocyte counts increase by 38%. Eosinophils and basophils are unchanged in pregnancy.[1] WBC counts peak in the third trimester, just before delivery, and then again during childbirth. This is considered part of the body's preparation for potential infection during childbirth.

Postpartum

In the immediate postpartum period, there is often an increase in the WBC count. This is a normal response to the stress of labor and delivery, as well as the natural inflammation associated with the healing process after childbirth. The peak in WBC count typically occurs around two to three days after birth. This increase, known as "postpartum leukocytosis," is primarily due to the release of white blood cells stored in the bone marrow during pregnancy. Levels remain high for a week postpartum, decreasing to normal ranges by four weeks postpartum. Individual variations can exist based on birth experience.

> Breastfeeding can have a transient effect on WBC counts. Prolactin, the hormone responsible for milk production, can slightly elevate WBC counts in breastfeeding individuals. This is generally considered a normal response.
>
> While it is common to observe an increase in WBC counts in the early postpartum period, a persistently high or rising count beyond the expected time frame could indicate an infection or other complications requiring medical attention.

White Blood Cell (WBC) Count

***STANDARD LAB RANGE: 4.5 – 11 × 10^9/L**

Trimester	Standard Pregnancy Ranges	**Functional Pregnancy Ranges**
Preconception	4.5 – 11	**5 – 8**
First Trimester	5.7 – 13.6	**6 – 11**
Second Trimester	5.6 – 14.8	**6 – 11**
Third Trimester	5.6 – 16.9	**9 – 15**
Postpartum	4.5 – 11	**5 – 11**

*All standard lab ranges taken from LabCorp 2024 unless otherwise noted.

WBC CONVERSION TABLE

× 10^9/L	Cells/μL
0.05	50
0.1	100
0.2	200
0.3	300
0.4	400
0.5	500
0.6	600
0.8	800
1	1,000
5	5,000
10	10,000
15	15,000

*Research studies used varied measurements of × 10^9/L and Cells/μL.

Causes of Elevated White Blood Cell (WBC) Count

Acute Infections: WBCs increase in cases of acute infection. Outside of pregnancy, acute illness can be assessed by changes in the lymphocyte and neutrophil differential (neutrophil-to-lymphocyte ratio). This becomes more difficult during pregnancy, when neutrophils naturally increase and lymphocytes decrease. Variations in the normal pregnancy presentation of the differential may help determine the underlying cause of the illness. (See the following differential analysis sections.)

In pregnancy, the most common causes of infection are viruses or bacteria (such as urinary tract infections). Additional testing and symptomology may help determine whether the presentation is due to acute illness or inflammation. A urinalysis can be run to rule out urinary tract infections (UTIs). Often UTIs are asymptomatic in pregnancy, with signs only found in the WBC and differential and in the urinalysis. Women with high WBC and a history of premature rupture of membranes (PROM), intrauterine growth restriction (IUGR), incompetent cervix, preterm labor, or placental dysfunction should be assessed for infections (urinary and/or stool).

Intestinal Parasite: The differential can be used to determine if there are possible gut pathologies at play. A comprehensive stool test can be used to rule parasites in or out. Treatment may not be possible during pregnancy due to fetal risk. Management and support are the primary treatment options in this case. Gut pathologies do carry their own risks for pregnancy, including an increased risk of certain nutrition deficiencies (fat-soluble vitamins and minerals primarily). A classic presentation for parasitic infections is elevated monocytes, eosinophils, and basophils.

Inflammation: There is an element of normal inflammation that occurs during pregnancy, but when there is too much, we have disease. Inflammation can cause both an increase and a decrease in WBC counts. C-reactive protein (CRP) can be elevated in cases of excess inflammation, although symptomatically assessing for signs of inflammation may be more accurate than testing CRP in pregnancy. Women with a high WBC, low platelets, high hemoglobin, and high liver enzymes should be assessed for HELLP syndrome. (The acronym stands for hemolysis, elevated liver enzymes, and low platelet

---

Studies have shown that a total WBC >10 × 10^9/L in the first trimester is associated with an increased risk of developing late-onset preeclampsia.[2] [3] The risk of preeclampsia in those with a mild increase of the normal pregnancy range is most likely not a predictive marker. Better studies should be conducted with greater variation in group ranges.

An elevated WBC >10 × 10^9/L in the first trimester increases the risk of miscarriage, preterm delivery, and preterm premature rupture of membranes (PPROM).[4]

Postpartum leukocytosis is common and varies based on the delivery method. It is common for total WBC counts to reach 20 to 30 × 10^9/L in the first 24 hours after delivery and slowly decrease over the next few weeks. These levels should return to normal by six weeks postpartum.

count.) Often a high WBC is the first sign of HELLP syndrome and preeclampsia before blood pressure rises.[5] Inflammation can be a cause of lower progesterone levels. If you suspect inflammation, check progesterone levels.

Adrenal Hyperfunction: Cortisol stimulates the production of WBCs, specifically neutrophils, while decreasing lymphocytes, eosinophils, and basophils.[6] In acute stress reactions or times of elevated cortisol, there can be a drastic increase in WBCs. Cortisol is our stress hormone; it is needed to regulate life functions, including immune responses. Symptoms of high cortisol may also include anxiety and insomnia. Note that it is normal to have an increase in cortisol during pregnancy. If a woman has symptoms of elevated cortisol, such as a sudden onset of anxiety and/or insomnia, check her progesterone.

Polycythemia: Polycythemia is a rare blood disorder where the bone marrow is overstimulated to produce more blood cells than normal. Typically, this would present with elevated red blood cell (RBC) counts, as well as elevated platelets, but not always. Women with polycythemia vera (PV) who have normal RBCs but elevated WBCs are at a higher risk of stroke, hypertension, placental abruption, IUGR, intrauterine fetal demise, and preterm labor. Polycythemia vera in pregnancy is very rare but does occur. This is a condition that needs proper medical management.

Iron Overload/Hemochromatosis: This is more common in those with hemochromatosis and those with high alcohol consumption prior to pregnancy. Iron is oxidative and increases reactive oxygen species (ROS) production in the body. It is associated with tissue damage, including placental damage and embryonic death.[7] (See Iron Section.)

Sedentary Lifestyles: Physical activity helps to regulate WBC production; some stress in the body is good. Those with a more sedentary lifestyle have higher WBC counts.

Irregular Sleep: Sleep apnea, insomnia, and other irregular sleep patterns (often due to poor sleep hygiene) can be a cause of higher WBC counts.

Cancer: This would be the most severe cause of elevated WBC and very rare, but I would be remiss not to add it here. Specific patterns in the differential can be used to assess. Referral to physician specialists would be required if cancer is suspected.

Mycotoxin Exposure: Inflammatory mycotoxins may stimulate the release of pro-inflammatory cytokines and increase WBC production, resulting in leukocytosis.

Other Possible Causes: dehydration, physical trauma, medications, autoimmune disease, hyperthyroidism, allergic reactions, certain medications (steroids), heavy metal exposure, environmental toxin exposure

Treatment Strategies for Elevated White Blood Cell (WBC) Count

Diet

Adequate hydration is important for maintaining healthy blood circulation and for supporting the immune cells. Water is needed for cellular respiration. Eliminate refined carbohydrates and hydrogenated oils, gluten, and caffeine. Highly processed foods, which often contain excessive sugar, unhealthy fats, and additives, can contribute to inflammation. Excessive processed sugar intake can lead to inflammation and may impact immune function. Incorporate a variety of fruits and vegetables into the diet. They are rich in vitamins, minerals, and antioxidants that support immune function and help reduce inflammation.

Foods rich in omega-3 fatty acids, like fatty fish (salmon, mackerel, sardines), flaxseeds, and walnuts, have anti-inflammatory properties that may help reduce inflammation. Foods containing probiotics, such as yogurt and kefir, can promote a healthy gut microbiome, which is essential for a well-functioning immune system. Fresh herbs that have antimicrobial properties can also be beneficial. These include ginger, garlic, lemongrass, thyme, rosemary, oregano, turmeric, cloves, and other culinary herbs.

Identify and manage any food allergies or sensitivities, as they can lead to inflammation and affect WBC counts. The goal in diet therapy is to reduce foods that are highly inflammatory and increase foods that provide anti-inflammatory or antimicrobial properties.

Lifestyle

Aerobic exercise can help lower high WBC counts.[8] In research studies, the greatest reduction was seen in those who participated in exercise equaling 8,000 steps three or four times per week. The best activity was walking/hiking. The reduction is seen over six months of continuous exercise. This is something that would be addressed in the preconception phase leading to pregnancy, and in those with higher levels in the first trimester. The higher the intensity of the workouts, the greater the decrease in WBC counts. Make sure that they are going to bed at a decent time. Not spending time on electronics before bed can help regulate sleep patterns. Sleep hygiene is the idea of cleaning habits and routines surrounding sleep. If they are struggling with restless sleep, a sleep study may be needed to assess for apnea.

Supplement

Antioxidant therapy may be a promising approach to prevention when risk factors are identified. N-acetyl cysteine and alpha-lipoic acid are two that studies have shown have a good safety profile and effectiveness. Omega-3 fatty acids impact hematopoietic differentiation by reducing myeloid progenitor cell frequency in the bone marrow and promoting progenitor cell differentiation.[9] Dosages may vary depending on the individual and their symptomology.

Additional Testing

c-reactive protein (CPR); ferritin; iron and total iron-binding capacity (TIBC); comprehensive metabolic panel (CMP); vitamin D, 25-hydroxy (25-hydroxycalciferol, 25OH-D); comprehensive thyroid profile II; thyroid peroxidase antibodies (TPOAb); thyroglobulin antibody (TgAb); thyroid receptor antibodies (TRAb); progesterone; urinalysis; toxin testing; sleep study; comprehensive stool testing

Causes of Low White Blood Cell (WBC) Count

Low WBC ($<9 \times 10^9$/L), low neutrophil count, and a decreased neutrophil-to-lymphocyte ratio are seen in women with cholestasis in the third trimester.[10]

Autoimmune Disease: Lupus, Hashimoto's thyroiditis, and other autoimmune diseases can be characterized by low WBC counts. In general, autoimmune diseases are five times more common in women, and the changes in maternal hormones and physiology can increase the onset of autoimmune disease presentation around reproduction. Systemic lupus erythematosus (SLE) may first appear in pregnancy. Women with a history of recurrent loss, unexplained second-trimester loss, IUGR, or unexplained preterm delivery with low WBCs and low platelets should be assessed for autoimmune disease.

Additional testing of antinuclear antibodies (ANA) is helpful in determining if autoimmune disease may be present. In the differential, you may see higher lymphocytes and lower neutrophils. In the comprehensive metabolic panel (CMP), you may see an increase in blood urea nitrogen (BUN). Autoimmune disease can be a cause of lower progesterone levels. If your patient has a preexisting autoimmune disease, it is important to monitor their progesterone levels throughout pregnancy.

Chronic Infections: Over time, chronic infections deplete the WBCs (too many soldiers dying in battle). In chronic infections, you may also see a decrease in neutrophils and an increase in monocytes as they clean up the damage. These infections could be bacterial but also long-standing or latent viral infections, such as Epstein-Barr virus, herpes simplex, human papillomavirus (HPV), or hepatitis. This can also be seen in chronic Lyme disease and mold exposure. A classic WBC pattern for mold exposure is low WBC counts, low lymphocytes, elevated eosinophils, elevated liver enzymes, and low kidney function.

Inflammation: Low WBC counts are seen in cases of chronic inflammation. This can be due to infection, oxidative stress, or other causes. This is often associated with low cortisol function.

Adrenal Hypofunction: When stress is long-term or the body is struggling to produce cortisol, it can change the production of WBCs. Chronic stress can cause lower progesterone levels. If you suspect chronic adrenal hypofunction, you should also test progesterone levels.

Medications: Certain medications, such as antibiotics, can cause lower WBCs. Always investigate medication use when a low WBC is present. Preconception history is important.

Age: Women over the age of 40 tend to have lower WBC counts, and this is physiologically normal. There are many reasons why older moms are at a higher risk of inflammation and immune-system-related complications. No matter how hard we try to ignore it, we do age, and our bodies age with us. Increased risk does not mean that problems are inevitable; it just means there is a higher likelihood. I know many advanced maternal age mothers who have amazing, beautiful, and uncomplicated pregnancies. Each pregnancy is different, and each mother is different. There are really no standards, and each patient should be treated as an individual.

Overexercising: Vigorous and strenuous exercise is a form of stress. These forms of exercise increase cortisol production and, over time, can cause a decrease in WBC production via chronic stress mechanisms. Professional athletes, those who train vigorously and continuously, have lower WBC counts.[11]

Mycotoxin Exposure: Immunosuppressive mycotoxins may impair immune function and decrease WBC production, leading to leukopenia. Mycotoxins significantly decline the total WBCs, granulocytes, lymphocytes, and platelets while increasing alanine aminotransferase (ALT)(SGPT) and alkaline phosphatase (ALP).

Vitamin B6 (Pyridoxine) Deficiency: Vitamin B6 is required for making interleukin-2 (IL-2), which directs the actions of white blood cells. Vitamin B6 is also involved in the synthesis of DNA, which is essential for the production and maturation of white blood cells in the bone marrow. A deficiency in vitamin B6 can result in a reduced ability to produce new and functional WBCs.

Vitamin B9 (Folate) Deficiency: Blast cells require vitamin B9 for proliferation during their differentiation via methylation and mitosis support. A deficiency in vitamin B9 can cause lower WBC counts. Vitamin B9 deficiency can also lead to megaloblastic anemia, and assessing the other indices in the CBC can help you determine whether vitamin B9 is a contributing factor.

Vitamin B12 (Cobalamin) Deficiency: Blast cells require vitamin B12 for proliferation during their differentiation via methylation and mitosis support in conjunction with vitamin B9 (folate). A deficiency in vitamin B12 can cause lower WBC counts. Looking at the rest of the CBC can give clues to assessing vitamin B12 levels. This is more common in women with digestive issues or those taking antacid medications. Vitamin B12 deficiency can also lead to megaloblastic anemia, and assessing the complete blood count can help you determine whether vitamin B12 is a contributing factor.

Copper Deficiency: Copper regulates the differentiation of WBC progenitor cells by regulating granulocyte colony-stimulating factor (G-CSF) production. Copper also regulates the maturation of neutrophils and is a structural component of superoxide dismutase (SOD). SOD is the most abundant antioxidant in blood cells and helps to protect against oxidative stress. Low copper causes low neutrophils. Copper levels should increase throughout pregnancy.

Zinc Deficiency: There is a balance between zinc and copper in stimulating CSF. It is also essential to enzyme systems that influence cell division and proliferation in mitosis. Low zinc causes higher neutrophils and lower lymphocytes. An element of a lower zinc level is normal in pregnancy, as long as it is not deficient.

Selenium Deficiency: Selenium regulates lymphocyte proliferation. Low WBC counts with extremely low lymphocyte counts may indicate selenium deficiency.

Vitamin C Deficiency: Vitamin C is actively transported into white blood cells and is required for T-cell lymphocyte differentiation, proliferation, and function. Vitamin C also helps to regulate interleukin production. Interleukins regulate the production and differentiation of WBCs.

Vitamin A Deficiency: Vitamin A stimulates the differentiation and maturation of promyelocytes to granulocytes, and with vitamin D3 it regulates monopoiesis, the formation of monocytes. Low vitamin A can cause low monocytes. Vitamin A is also required for lymphocyte differentiation and growth.

Vitamin D Deficiency: Vitamin D3 inhibits interleukin-4 (IL-4) and granulocyte/monocyte colony-stimulating factor (GM-CSF), which stimulates monocyte-to-dendrite cell maturation. Deficiencies in vitamin D can cause higher monocyte counts by decreasing the conversion of monocytes to dendrites.

Vitamin K Deficiency: Studies have shown a connection between vitamin K2 and changes in WBC counts and function, but no mechanism is currently elucidated. MK-4, a specific form of vitamin K, promotes healthy stem-cell production and is found in high amounts in bone marrow.

Other Possible Causes: environmental toxin exposure, hypothyroidism, genetic anemias, cancer

Treatment Strategies for Low White Blood Cell (WBC) Count

Diet

This may depend on the underlying cause. Focusing on increasing antioxidant-rich foods is always important in the presence of both acute and chronic infections and inflammation. Removing highly inflammatory foods is also important. Increasing dietary consumption of identified nutritional deficiencies is essential. Include sources of omega-3 fatty acids, like fatty fish (salmon, mackerel), flaxseeds, chia seeds, and walnuts. Omega-3s have anti-inflammatory properties and support immune function. Consuming probiotic-rich foods like yogurt, kefir, and fermented foods may help maintain a healthy gut microbiome, which plays a role in overall immune function. Culinary herbs such as oregano, thyme, basil, rosemary, sage, turmeric, cilantro, parsley, ginger, and garlic all offer antioxidant and antimicrobial benefits.

Lifestyle

Anaerobic exercise is best for those with low WBC counts, as high-impact aerobic activity can decrease WBC counts. Lower WBC counts are seen in professional athletes or those who overtrain. Yoga and Pilates are better exercise options for those with low WBC counts. Adequate quality sleep is crucial for maintaining a healthy immune system. During sleep, especially deep and restorative sleep stages, the immune system actively engages in processes that help maintain and restore immune health. This includes the production and activity of white blood cells. The body's circadian rhythms, including sleep-wake cycles, have a significant influence on immune function. Disrupted sleep patterns or irregular sleep-wake schedules can lead to immune dysfunction.

Resetting the natural sleep-wake cycle, also known as the circadian rhythm, is essential for improving sleep quality and overall well-being. A few strategies for this reset include setting a bedtime, waking up at the same time every day (even on weekends), and increasing the exposure to natural sunlight in the morning and natural darkness in the evenings. This may involve dimming interior lighting at a specific time and reducing exposure to artificial light in the evening, especially from screens (computers, smartphones, TVs). This may mean setting a TV bedtime, turning off the electronics at a specific time, and creating a relaxing evening routine. Stress and anxiety can disrupt the sleep-wake cycle. Practicing stress-reduction techniques such as meditation, yoga, or progressive muscle relaxation may help.

Supplements

When risk factors are identified, antioxidant therapy may be a promising approach to prevention. Studies have shown that N-acetyl cysteine and alpha-lipoic acid have good safety profiles and effectiveness. Individual supplements may be needed based on the diagnosis of nutritional deficiencies associated with poor white blood cell formation and function.

Additional Testing

antinuclear antibodies (ANA); vitamin B12 (cobalamin); methylmalonic acid; homocysteine; comprehensive metabolic panel (CMP); bile acid, serum; c-reactive protein (CRP); ferritin; iron and TIBC; vitamin D, 25-hydroxy (25-hydroxycalciferol, 25OH-D); comprehensive thyroid profile II; thyroid peroxidase antibodies (TPOAb); thyroglobulin antibody (TgAb); ceruloplasmin; oral zinc tolerance test; prothrombin time (PT)

References

1. Dockree S, Shine B, Pavord S, Impey L, Vatish M. White blood cells in pregnancy: reference intervals for before and after delivery. EBioMedicine. 2021 Dec;74:103715. doi: 10.1016/j.ebiom.2021.103715. Epub 2021 Nov 23. PMID: 34826802; PMCID: PMC8626574.

2. Wu K, Gong W, Ke HH, Hu H, Chen L. Impact of elevated first and second trimester white blood cells on prevalence of late-onset preeclampsia. Heliyon. 2022 Nov 23;8(11):e11806. doi: 10.1016/j.heliyon.2022.e11806. PMID: 36458313; PMCID: PMC9706692.

3. Örgül G, Aydın Haklı D, Özten G, Fadiloğlu E, Tanacan A, Beksaç MS. First-trimester complete blood cell indices in early and late-onset preeclampsia. Turk J Obstet Gynecol. 2019;16(2):112–117. doi:10.4274/tjod.galenos.2019.93708

4. Al-Husban, N., Al-Atrash, H., Alhayek, N. et al. Platelet and White Blood Cell (WBC) Counts in the First Trimester and Pregnancy Outcome: Prospective Controlled Study. J. Fetal Med. 6, 89–94 (2019). doi.org/10.1007/s40556–019-00202–0

5. Liao D, Chen L, Li Q, Liu G, Wang W, Li J, Deng S. Predictive Value of the Peripheral Blood Parameters for Preeclampsia. Clin Lab. 2022 Mar 1;68(3). doi: 10.7754/Clin.Lab.2021.210726. PMID: 35254028.

6. McKay LI, Cidlowski JA. Physiologic and Pharmacologic Effects of Corticosteroids. In: Kufe DW, Pollock RE, Weichselbaum RR, et al., editors. Holland-Frei Cancer Medicine. 6th edition. Hamilton (ON): BC Decker; 2003. www.ncbi.nlm.nih.gov/books/NBK13780

7. Fisher, A.L., Sangkhae, V., Balušíková, K. et al. Iron-dependent apoptosis causes embryotoxicity in inflamed and obese pregnancy. Nat Commun 12, 4026 (2021). doi.org/10.1038/s41467–021-24333-z

8. Johannsen NM, Swift DL, Johnson WD, Dixit VD, Earnest CP, Blair SN, Church TS. Effect of different doses of aerobic exercise on total white blood cell (WBC) and WBC subfraction number in postmenopausal women: results from DREW. PLoS One. 2012;7(2):e31319. doi: 10.1371/journal.pone.0031319. Epub 2012 Feb 17. PMID: 22363616; PMCID: PMC3281960.

9. Varney ME, Hardman WE, Sollars VE. Omega 3 fatty acids reduce myeloid progenitor cell frequency in the bone marrow of mice and promote progenitor cell differentiation. Lipids Health Dis. 2009 Mar 18;8:9. doi: 10.1186/1476–511X-8–9. PMID: 19296839; PMCID: PMC2669087.

10. Silva J, Magenta M, Sisti G, Serventi L, Gaither K. Association Between Complete Blood Count Components and Intrahepatic Cholestasis of Pregnancy. Cureus. 2020;12(12):e12381. Published 2020 Dec 30. doi:10.7759/cureus.12381

11. Horn PL, Pyne DB, Hopkins WG, Barnes CJ. Lower white blood cell counts in elite athletes training for highly aerobic sports. Eur J Appl Physiol. 2010 Nov;110(5):925–32. doi: 10.1007/s00421–010-1573–9. Epub 2010 Jul 17. PMID: 20640439.

Neutrophils

The absolute neutrophil count measures the total count of neutrophils in a sample. The neutrophil percentage tells you what percentage of the white blood cell count is made up of neutrophils. It is found in the complete blood count (CBC) with differential panel.

Neutrophils are a type of granulated white blood cell. They originate in bone marrow from myeloid progenitor cells. Neutrophils are either segmented or banded (nonsegmented). Banded neutrophils are young and are increased in acute infection, with or without an increase in total WBC count. Segmented neutrophils are mature blood cells. The primary job of neutrophils is to identify microbial infections then trap, neutralize, and kill them through phagocytosis.

Neutrophils, like other blood cells, are derived from hematopoietic stem cells in the bone marrow. They belong to the myeloid lineage of blood cells. Myeloblasts, which are committed progenitor cells, develop into promyelocytes, myelocytes, and metamyelocytes, and then mature into neutrophils. During their development, neutrophils accumulate specific granules in their cytoplasm. These granules contain enzymes and antimicrobial proteins that help neutrophils combat infections. This is the reason they are also known as granulocyte white blood cells. This group also includes basophils and eosinophils.

Neutrophils are the first line of defense in the immune system. They are phagocytic cells, meaning they can engulf and digest microorganisms such as bacteria and fungi. Once a neutrophil recognizes a pathogen, it engulfs the invader, forming a phagosome, fusing with granules to create a phagolysosome. The enzymes and antimicrobial proteins contained in the granules work to destroy the microorganism. As part of their defense mechanisms, they produce reactive oxygen species (ROS). This process, known as the respiratory burst, helps kill or neutralize pathogens within the phagolysosome. If not regulated by antioxidants, this can increase oxidative stress in the body. When neutrophils encounter pathogens, they can release their DNA, along with antimicrobial proteins, into the extracellular space. This results in the formation of neutrophil extracellular traps (NETs). NETs are weblike structures that ensnare and immobilize pathogens, preventing their spread. This process is called NETosis.

NETosis

Neutrophils are activated by pathogen-associated molecular patterns (PAMPs) or damage-associated molecular patterns (DAMPs). This activation triggers the release of ROS and granules. As the neutrophil's chromatin (DNA) begins to decondense, the nuclear envelope and cell membrane rupture, allowing the chromatin to mix with granule proteins. The cell releases a weblike structure composed of chromatin, granule proteins, and antimicrobial enzymes, forming NETs. NETosis is a double-edged sword. While it helps combat infections, excessive NET formation can contribute to inflammation and tissue damage, which is seen in various inflammatory diseases, including diseases of the placenta.

Pregnancy

In pregnancy, there is an increase in neutrophil production and a decrease in neutrophil apoptosis. Total neutrophil counts increase by 55% within the first two months of pregnancy. The neutrophil count begins to increase in the second month of pregnancy and reaches a plateau in the second or third trimester, when the white blood cell counts range from 9 to 15 $\times 10^9$/L.[1] Studies have shown that these WBCs help with placental development and maintaining maternal-fetal tolerance.[2] However, excess neutrophil production is associated with placental cell damage. Balance is key.

Chemotaxis, the ability of neutrophils to migrate toward sites of infection or inflammation, may be somewhat impaired during pregnancy. This adaptation helps prevent an overly aggressive immune response to the developing fetus. This change is primarily driven by progesterone. Progesterone also reduces NETosis. The overall immune response during pregnancy is shifted toward a state of immune tolerance, allowing the maternal immune system to coexist with the semi-allogeneic fetus. This balance is essential to prevent the rejection of the fetus as a foreign entity. However, the altered immune response can render pregnant individuals more susceptible to some infections.

Postpartum

In the immediate hours after childbirth, neutrophil counts may temporarily increase. This increase is a normal response to the stress of labor and delivery. Over the course of the postpartum weeks, neutrophil counts gradually return to pre-pregnancy levels. The speed of this normalization can vary among individuals. Neutrophil function returns to its normal state, with the ability to efficiently combat infections and respond to inflammation.

> I prefer looking at percentages when analyzing the differential. The absolutes are variable based on the total WBC count. You can do the math yourself if needed to identify the percentage of WBC type.

STANDARD LAB RANGE: 1.4 – 7 × 10^9/L

Trimester	Standard Pregnancy Ranges	**Functional Pregnancy Ranges**
Preconception	1.4 – 7	**1.4 – 4.6**
First Trimester	3.6 – 10.1	**3.6 – 6**
Second Trimester	3.8 – 12.3	**3.8 – 8**
Third Trimester	3.9 – 13.1	**3.9 – 10**
Postpartum	1.4 – 7	**1.4 – 7**

STANDARD LAB RANGE: 30% – 70%

Trimester	Standard Pregnancy Ranges	**Functional Pregnancy Ranges**
Preconception	30 – 70%	**40 – 60%**
First Trimester	Not Established	**60 – 80%**
Second Trimester	Not Established	**60 – 80%**
Third Trimester	Not Established	**60 – 80%**
Postpartum	30 – 70%	**40 – 60%**

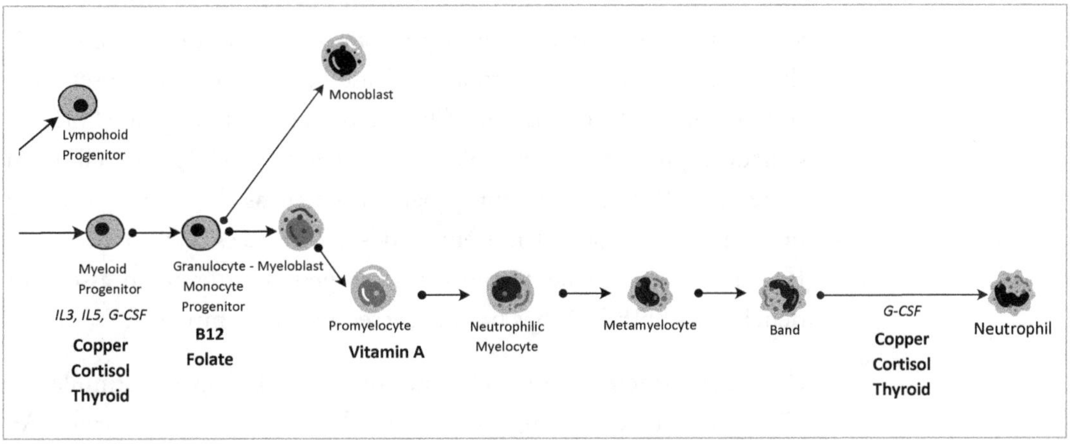

Figure 1: Neutrophil Maturation

Stem-cell production is stimulated by MK-4. Myeloblast differentiation is stimulated by IL-3, IL-5, and G-CSF. Copper regulates G-CSF in myeloid progenitor maturation. Vitamin A stimulates the differentiation and maturation of promyelocytes to granulocytes. Vitamin B12 (cobalamin) and vitamin B9 (folate) are required for DNA methylation during early cellular development. Vitamin C, selenium, and other nutrients are accumulated in cells during development. Vitamin A stimulates the differentiation and maturation of promyelocytes to granulocytes. Copper regulates G-CSF in neutrophil maturation.

Causes of Elevated Neutrophils

See White Blood Cell (WBC) Count Section.

Neutrophil counts >6 × 10^9/L in the first trimester have been identified as a predictive marker for gestational diabetes and late-pregnancy preeclampsia.[3 4]

Elevated neutrophils in the third trimester have been associated with an increased risk of placental dysfunction, leading to small-for-gestational-age fetal growth.[5]

Acute Bacterial/Fungal Infection: Acute bacterial infections commonly cause elevated neutrophils. The increased demand for neutrophils during an infection can cause a rise in their numbers in the bloodstream, resulting in neutrophilia. This could be an asymptomatic urinary tract infection or candida overgrowth, both of which can increase the risk of PROM.

Inflammation: In acute infections and inflammatory reactions, neutrophils are the first WBCs to arrive to fight infection and reduce inflammation. In chronic inflammation, high neutrophils can cause more harm than good, increasing inflammation and causing tissue damage, such as in cases of asthma. This is due to the production of ROS as a normal part of their mechanism of action in fighting pathogens.

Low Progesterone: In early pregnancy, the rise in neutrophils is stimulated by a higher increase of G-CSF, stimulated by copper, cortisol, and thyroid hormones. One of the roles of progesterone is to regulate this function, creating balance. NETs are net-like structures that are released by activated neutrophils. NETs have been associated with autoimmune diseases and pregnancy complications. NETosis is the process by which neutrophils release NETs. NETosis causes ROS production and cell death. While estrogen and human chorionic gonadotrophin (hCG) stimulate an increase in NETs, as well as an increase in ROS production, progesterone curbs this effect—keeping neutrophils primed but not engaged—and reduces ROS production. If you see elevated neutrophils, test progesterone levels to assess for deficiencies.[6] NETosis has been observed in preeclampsia.

Zinc Deficiency: There is a balance of zinc and copper in stimulating CSF. Low zinc causes higher neutrophils and lower lymphocytes. An element of a lower zinc level is normal in pregnancy, but it should not be deficient. Zinc has also been shown to decrease the NET actions of neutrophils like progesterone.

Magnesium Deficiency: Neutrophilia is a common finding during hypomagnesemia.[7] Magnesium is required for hemopoiesis on many levels. Magnesium deficiency has been associated with higher neutrophil counts, lower lymphocyte counts, and lower red blood cell (RBC) counts. The exact mechanism for this is unclear but is measurable in studies. It is theorized that magnesium plays a role in the regulation of stem cell factor (SCF).

Graves' Disease: Thyroid hormones affect the production of G-CSF. It is well established that an increase in G-CSF and granulocytes is found in those with hyperthyroidism.[8] In the first few weeks of pregnancy, there is a significant increase in the production of thyroid hormones in response to hCG production. This helps to stimulate the normal increase in neutrophils that we see in early pregnancy.

Other Possible Causes: some autoimmune diseases, preeclampsia, chronic emotional stress, high cortisol, certain medications (lithium, antibiotics, clozapine), physical trauma, polycythemia, diabetic ketoacidosis, dehydration, cancer

Treatment Strategies for Elevated Neutrophils

See White Blood Cell (WBC) Count Section.

Diet

Focus on increasing zinc-rich foods. Good dietary sources of zinc include meat, poultry, beans, nuts, and dairy products. Antioxidant-rich foods can help reduce inflammation and support immune function. Include foods like fruits (berries, citrus), vegetables (spinach, kale, bell peppers), and nuts (almonds, walnuts) in the diet. Consuming probiotic-rich foods like yogurt and fermented foods can help maintain a healthy gut microbiome, which may help with gut or urinary bacterial infections. Reducing neutrophil counts by addressing bacterial overgrowth generally involves improving the overall health of the gut and addressing any underlying issues contributing to the overgrowth.

While specific foods and herbs may not directly reduce neutrophil counts, they can help promote a balanced gut microbiome and maintain overall health. Garlic has natural antibacterial properties and can help control harmful bacteria. Ginger may have antibacterial and anti-inflammatory effects that can support gut health. Fiber-rich foods, including fruits, vegetables, and whole grains, support the growth of beneficial gut bacteria, specifically the lactobacillus spp. Some herbal teas, such as peppermint and ginger, may have antibacterial properties and can soothe the digestive system. Other culinary herbs such as thyme, oregano, rosemary, lemongrass, and basil can be added to meals to boost antimicrobial properties. Quercetin is a flavonoid, a type of plant compound with antioxidant properties. It is found in various fruits and vegetables. Some common sources include onions, apples, berries, citrus fruits, leafy greens, tomatoes, broccoli, red grapes, cherries, and capers.

Lifestyle

If a urinary tract infection is the cause of elevated neutrophils, sitz baths can provide relief. This involves sitting in warm, shallow water that is filled with salts and herbs, and can promote healing and reduce discomfort in the pelvic area.

Supplements

Vaginal progesterone, but not other forms of progesterone, has been shown to reduce inflammation in the maternal-fetal interface and have effects on WBC parameters.[9] Your patient can try zinc picolinate in lozenge form. Have them consume it daily until a metallic taste is experienced with dosing. Use caution with zinc supplementation, as it can decrease copper levels, and copper naturally increases in pregnancy. N-acetyl cysteine has been shown to help protect tissues from the damaging effects of elevated neutrophils.[10] Quercetin has been shown to decrease NETs, but supplementation may cause potential harm to fetuses. Therefore, dietary quercetin is a more appropriate application in pregnancy.[11]

Additional Testing

urinalysis; comprehensive thyroid profile II; reverse T3 (rT3); thyroid peroxidase antibodies (TPOAb); thyroglobulin antibody (TgAb); thyroid receptor antibodies (TRAb); c-reactive protein (CRP); comprehensive metabolic panel (CMP); progesterone; oral zinc tolerance test; comprehensive stool testing

Causes of Low Neutrophils

See White Blood Cell (WBC) Count Section.

Neutropenia in pregnancy has been associated with preterm birth.

Dysbiosis: The microbiome plays a role in neutrophil production and function.[12] The reduction or absence of commensal bacteria in the gut through chronic antibiotic use or excessive sanitation (cleaning products, hand sanitizers) has been shown to reduce neutrophils and their progenitor cells. In acute gut-inflammation reactions, there may be an increase in neutrophils, leading to an eventual decrease.

Chronic Infections: Like dysbiosis, chronic bacterial infections can cause neutrophils to decrease.

Copper Deficiency: A neutrophil percentage less than 60% in pregnancy can be a biomarker of copper deficiency. Neutropenia is a unique presentation of copper deficiency. Copper regulates the differentiation of WBC progenitor cells by regulating G-CSF production.[13] Additionally, looking at other values in the CBC, such as the mean corpuscular hemoglobin (MCH) and mean corpuscular hemoglobin concentration (MCHC), can also help identify copper deficiency as a cause of neutropenia.

Other Possible Causes: hypothyroidism, aplastic anemia, autoimmune disease, certain medications (antiseizure medications, carbimazole, and propylthiouracil), vitamin B9 (folate) deficiency, vitamin B12 (cobalamin) deficiency, cancer

Treatment Strategies for Low Neutrophils

See White Blood Cell (WBC) Count Section.

Diet

Focus on increasing copper-rich foods, as well as antioxidant-rich foods that help to extend the life of neutrophils, such as vitamin C, manganese, omega-3 fatty acids, vitamin E, and other phytonutrient antioxidants like phenols and flavonoids. Dysbiosis is an imbalance in the gut microbiota, with an overgrowth of harmful bacteria or a decrease in beneficial ones. A diet high in fiber supports the growth of beneficial gut bacteria. This includes plenty of fruits, vegetables, whole grains, legumes, and seeds. Prebiotics are nondigestible fibers that nourish beneficial gut bacteria. Foods like garlic, onions, leeks, asparagus, and bananas are good sources of prebiotics.

Incorporate foods containing live probiotic cultures, such as yogurt, kefir, sauerkraut, kimchi, and kombucha. Include sources of healthy fats, like avocados, nuts, seeds, and olive oil, which may help reduce inflammation in the gut. Bone broth contains collagen and amino acids that can help support gut health and may be beneficial for those with leaky gut syndrome. High-sugar diets can promote the growth of harmful gut bacteria. Limit the intake of sugary foods and beverages. Some artificial sweeteners, like aspartame, may disrupt the gut microbiota. Include anti-inflammatory foods like turmeric, ginger, and fatty fish in your diet to help reduce gut inflammation.

Supplements

Studies have shown that selenium supplementation can increase neutrophil production.[14] Study dosages range from 50 μg over two to three months to 200 μg over one month to increase neutrophil production. Vitamin B3 (niacin) supplements have also been shown to increase neutrophil production.[15]

Additional Testing

antinuclear antibodies (ANA); vitamin B12 (cobalamin); comprehensive metabolic panel (CMP); c-reactive protein (CRP); ferritin; iron and TIBC; homocysteine; vitamin D, 25-hydroxy (25-hydroxycalciferol, 25OH-D); comprehensive thyroid profile II; thyroid peroxidase antibodies (TPOAb); thyroglobulin antibody (TgAb); copper, total; ceruloplasmin

References

1. Al-Husban, N., Al-Atrash, H., Alhayek, N. et al. Platelet and White Blood Cell (WBC) Counts in the First Trimester and Pregnancy Outcome: Prospective Controlled Study. J. Fetal Med. 6, 89–94 (2019). doi.org/10.1007/s40556–019-00202–0

2. Bert S, Ward EJ, Nadkarni S. Neutrophils in pregnancy: New insights into innate and adaptive immune regulation. Immunology. 2021 Dec;164(4):665–676. doi: 10.1111/imm.13392. Epub 2021 Jul 29. PMID: 34287859; PMCID: PMC8561097.

3. Tiange Sun, Fanhua Meng, Hongmei Zhao, Min Yang, Rui Zhang, Zhiyan Yu, Xinmei Huang, Heyuan Ding, Jun Liu, Shufei Zang; Elevated First-Trimester Neutrophil Count Is Closely Associated With the Development of Maternal Gestational Diabetes Mellitus and Adverse Pregnancy Outcomes. Diabetes 1 July 2020; 69 (7): 1401–1410.

4. Sahin M, Oguz A, Tüzün D, et al. A new marker predicting gestational diabetes mellitus: First trimester neutrophil/lymphocyte ratio. Medicine (Baltimore). 2022;101(36):e30514. doi:10.1097/MD.0000000000030511

5. Harita N, Kariya M, Hayashi T, Sato KK, Nakamura K, Endo G, Narimoto K. Increment of absolute neutrophil count in the third trimester and increased risk of small-for-gestational-age birth: Hirakata Risk Associated with Pregnancy Assessment Research (HIRAPAR). Eur J Obstet Gynecol Reprod Biol. 2012 Sep;164(1):30–4. doi: 10.1016/j.ejogrb.2012.05.039. Epub 2012 Jul 3. PMID: 22762842.

6. Giaglis S, Stoikou M, Sur Chowdhury C, et al. Multimodal Regulation of NET Formation in Pregnancy

7. Progesterone Antagonizes the Pro-NETotic Effect of Estrogen and G-CSF. Front Immunol. 2016;7:565. Published 2016 Dec 5. doi:10.3389/fimmu.2016.00565

8. Lima FDS, Fock RA. A Review of the Action of Magnesium on Several Processes Involved in the Modulation of Hematopoiesis. Int J Mol Sci. 2020;21(19):7084. Published 2020 Sep 25. doi:10.3390/ijms21197084

9. Iitaka M, Noh JY, Kitahama S, et al. Elevated serum granulocyte colony-stimulating factor levels in patients with Graves' disease. Clin Endocrinol (Oxf). 1998;48(3):275–280. doi:10.1046/j.1365–2265.1998.00422.x

10. Furcron AE, Romero R, Plazyo O, et al. Vaginal progesterone, but not 17α-hydroxyprogesterone caproate, has antiinflammatory effects at the murine maternal-fetal interface. Am J Obstet Gynecol. 2015;213(6):846.e1–846.e19. doi:10.1016/j.ajog.2015.08.010

11. Mottahedin A, Blondel S, Ek J, et al. N-acetylcysteine inhibits bacterial lipopeptide-mediated neutrophil transmigration through the choroid plexus in the developing brain. Acta Neuropathol Commun. 2020;8(1):4. Published 2020 Jan 23. doi:10.1186/s40478–019-0877–1

12. Pereira GS, Percebom I, Mendes S, et al. Quercetin inhibits neutrophil extracellular traps release and their cytotoxic effects on A549 cells, as well the release and enzymatic activity of elastase and myeloperoxidase. Braz J Biol. 2022;84:e252936. Published 2022 Apr 20. doi:10.1590/1519–6984.252936

13. Zhang D, Frenette PS. Cross talk between neutrophils and the microbiota. Blood. 2019;133(20):2168–2177. doi:10.1182/blood-2018–11-844555

14. Percival SS. Neutropenia caused by copper deficiency: possible mechanisms of action. Nutr Rev. 1995;53(3):59–66. doi:10.1111/j.1753–4887.1995.tb01503.x

15. Masri DS. Microquantity for macroquality: case study on the effect of selenium on chronic neutropenia. J Pediatr Hematol Oncol. 2011;33(8):e361-e362. doi:10.1097/MPH.0b013e31822d4d39

16. Bird, L. Vitamin B3: a neutrophil supplement. Nat Rev Immunol 9, 149 (2009). doi.org/10.1038/nri2521

Lymphocytes

The absolute lymphocyte count measures the total count of lymphocytes in a sample. The lymphocyte percentage tells you what percentage of the white blood cell count is made up of lymphocytes. It is found in the complete blood count (CBC) with differential panel.

Lymph is Latin for "water." Lymphocytes are a type of nongranulated white blood cell. They originate from lymphoblasts in the spleen, lymph nodes, tonsils, thymus, intestines, bone marrow, and appendix. The primary job of lymphocytes is to produce antibodies in response to bacteria, viruses, or any other potentially pathogenic antigen, including cancer.

Lymphocytes include β cells, T cells, and natural killer (NK) cells—all crucial components of the immune system, each with unique formation processes and functions.

T cells, or T lymphocytes, also originate from hematopoietic stem cells in the bone marrow. However, they migrate to the thymus gland, where they undergo maturation and selection processes. T-cell development is regulated by various thymic hormones and cytokines. T cells play a central role in cell-mediated adaptive immunity or acquired immunity. They include cytotoxic T cells (CD8+), which can directly kill infected or abnormal host cells, and helper T cells (CD4+), which coordinate immune responses. Regulatory T cells (Tregs) control and modulate immune responses, while memory T cells "remember" previous encounters with pathogens. T cells recognize antigens and activate the β cells. They can also kill viruses and cancer cells.

β cells are formed in the bone marrow from hematopoietic stem cells. In the bone marrow, they undergo a process called B lymphopoiesis. During this process, genes are rearranged to generate a diverse range of β-cell receptors (antibodies). β-cell development is influenced by various cytokines and growth factors, including interleukin-7 (IL-7). These factors support β-cell proliferation and differentiation. β cells are primarily responsible for humoral immunity, a component of the adaptive immune system. Once activated by an antigen, they differentiate into plasma cells, which produce antibodies. Antibodies can neutralize pathogens and tag them for destruction by other immune cells. Plasma cells are differentiated from antigen-activated β cells in secondary lymphoid organs such as the spleen and lymph nodes.

Plasma cells compose between 2% and 3% of all lymphocytes. Plasma cells engulf antigens, present them to T cells, and produce large amounts of antibodies in response to antigens. Antibodies can neutralize pathogens by blocking their ability to infect host cells. This can prevent the spread of infection. Antibodies tag pathogens for destruction by other immune cells, such as phagocytes. This process enhances the recognition and elimination of the pathogen. Some antibodies can trigger the complement system, a group of proteins that enhance the immune response by causing cell lysis (bursting) of the pathogen. Plasma cells produce antibodies specific to the encountered antigen. Some β cells also differentiate into memory β cells, which "remember" the antigen. This provides a quicker and more robust immune response upon re-encounter with the same antigen in the future. Long-lived plasma cells (LLPC) live for longer and secrete antibodies. They do not need continued antigen exposure to produce antibodies.

Natural killer (NK) cells play a role in our innate immune responses. NK cells form in the bone marrow from common lymphoid progenitor cells. NK cells attack any foreign cell, including cancer cells. The development of NK cells is regulated by various cytokines, including interleukin-15 (IL-15). They can recognize cells that lack self-antigens and induce apoptosis in these cells. NK cells provide rapid immune responses in the absence of prior exposure to the pathogen.

Pregnancy

In pregnancy, there is a 36% decrease in lymphocyte production. This helps to protect the placenta and fetus from immune-system attacks, as they are foreign cells. These levels are decreased through the second trimester and increase again during the third trimester in preparation for childbirth.[1] To prevent the rejection of the developing fetus, the maternal immune system becomes more tolerant. Tregs suppress immune responses against fetal antigens. Pregnancy induces a shift in the immune response, favoring a type 2 helper T-cell (Th2) response. This shift is thought to support the maintenance of pregnancy. Th2 responses are associated with antibody production and tissue repair.

Postpartum

During the first few days after childbirth, it's common for lymphocyte counts to decrease. This is partly due to the physiological changes associated with childbirth and the shift in hormone levels. In the weeks following childbirth, lymphocyte counts typically return to pre-pregnancy levels. This process is part of the body's recovery and rebalancing phase. If a woman is breastfeeding, her immune system may continue to adapt to provide immune protection for both her and her infant, causing an increase in lymphocyte counts. Breast milk contains antibodies that are passed on to the baby, further impacting lymphocyte activity.

The neutrophil-to-lymphocyte ratio (NLR) has been a controversial biomarker for predicting preeclampsia. A review of research in 2020 concluded that this measure is a useful marker for predicting the severity of preeclampsia in pregnancy.[2]

The NLR is used as a biomarker of systemic inflammation. Outside of pregnancy, this ratio is used to help with the management of inflammatory conditions. In pregnancy, it may be used to help identify systemic inflammation. The NLR is calculated by dividing the number of neutrophils by the number of lymphocytes. The higher the number, the greater the risk of inflammation...and in pregnancy, the greater the risk of preeclampsia.

Another important ratio is the platelet-to-lymphocyte ratio (PLR). The PLR is calculated by dividing the absolute platelet count by the lymphocyte count. Monocyte to lymphocyte ratio (MLR) is another marker that can be used to assess systemic inflammation, specifically for coagulation dysfunction in preeclampsia patients. This ratio is naturally elevated in pregnancy, but a significant increase could signal systemic inflammation.[3] These are tools that providers can use to assess for systemic inflammation that may predict pregnancy complications in the first-trimester obstetric panel.

Lymphocytes indicate the ability of the body to handle toxins and infections. When increased, acute exposure is possible (viral or toxins), and when decreased, a woman is more susceptible to severe infection or reactions to toxins.

The reference ranges for lymphocytes are quite variable between sources. The ranges I've presented are an average of these intervals and related research surrounding ranges and increased risks of complications. You will see inconsistencies in reports from many trusted sources. Again, patterns in the differential are more important than single values, and percentages may be a better use of differential than absolutes, as the ranges will vary based on the total WBC counts.

STANDARD LAB RANGE: 0.7 – 3.1 × 10⁹/L

Trimester	Standard Pregnancy Ranges	**Functional Pregnancy Ranges**
Preconception	0.7 – 4.6	**1.4 – 4.6**
First Trimester	1.1 – 3.6	**1.1 – 2.9**
Second Trimester	0.9 – 3.9	**0.9 – 2.9**
Third Trimester	1.1 – 3.9	**1.1 – 2.9**
Postpartum	0.7 – 4.6	**1.4 – 4.6**

STANDARD LAB RANGE: 20% – 40%

Trimester	Standard Pregnancy Ranges	**Functional Pregnancy Ranges**
Preconception	20 – 40%	**20 – 40%**
First Trimester	Not Established	**12 – 20%**
Second Trimester	Not Established	**12 – 20%**
Third Trimester	Not Established	**12 – 20%**
Postpartum	20 – 40%	**20 – 40%**

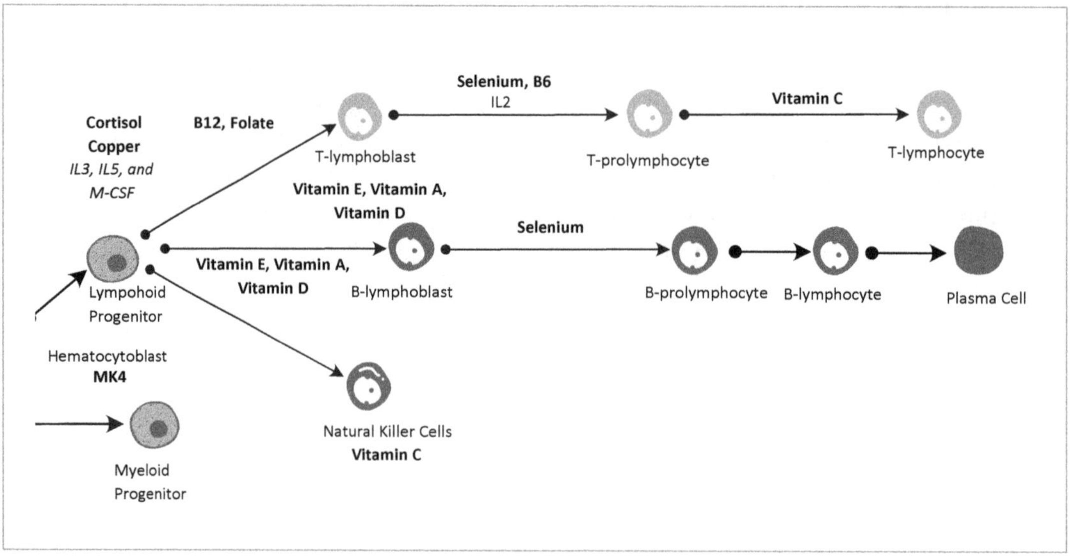

Figure 2: Lymphocyte Maturation

Stem-cell production is stimulated by MK-4. Cortisol regulates T-cell and β-cell proliferation; they are inversely related. Vitamin B12 (cobalamin) and vitamin B9 (folate) are required for DNA methylation during early cellular development. Selenium and vitamin B6 (pyridoxine) regulate T-lymphocyte proliferation by enhancing IL-2 production. Selenium inhibits the activation, differentiation, and maturation of β cells. Vitamin C is needed for T-cell differentiation and development, and is also needed for MK-cell proliferation. Vitamin E activates genes for lymphocyte proliferation regulation. Vitamin A and vitamin D3 modulate the differentiation between β cells and T cells.

Causes of Elevated Lymphocytes

See White Blood Cell (WBC) Count Section.

There is an inverse relationship between cortisol and lymphocyte production.[4]

Elevated lymphocytes are associated with an increased risk of miscarriage and implantation failure. This may be seen in those with repeated failed in vitro fertilization (IVF) transfers.

Acute Viral Infection: Acute viral infections will increase lymphocyte counts as they attack antigens; lymphocyte counts can drop after the infection.

Acute Toxin Exposure: In severe acute toxic exposure or viral infections, lymphocytes can increase, and neutrophils decrease to be almost equal in absolute and percentage.

Autoimmune Hypothyroidism: There is a cyclical relationship between lymphocyte production and hypothyroid presentations. Thyroid hormones help to regulate immune responses. When thyroid hormones are low, there is an increase in immune response to antigens. This increase in lymphocytes can cause lymphocytic thyroiditis, which can cause both hyper- and hypothyroid presentations. This typically presents with increased thyroid hormone secretion, followed by burnout of the gland and a subsequent decrease in thyroid hormone production due to inflammation.

Placental Dysfunction: Lymphocytes are one of the fetal-blood-cell types that can be found in maternal circulation. In cases where the placenta allows more fetal-blood-cell leakage into circulation, lymphocyte values may increase.

Vitamin D deficiency: Vitamin D regulates the proliferation and differentiation of β cells and T cells. It helps to suppress the proliferation of T cells.[5] If lymphocytes are elevated, testing vitamin D is a good next step.

Cancer: Specific lymphoma cancers can cause elevations in lymphocytes. This is rare and, if identified, should be treated by medical specialists.

Other Possible Causes: adrenal hypofunction, autoimmune disease, hyperthyroidism, chronic inflammatory diseases (inflammatory bowel disease, asthma), allergies, liver damage, enlarged spleen, dehydration

Treatment Strategies for Elevated Lymphocytes

See White Blood Cell (WBC) Count Section.

Diet

While specific dietary recommendations may not directly lower elevated lymphocyte counts, they can help maintain a healthy immune system and manage any underlying conditions contributing to lymphocytosis. Increasing antioxidant-rich foods like blueberries, strawberries, raspberries, citrus, leafy greens such as parsley and kale, and other colorful vegetables help the immune system fight infections. Antiviral herbs are a good addition to meals and teas. These include green tea, garlic, honey, ginger, and turmeric.

Supplements

Although they do not lower elevated lymphocytes, supplements such as resveratrol, epigallocatechin-3-gallate (EGCG), vitamin D, and vitamin E have been shown to have regulatory effects on lymphocyte function. Progesterone should also be assessed, if lymphocytes are elevated. Although progesterone doesn't seem to influence the production of lymphocytes directly, it does decrease the cytotoxic activity of lymphocytes.[6]

Additional Testing

comprehensive thyroid profile II; thyroid peroxidase antibodies (TPOAb); thyroglobulin antibody (TgAb); thyroid receptor antibodies (TRAb); vitamin D, 25-hydroxy (25-hydroxycalciferol, 25OH-D); nucleated red blood cells (nRBC)

Causes of Low Lymphocytes

See White Blood Cell (WBC) Count Section.

Lymphocytopenia is a normal presentation in pregnancy. Levels that are excessively low, or below normal ranges, can increase the risk of infections in pregnancy.[7]

Chronic Viral Infection: Chronic viral infections will decrease lymphocyte counts as they continue to attack the antigens. This can be seen in respiratory viruses, herpes, hepatitis, HIV/AIDS (human immunodeficiency virus/acquired immunodeficiency syndrome), Epstein-Barr virus, and other latent viral infections.

Autoimmune Diseases: Lymphocytopenia is not uncommon in certain autoimmune conditions, such as lupus and rheumatoid arthritis.

Testing for antinuclear antibodies (ANA) can help identify autoimmune conditions in pregnancy.

Iron Overload/Hemochromatosis: Studies show an inverse relationship between iron and lymphocyte production in patients with hemochromatosis.[8] (See Iron Section.)

Zinc Deficiency: There is a balance of zinc and copper in stimulating CSF. Low zinc causes higher neutrophils and lower lymphocytes. An element of a lower zinc level is normal in pregnancy, but it should not be deficient. Zinc blocks viral replicase enzymes. This requires flavonoids to function.

Selenium Deficiency: Selenium can enhance T-lymphocyte proliferation.[9]

Other Possible Causes: adrenal hyperfunction, progesterone deficiency, magnesium deficiency, aplastic anemia, certain medications (corticosteroids and anticonvulsants), malnutrition, mycotoxin exposure, sleep disorders, cancer

Treatment Strategies for Low Lymphocytes

See White Blood Cell (WBC) Count Section.

Diet

Increase flavonoid-rich foods such as green tea, red grapes, berries, green leafy vegetables, red cabbage, citrus, and fermented soy. Focus on increasing zinc-rich foods. Good dietary sources of zinc include meat, poultry, beans, nuts, and dairy products. Seafood, nuts, and seeds can provide both zinc and selenium, which can have a regulatory effect on lymphocyte proliferation and function. Additionally, avoiding trans-fatty acids, which have been shown to thicken lymphocytes and reduce their functionality, can help keep the existing lymphocytes functioning properly.

Lifestyle

Sleep deprivation is known to cause a reduction in lymphocyte production. Increasing the onset of sleep by just one hour can have a drastic positive effect on lymphocyte and WBC production and inflammation reduction. Instruct patients to fall asleep earlier in the evenings, avoiding late-night electronics. This may mean creating new daily routines or recognizing stress triggers that may be causing sleep disruption.

Supplements

Selenium dosed at 200 μg/day was shown to reduce the cytotoxicity of lymphocytes as well as increase proliferation.[10] Flavonoids, such as EGCG found in green tea, can be used to improve lymphocyte function and regulate cytotoxicity. Supplementing with zinc in lozenge form may be useful if zinc deficiency is identified. Have them consume it daily until a metallic taste is experienced with dosing. Use caution with zinc supplementation, as it can decrease copper levels, and copper naturally increases in pregnancy.

Additional Testing

ferritin; iron and TIBC; progesterone; antinuclear antibodies (ANA); oral zinc tolerance test

References

1. Chandra S, Tripathi AK, Mishra S, Amzarul M, Vaish AK. Physiological changes in hematological parameters during pregnancy. Indian J Hematol Blood Transfus. 2012 Sep;28(3):144–6. doi: 10.1007/s12288–012-0175–6. Epub 2012 Jul 15. PMID: 23997449; PMCID: PMC3422383.

2. Kang Q, Li W, Yu N, et al. Predictive role of neutrophil-to-lymphocyte ratio in preeclampsia: A meta-analysis including 3982 patients. Pregnancy Hypertens. 2020;20:111–118. doi:10.1016/j.preghy.2020.03.009

3. Cui, H.X., Chen, C., Jung, Y.M. et al. Neutrophil-to-lymphocyte ratio (NLR) as a predictive index for liver and coagulation dysfunction in preeclampsia patients. BMC Pregnancy Childbirth 23, 4 (2023). doi.org/10.1186/s12884–022-05335–1

4. Hwang KH, Jang K, Nam SY, Kim YJ. Cortisol Secretion and Subsequent Impaired Lymphopoiesis after Starvation Can Be Reduced by Moxibustion Treatment. Evid Based Complement Alternat Med. 2021;2021:8856687. Published 2021 Feb 3. doi:10.1155/2021/8856687

5. Charoenngam N, Holick MF. Immunologic Effects of Vitamin D on Human Health and Disease. Nutrients. 2020;12(7):2097. Published 2020 Jul 15. doi:10.3390/nu12072097

6. Szekeres-Bartho J, Hadnagy J, Pacsa AS. The suppressive effect of progesterone on lymphocyte cytotoxicity: unique progesterone sensitivity of pregnancy lymphocytes. J Reprod Immunol. 1985;7(2):121–128. doi:10.1016/0165–0378(85)90066-x

7. Abu-Raya B, Michalski C, Sadarangani M, Lavoie PM. Maternal Immunological Adaptation During Normal Pregnancy. Front Immunol. 2020;11:575197. Published 2020 Oct 7. doi:10.3389/fimmu.2020.575197

8. Barton JC, Wiener HW, Acton RT, Go RC. Total blood lymphocyte counts in hemochromatosis probands with HFE C282Y homozygosity: relationship to severity of iron overload and HLA-A and -B alleles and haplotypes. BMC Blood Disord. 2005;5:5. Published 2005 Jul 25. doi:10.1186/1471–2326-5–5

9. Wang RD, Wang CS, Feng ZH, Luo Y. Investigation on the effect of selenium on T lymphocyte proliferation and its mechanisms. J Tongji Med Univ. 1992;12(1):33–38. doi:10.1007/BF02887756

10. Hoffmann PR, Berry MJ. The influence of selenium on immune responses. Mol Nutr Food Res. 2008;52(11):1273–1280. doi:10.1002/mnfr.200700330

Monocytes

The absolute monocyte count measures the total count of monocytes in a sample. The monocyte percentage tells you what percentage of the white blood cell count is made up of monocytes. It is found in the complete blood count (CBC) with a differential panel.

Monocytes, lacking granules, fall under the category of agranulocytes. Accounting for between 2% and 10% of all leukocytes in the human body, monocytes play a crucial role in mitigating damage caused by inflammation and diseases. This involves the elimination of host cells through the process of phagocytosis. During the acute immune response, neutrophils take the lead, with monocytes following to clean up damaged cells. Elevated levels of monocytes are observed during the recovery phase of a disease.

Further differentiation of monocytes results in the formation of macrophages and dendrites. Macrophages, originating from monocytes in the bloodstream, migrate to the tissues to fulfill their functions. Dendrites regulate the adaptive immune system, initiating responses related to immune-system memory and promoting tolerance to pathogens.

The production of monocytes involves a series of intricate steps regulated by various factors crucial for their differentiation and maturation. Initially, monocyte progenitor cells undergo transformation into monoblasts under the influence of granulocyte-monocyte colony-stimulating factor (GM-CSF), with this process dependent on the presence of zinc. Subsequently, monoblasts progress into promonocytes, and this stage of monopoiesis is modulated by vitamins D and A. The conversion of promonocytes to mature monocytes is the final step, and it is influenced by vitamin C, which plays a role in the regulation of monocytes transitioning into dendrites. Moreover, iron affects the differentiation of monocytes into macrophages.

Pregnancy

In pregnancy, monocytes increase by approximately 38%. Serum monocyte levels remain elevated until 20 weeks and then decrease slightly in the third trimester. It is normal for there to be a slight increase in the pro-inflammatory pattern in pregnancy. Macrophages can be found in the maternal-fetal interface and positively influence embryo implantation, placental formation, embryonic development, and delivery processes.[1] Dendritic cells play an immuno-modulating role in pregnancy, which requires the maternal immune system to tolerate the fetus and, at the same time, to maintain adequate defense against pathogens.[2]

Postpartum

Monocytes can stay elevated postpartum in response to tissue damage caused by childbirth. These levels may stay elevated for three months postpartum but should not be outside of normal ranges. These levels may be abnormally elevated in women with gestational hypertensive disorders or postpartum preeclampsia.

Outside of normal rises, elevated monocytes are associated with increased preeclampsia risk. Interestingly, you'll also see low monocytes with preeclampsia, as more monocytes are converted to macrophage and dendrite lineages.[3]

An increased monocyte-to-lymphocyte ratio is a common finding in pregnancy.

STANDARD LAB RANGE: 0.1 – 0.9 × 10^9/L

Trimester	Standard Pregnancy Ranges	**Functional Pregnancy Ranges**
Preconception	0.1 – 0.7	**0.1 – 0.7**
First Trimester	0.1 – 1.1	**0.1 – 1.1**
Second Trimester	0.1 – 1.1	**0.2 – 1.1**
Third Trimester	0.1 – 1.4	**0.3 – 1.4**
Postpartum	0.1 – 1.4	**0.3 – 1.4**

STANDARD LAB RANGE: 2% – 10%

Trimester	Standard Pregnancy Ranges	**Functional Pregnancy Ranges**
Preconception	2 – 10%	**2 – 8%**
First Trimester	Not Established	**2 – 9%**
Second Trimester	Not Established	**2 – 9%**
Third Trimester	Not Established	**2 – 9%**
Postpartum	2 – 10%	**2 – 8%**

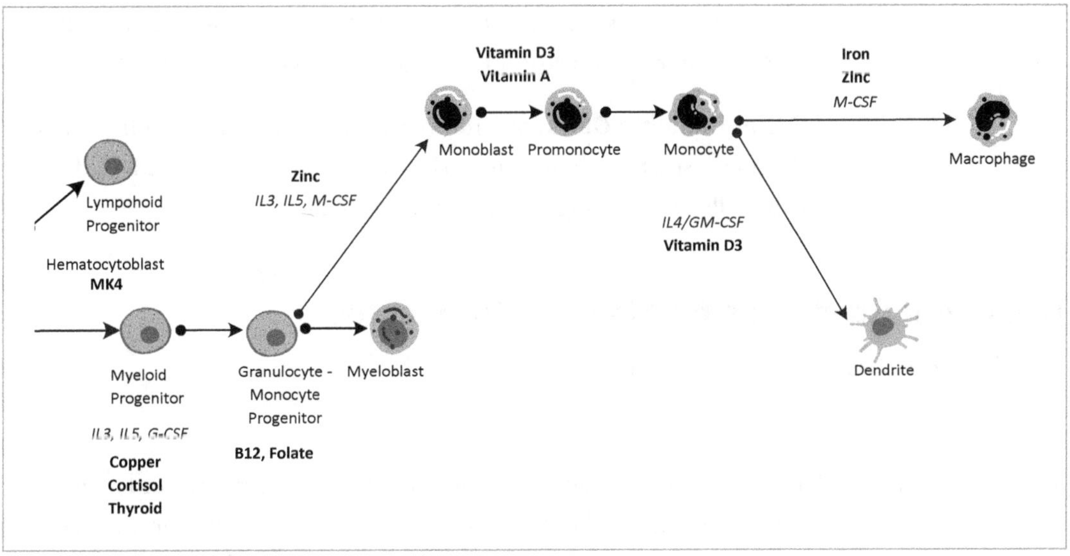

Figure 4: Monocytes Maturation:

Stem cell production is stimulated by MK4; Myeloblast differentiation is stimulated by IL3, IL5 and G-CSF; G-CSF is affected by copper and thyroid hormones; Zinc regulates M-CSF; B12 and folate are required for DNA methylation during early cellular development; Vitamin D3 & Vitamin A Modulation Monopoiesis; IL4/GM-CSF stimulates dendrite formation - regulated by Vitamin D3; Iron regulates Macrophage differentiation.

Causes of Elevated Monocytes

See White Blood Cell (WBC) Count Section.

Acute Infection Recovery: Monocytes are the cleanup crew of tissue damage. Elevations in monocytes indicate a recovery phase of illness or increased tissue damage recovery.

Liver Damage: In cases of liver damage or liver inflammation, monocytes increase. You will also typically see an overall increase in WBC production as well as higher lymphocyte production.

Ovarian Dysfunction: It has been well established that there is a pattern of elevated monocyte production and function in diminished ovarian reserve presentations. It has been theorized that some cases may belong to the category of autoimmune pathologies. Changes in monocyte levels may indicate the initial stages of autoimmune ovarian disease.[4]

Preeclampsia: During preeclampsia, the stressed placenta produces various pro-inflammatory factors, which further activate the monocytes and increase monocyte maturation toward nonclassical monocytes. Monocyte activation results in monocyte cytokine production.[5]

Other Possible Causes: autoimmune disease, chronic inflammatory diseases, stress, adrenal hyperfunction, myeloproliferative disease, tuberculosis, smoking, physical trauma, cancer

Treatment Strategies for Elevated Monocytes

See White Blood Cell (WBC) Count Section.

Diet

Incorporating foods rich in antioxidants, such as fruits (berries, citrus fruits) and vegetables (spinach, kale), can help neutralize oxidative stress and support overall immune health. Calcium and vitamin D are essential for immune regulation and can aid in maintaining a healthy balance of monocytes. Fatty acids, present in fatty fish, nuts and seeds, and bone-in/skin-on chicken, possess anti-inflammatory properties that may assist in modulating immune responses and potentially lowering elevated monocyte levels.

Lifestyle

During sleep, the body undergoes crucial repair and regeneration processes, enhancing its ability to combat infections and manage inflammation effectively. Consistent and restorative sleep patterns support the production of immune cells, including monocytes, while also facilitating their proper functioning. Insufficient sleep, on the other hand, can lead to elevated stress hormones and increased inflammation, potentially contributing to higher levels of monocytes. Integrating good sleep hygiene practices, such as maintaining a consistent sleep schedule and creating a conducive environment, can be instrumental in optimizing immune-system function and aiding in the recovery from infections and inflammation.

Additional Testing

comprehensive metabolic panel (CMP); c-reactive protein (CRP); lactate dehydrogenase (LDH); gamma-glutamyl transpeptidase (GGT)

Causes of Low Monocytes

See White Blood Cell (WBC) Count Section.

Vitamin D Deficiency: Vitamin D inhibits interleukin-4 (I-L4) and GM-CSF, which stimulates monocyte-to-dendrite cell maturation. When vitamin D is deficient, more monocytes are converted to

Decreased monocyte count throughout pregnancy is closely

associated with the development of gestational diabetes mellitus (GDM), macrosomia, and the chronic inflammatory state of GDM. First-trimester monocyte count has been shown to have great potential as an early diagnostic marker of GDM.[6]

dendrites, and thus there can be a decrease in monocytes in certain presentations.

Vitamin A Deficiency: Vitamin A is essential for the normal development and differentiation of immune cells, including monocytes. Vitamin A deficiency affects the maturation of monocytes in the bone marrow, leading to lower levels of circulating monocytes. It can also impair monocyte phagocytic activity.

Other Possible Causes: zinc deficiency, autoimmune disease, chronic inflammation, chronic viral disease (HIV), adrenal hypofunction, certain medicines (antibiotics and antivirals), preeclampsia

Treatment Strategies for Low Monocytes

See White Blood Cell (WBC) Count Section.

Diet

Zinc is particularly vital for the conversion of monocyte progenitor cells into monoblasts through the action of M-CSF. Ensuring an adequate intake of zinc-rich foods such as meat, seafood, nuts, and seeds can contribute to healthier monocyte development. Additionally, vitamins D and A modulate monopoiesis, guiding the progression of monoblasts to promonocytes. Foods rich in vitamin D, such as fatty fish, mushrooms, pork lard, and eggs, as well as those abundant in vitamin A, like liver, carrots, and sweet potatoes, can support monocyte maturation.

Supplements

If other biomarkers indicate zinc or vitamin D deficiency, supplementation may be beneficial.

Additional Testing

vitamin D, 25-hydroxy (25-hydroxycalciferol, 25OH-D); comprehensive metabolic panel (CMP); c-reactive protein (CRP); oral zinc tolerance test

References

1. Yao Y, Xu XH, Jin L. Macrophage Polarization in Physiological and Pathological Pregnancy. Front Immunol. 2019;10:792. Published 2019 Apr 15. doi:10.3389/fimmu.2019.00792

2. Wei R, Lai N, Zhao L, et al. Dendritic cells in pregnancy and pregnancy-associated diseases. Biomed Pharmacother. 2021;133:110921. doi:10.1016/j.biopha.2020.110921

3. Faas MM, de Vos P. Maternal monocytes in pregnancy and preeclampsia in humans and in rats. J Reprod Immunol. 2017;119:91–97. doi:10.1016/j.jri.2016.06.009

4. Zhang Z, Huang L, Brayboy L. Macrophages: an indispensable piece of ovarian health. Biol Reprod. 2021;104(3):527–538. doi:10.1093/biolre/ioaa219

5. Faas MM, Spaans F, De Vos P. Monocytes and macrophages in pregnancy and preeclampsia. Front Immunol. 2014;5:298. Published 2014 Jun 30. doi:10.3389/fimmu.2014.00298

6. Huang X, Zha B, Zhang M, et al. Decreased Monocyte Count Is Associated With Gestational Diabetes Mellitus Development, Macrosomia, and Inflammation. J Clin Endocrinol Metab. 2022;107(1):192–204. doi:10.1210/clinem/dgab657

Eosinophils

The absolute eosinophil count measures the total count of eosinophils in a sample. The eosinophil percentage tells you what percentage of the white blood cell count is made up of eosinophils. It is found in the complete blood count (CBC) with a differential panel.

Eosinophils compose between 1% and 3% of all white blood cells in the human body. They help control inflammation and allergic reactions, attack and destroy certain parasites, and play a role in detoxification and protein breakdown.

Eosinophils are granulocytes and contain granules that secrete substances that destroy allergens and parasites. The highest amounts of eosinophils are often found in mucosal tissues, such as the gastrointestinal (GI) tract and the respiratory system.

The production of eosinophils, like other blood cells, occurs through hematopoiesis, which takes place primarily in the bone marrow. Myeloid progenitor cells commit to the eosinophil lineage under the influence of specific cytokines, including interleukin-5 (IL-5) and granulocyte colony-stimulating factor (G-CSF). Copper regulates G-CSF in myeloid progenitor maturation. Vitamin D regulates the final steps in eosinophil maturation. Mature eosinophils are released from the bone marrow into the peripheral blood.

Pregnancy

There is a mild suppression of eosinophil production in pregnancy, but it should not be suppressed below normal ranges. This suppression can make it difficult to identify parasite infections in pregnancy and may reduce the immune-system response to parasites.[1]

Postpartum

There can be an increase of 90% in eosinophil production on days three to five postpartum.

> It has been observed that eosinophil levels increase and decrease at unique times in pregnancy. At 10 days gestation, there can be an increase in eosinophil production that returns to normal quickly. A sharp drop in eosinophils at the onset of labor is also associated with longer and more difficult labors.[2]
>
> A classic presentation of parasitic infection is monocytes >9%, eosinophils >3%, and basophils >1% in a preconception period.

STANDARD LAB RANGE: 0.0 – 0.4 × 10^9/L

Trimester	Standard Pregnancy Ranges	**Functional Pregnancy Ranges**
Preconception	0.0 – 0.6	**0.0 – 0.6**
First Trimester	0.0 – 0.6	**0.0 – 0.6**
Second Trimester	0.0 – 0.6	**0.0 – 0.6**
Third Trimester	0.0 – 0.6	**0.0 – 0.6**
Postpartum	0.0 – 0.6	**0.0 – 0.6**

STANDARD LAB RANGE: 0% – 7%

Trimester	Standard Pregnancy Ranges	**Functional Pregnancy Ranges**
Preconception	0 – 7%	**0 – 3%**
First Trimester	Not Established	**0 – 3%**
Second Trimester	Not Established	**0 – 3%**
Third Trimester	Not Established	**0 – 3%**
Postpartum	Not Established	**0 – 3%**

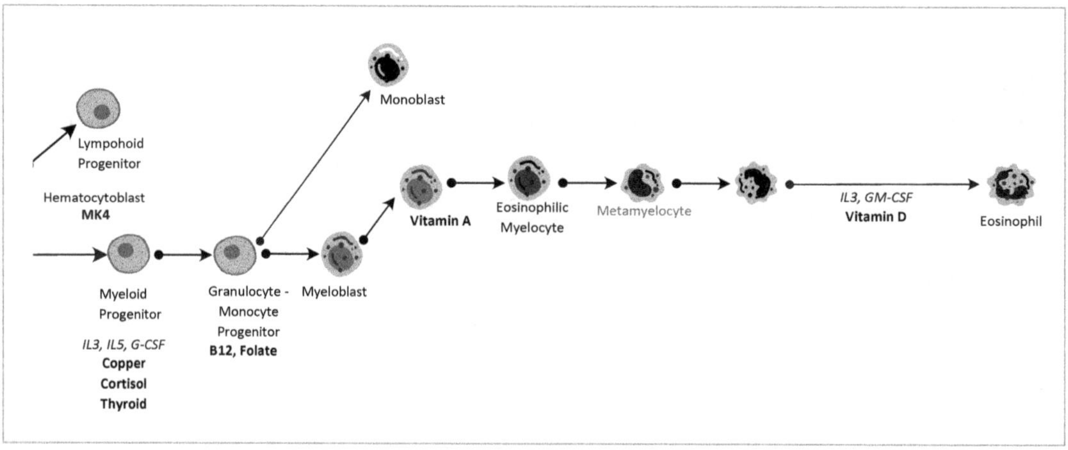

Figure 3: Eosinophil Maturation

Stem-cell production is stimulated by MK-4. Myeloblast differentiation is stimulated by IL-3, IL-5, and G-CSF. Copper regulates G-CSF in myeloid progenitor maturation. Vitamin A stimulates the differentiation and maturation of promyelocytes to granulocytes. Vitamin B12 (cobalamin) and vitamin B9 (folate) are required for DNA methylation during early cellular development. Vitamin C, selenium, and other nutrients are accumulated in cells during development. Vitamin A stimulates the differentiation and maturation of promyelocytes to granulocytes. Vitamin D3 modulates GM-CSF in eosinophil maturation.

Causes of Elevated Eosinophils

See White Blood Cell (WBC) Count Section.

Women with preterm labor and intact membranes who have a large proportion of eosinophils in the amniotic fluid are at an increased risk for spontaneous preterm delivery.[3]

Parasitic Infections: It is estimated that 60% of Americans have parasites but have not had proper diagnostics. Risk factors for parasitic infections include:

- farm animals
- foreign travel
- history of food-borne illness (food poisoning)
- house pets
- household family member with a previous parasite diagnosis
- increased consumption of raw and uncooked vegetables (particularly lettuce)
- increased consumption of raw meat/fish
- well-water use

Symptoms of parasitic infections may include:

- ADHD (attention-deficit/hyperactivity disorder) symptoms in adulthood
- burning or itching anus
- chronic allergies
- chronic anemia
- chronic fatigue
- difficulty gaining weight in pregnancy
- dry or scaly skin
- pallid complexion
- reduced appetite
- skin disorders (especially rashes along the jawline and neck)

Parasitic infections become difficult to treat in pregnancy. Many medications and herbal therapies are not safe in the pregnancy state. Management is the correct course of action until the woman is in a place in which it is safe to do proper treatment. Additional testing in cases of elevated eosinophils would include a comprehensive stool analysis. Additionally, you may see anemia due to malabsorption.

Asthma: Shortness of breath and an increase in mucus production are often normal presentations in pregnancy. Many of the lab ranges you would see in pre-pregnancy individuals with asthma become normal presentations in pregnancy, such as increased neutrophils, decreased lymphocytes, and increased serum copper and ceruloplasmin. Women with preexisting asthma may present with elevated eosinophils.

Inflammatory Bowel Diseases: Crohn's, ulcerative colitis, and celiac disease can all present with elevated eosinophils.

Food and Environmental Allergies: In cases of food allergies causing elevated eosinophils, basophils may be normal or elevated as well, with a normal monocyte presentation. The comprehensive metabolic panel (CMP) can also show a higher blood urea nitrogen (BUN).

Other Possible Causes: polycythemias, hyperthyroidism, edema, autoimmune disease, certain medications (antibiotics), environmental toxin exposure, heavy metal exposure, cancer

Treatment Strategies for Elevated Eosinophils

See White Blood Cell (WBC) Count Section.

Diet

Since eosinophils play a significant role in allergic responses, reducing allergens may be important. This involves identifying and avoiding common allergens such as certain foods, airborne particles, or environmental triggers. Additionally, supporting gut health and encouraging a well-balanced and diverse microbiome can contribute to immune system regulation. Consuming fiber-rich foods, prebiotics, and probiotics promotes a flourishing gut microbiota, potentially mitigating inflammation and allergic responses associated with elevated eosinophils.

Fermented foods and bone broth are renowned for their potential to reduce gut inflammation and promote digestive health. This may include foods such as yogurt, kefir, sauerkraut, and kimchi, which contain beneficial probiotics that contribute to a diverse and balanced gut microbiome. These probiotics support the growth of beneficial bacteria in the digestive tract, helping to maintain a healthy gut lining and modulate the immune response, ultimately reducing inflammation. Bone broth, rich in collagen and amino acids, provides essential nutrients that support gut integrity and may help soothe and repair the digestive lining.

Supplements

N-acetyl cysteine (NAC) has shown promise in providing relief for conditions involving elevated eosinophils. NAC has been studied for its therapeutic effects in respiratory conditions such as asthma and chronic obstructive pulmonary disease (COPD), where elevated eosinophils are often seen. This can also be used in pregnancy for acute upper respiratory infections. The standard dose for NAC is between 500 mg and 600 mg twice a day.

Additional Testing

comprehensive metabolic panel (CMP); comprehensive thyroid profile II; reverse T3 (rT3); thyroid peroxidase antibodies (TPOAb); thyroglobulin antibody (TgAb); thyroid receptor antibodies (TRAb); antinuclear antibodies (ANA); c-reactive protein (CRP); toxin testing; comprehensive stool testing

Causes of Low Eosinophils

See White Blood Cell (WBC) Count Section.

Other Possible Causes: hypothyroidism, vitamin D deficiency, long-term gut inflammation, adrenal dysfunction, systemic inflammatory response syndrome (SIRS)

Eosinophil counts <55 cells/μL may be used as a diagnostic marker for preeclampsia.[4]

Treatment Strategies for Low Eosinophils

See White Blood Cell (WBC) Count Section.

Diet

Vitamin A, found in foods like eggs, liver, carrots, sweet potatoes, and leafy greens, contributes to the development and maturation of eosinophils. Likewise, vitamin D, obtained through sunlight exposure and dietary sources such as fatty fish, eggs, pork lard, mushrooms, and dairy products, plays a crucial role in regulating the immune system, including the synthesis of eosinophils. These vitamins contribute to the maturation and activation of eosinophils.

Additional Testing

comprehensive metabolic panel (CMP); vitamin D, 25-hydroxy (25-hydroxycalciferol, 25OH-D); comprehensive thyroid profile II; c-reactive protein (CRP); comprehensive stool testing

References

1. Yae-Jean Kim, Thomas B. Nutman,CHAPTER 21—Eosinophilia, Editor(s): Patricia Frye Walker, Elizabeth D. Barnett, Immigrant Medicine, W.B. Saunders, 2007, Pages 309–319, ISBN 9780323034548, doi.org/10.1016/B978–0-323–03454-8.50025–5. (www.sciencedirect.com/science/article/pii/B9780323034548500255)

2. MARCUS MB, CIBLEY LJ, BRANDT ML, MILLMAN L, BARLAS D. Circulating eosinophils in labor and puerperium. Am J Obstet Gynecol. 1958;75(1):11–15. doi:10.1016/0002–9378(58)90543-x

3. Romero R, Kusanovic JP, Gomez R, et al. The clinical significance of eosinophils in the amniotic fluid in preterm labor. J Matern Fetal Neonatal Med. 2010;23(4):320–329. doi:10.3109/14767050903168465

4. Gelaw Y, Asrie F, Walle M, Getaneh Z. The value of eosinophil count in the diagnosis of preeclampsia among pregnant women attending the University of Gondar Comprehensive Specialized Hospital, Northwest Ethiopia, 2021. BMC Pregnancy Childbirth. 2022;22(1):557. Published 2022 Jul 12. doi:10.1186/s12884–022-04892–9

Basophils

The absolute basophil count measures the total count of basophils in a sample. The basophil percentage tells you what percentage of the white blood cell count comprises basophils. It is found in the complete blood count (CBC) with differential panel.

Basophils compose between 0.5% and 1% of all leukocytes in the human body. Basophils react in all cases of inflammation, especially allergic reactions. They also play a role in both internal and external parasitic infections. During an inflammatory response, basophils produce histamines and heparin. Histamines enlarge your blood vessels in affected areas, while heparin prevents clotting.

Basophils are granulocytes that originate from myeloid progenitors stimulated by interleukins IL-3 and IL-5 and G-CSF. The production of basophils is regulated by magnesium. Basophil progenitors mature in the bone marrow before being released into the bloodstream.

Pregnancy

Basophil levels slightly decrease during pregnancy and return to normal four to six weeks postpartum. This decrease should not be evident in the blood work.

Postpartum

There can be a decrease in basophil production toward the end of pregnancy and into the postpartum phase. These levels will return to normal by four months postpartum.[1]

STANDARD LAB RANGE: 0.0 – 0.2 × 10^9/L

Trimester	Standard Pregnancy Ranges	**Functional Pregnancy Ranges**
Preconception	0.0 – 0.1	**0.0 – 0.1**
First Trimester	0.0 – 0.1	**0.0 – 0.1**
Second Trimester	0.0 – 0.1	**0.0 – 0.1**
Third Trimester	0.0 – 0.1	**0.0 – 0.1**
Postpartum	0.0 – 0.1	**0.0 – 0.1**

STANDARD LAB RANGE: 0% – 3%

Trimester	Standard Pregnancy Ranges	**Functional Pregnancy Ranges**
Preconception	0 – 3%	**0 – 1%**
First Trimester	Not Established	**0 – 1%**
Second Trimester	Not Established	**0 – 1%**
Third Trimester	Not Established	**0 – 1%**
Postpartum	0 – 3%	**0 – 1%**

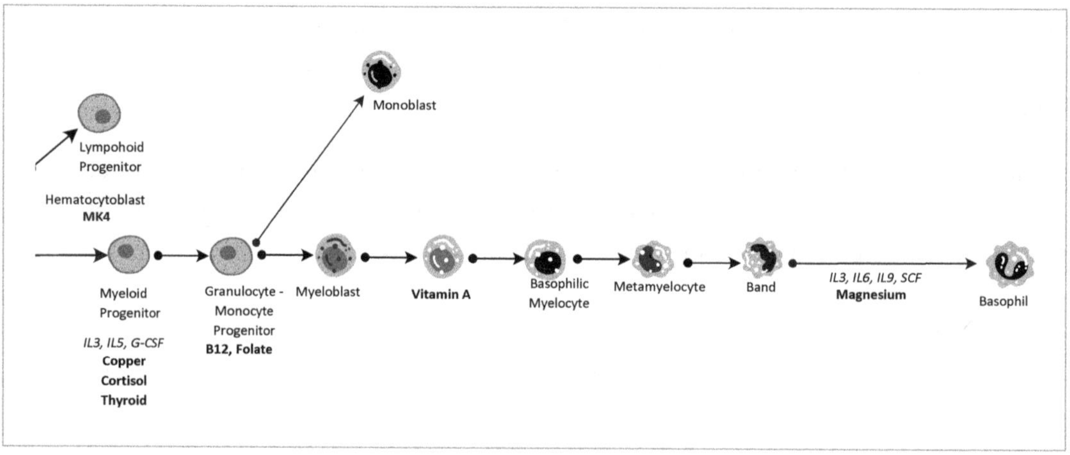

Figure 4: Basophil Maturation

Stem-cell production is stimulated by MK-4. Myeloblast differentiation is stimulated by IL-3, IL-5, and G-CSF. Copper regulates G-CSF in myeloid progenitor maturation. Vitamin A stimulates the differentiation and maturation of promyelocytes to granulocytes. Vitamin B12 (cobalamin) and vitamin B9 (folate) are required for DNA methylation during early cellular development. Vitamin C, selenium, and other nutrients are accumulated in cells during development. Vitamin A stimulates the differentiation and maturation of promyelocytes to granulocytes. Magnesium modulates SCF in basophil maturation.

Causes of Elevated Basophils

See White Blood Cell (WBC) Count Section.

Parasitic Infections: Basophils will be elevated with eosinophils and monocytes. Basophils contribute to the elimination of parasites by releasing substances that can damage or immobilize them. Histamine, for example, enhances vascular permeability, facilitating the entry of other immune cells to the infection site.

Allergies: Acute allergic reactions will increase basophil production. β cells produce immunoglobin E (IgE) antibodies. Basophils, like mast cells, are equipped with receptors that specifically recognize IgE antibodies and become activated. Activated basophils release inflammatory mediators including histamine, leukotrienes, and cytokines. Histamine is a particularly important mediator in allergic reactions.

Systemic Inflammation: When basophils are elevated greater than 1%, systemic inflammation should be considered. CRP can be a useful additional biomarker. (See C-Reactive Protein (CRP) Section.)

Autoimmune Hypothyroidism: Autoimmune hypothyroidism is associated with a state of chronic inflammation. The inflammatory environment may contribute to alterations in white blood cell populations, including increased basophils. Thyroid hormones have immunomodulatory effects, influencing the balance of pro-inflammatory and anti-inflammatory responses. In hypothyroidism, this balance may be disrupted. Basophils can be elevated when autoimmune hypothyroidism is present. In this scenario, you would also see a decrease in red blood cell (RBC) counts, hemoglobin (HB), hematocrit (HCT), mean corpuscular hemoglobin (MCH), and mean corpuscular hemoglobin concentration (MCHC), with an increase in mean corpuscular volume (MCV).

Hyperthyroidism: Thyroid hormones influence hematopoiesis, and changes in thyroid hormone levels can affect the production and maturation of white blood cells, potentially leading to an increase in basophils. In this case, you will also see elevated red blood cell (RBC) counts, hemoglobin (HGB), hematocrit (HCT), mean corpuscular hemoglobin (MCH), and mean corpuscular hemoglobin concentration (MCHC).

Pesticide Exposure: Studies have shown that exposure to high amounts of pesticides can cause elevated basophils, as well as neutrophils and platelets.[2]

Other Possible Causes: polycythemias, influenza, adrenal dysfunction, autoimmune disease, environmental chemical exposure, heavy metal exposure, cancer

Treatment Strategies for Elevated Basophils

See White Blood Cell (WBC) Count Section.

Diet

Increase flavonoid-rich foods such as green tea, red grapes, berries, green leafy vegetables, red cabbage, citrus, and fermented soy. Foods high in vitamin C such as citrus fruits, strawberries, and bell peppers may have anti-allergic properties and act as natural antihistamines. Choose locally grown and seasonal fruits and vegetables. These may be less likely to contain high levels of pesticides, which can trigger allergic and immune-system reactions. Not everyone can afford local and organic produce. Rinsing in tap water alone has been shown to remove a significant amount of pesticide residues. Some studies have shown that washing in a vinegar and water mix can remove up to 65% of the pesticide residues.[3]

Following a low-histamine diet may also have a positive effect on basophil counts. The histamine diet is not designed to remove all dietary histamines but to reduce high exposure. This would include consuming foods that are fresh and not eating overly ripe foods or leftovers. Avoid highly processed foods. Avoid aged cheeses, fermented vegetables, stored nuts and seeds, and legumes and grains. A true low-histamine diet can be overwhelming, as it limits many foods.

Supplements

Quercetin is one of the most potent flavonoids for regulating histamine and basophil reactions, but studies show that it is also an iron chelator and may not be safe to use in pregnancy.[4]

Diamine oxidase (DAO) is an enzyme that helps the body break down histamines in the digestive tract. DAO is produced in high amounts by the placenta during pregnancy, with lower levels being associated with higher-risk pregnancies. The initial rise is seen around five to six weeks gestational age. Although there is adequate data on the function and production of DAO in pregnancy, there is little research on the use of it in supplementation. That being said, no adverse health effects have been reported in studies on DAO supplements to date. Some studies have suggested that supplementing with copper, vitamin B6 (pyridoxine), and vitamin C can help lower histamine levels. This should only be done when insufficiency or deficiency is suspected.

Additional Testing

c-reactive protein (CRP); comprehensive thyroid profile II; reverse T3 (rT3); thyroid peroxidase antibodies (TPOAb); thyroglobulin antibody (TgAb); thyroid receptor antibodies (TRAb); comprehensive stool testing; allergy testing; antinuclear antibodies (ANA)

Causes of Low Basophils

See White Blood Cell (WBC) Count Section.

Magnesium Deficiency: The production of basophils is regulated by magnesium, via its connection to stem cell factor (SCF), which is needed in the maturation process of basophils.

Other Possible Causes: hypothyroidism, adrenal dysfunction, chronic inflammation, adrenal hyperfunction, progesterone deficiency

Treatment Strategies for Low Basophils

See White Blood Cell (WBC) Count Section.

Diet

Boosting magnesium intake through diet may help if magnesium deficiency is suspected. Leafy green vegetables like spinach and kale, nuts such as almonds and cashews, seeds like pumpkin and sunflower, and whole grains like brown rice and quinoa are excellent sources of magnesium. Fatty fish like salmon, dark chocolate with high cocoa content, avocados, bananas, and herbs like coriander and parsley also contribute to magnesium intake.

Additional Testing

comprehensive thyroid profile II; comprehensive metabolic panel (CMP); c-reactive protein (CRP); progesterone

References

1. Nasu M, Fujiyasu S, Iwatani Y, Amino N, Tanizawa O, Miyai K. Rinsho Byori. 1992;40(12):1292–1296

2. Nejatifar F, Abdollahi M, Attarchi M, et al. Evaluation of hematological indices among insecticides factory workers. Heliyon. 2022;8(3):e09040. Published 2022 Mar 3. doi:10.1016/j.heliyon.2022.e09040

3. Yang SJ, Mun S, Kim HJ, et al. Effectiveness of Different Washing Strategies on Pesticide Residue Removal: The First Comparative Study on Leafy Vegetables. Foods. 2022;11(18):2916. Published 2022 Sep 19. doi:10.3390/foods11182916

4. Vanhees K, Godschalk RW, Sanders A, van Waalwijk van Doorn-Khosrovani SB, van Schooten FJ. Maternal quercetin intake during pregnancy results in an adapted iron homeostasis at adulthood. *Toxicology*. 2011;290(2–3):350–358. doi:10.1016/j.tox.2011.10.017

Immature Granulocytes

The absolute immature granulocyte count measures the total count of young granulocytes in a sample. The immature granulocyte percentage tells you what percentage of the white blood cell count is made up of young granulocytes. It is often found in the complete blood count (CBC) with differential panel but not always.

Granulocytes are white blood cells with granules. They include neutrophils, eosinophils, and basophils. Generally, immature granulocytes are found only in the bone marrow; in certain situations, these immature cells are released into circulation to finish maturing.

Pregnancy

Outside of pregnancy, having immature granulocytes in the bloodstream is a sign of disease. It is commonly seen in allergic reactions, acute infections, and inflammation. In pregnancy, having immature granulocytes is a normal presentation.[1] Immature granulocytes increase in pregnancy, becoming significantly higher in the second and third trimesters. These ranges also increase with age. This increase is due to a higher cell turnover of neutrophils.

Postpartum

Immature granulocyte release into the bloodstream continues for up to eight weeks postpartum.

STANDARD LAB RANGE: 0.0 – 0.1 × 10^9/L

Trimester	Standard Pregnancy Ranges	**Functional Pregnancy Ranges**
Preconception	0.0 – 0.1	**0.0 – 0.05**
First Trimester	0.003 – 0.09	**0.003 – 0.09**
Second Trimester	0.007 – 0.247	**0.007 – 0.247**
Third Trimester	0.018 – 0.456	**0.018 – 0.456**
Postpartum	0.018 – 0.456	**0.018 – 0.456**

STANDARD LAB RANGE: 0% – 1%

Trimester	Standard Pregnancy Ranges	**Functional Pregnancy Ranges**
Preconception	0–1%	**0–1%**
First Trimester	0–1%	**0–1%**
Second Trimester	0.1–2%	**0.1–2%**
Third Trimester	0.2–3.8%	**0.2–3.8%**
Postpartum	0.2–3.8%	**0.2–3.8%**

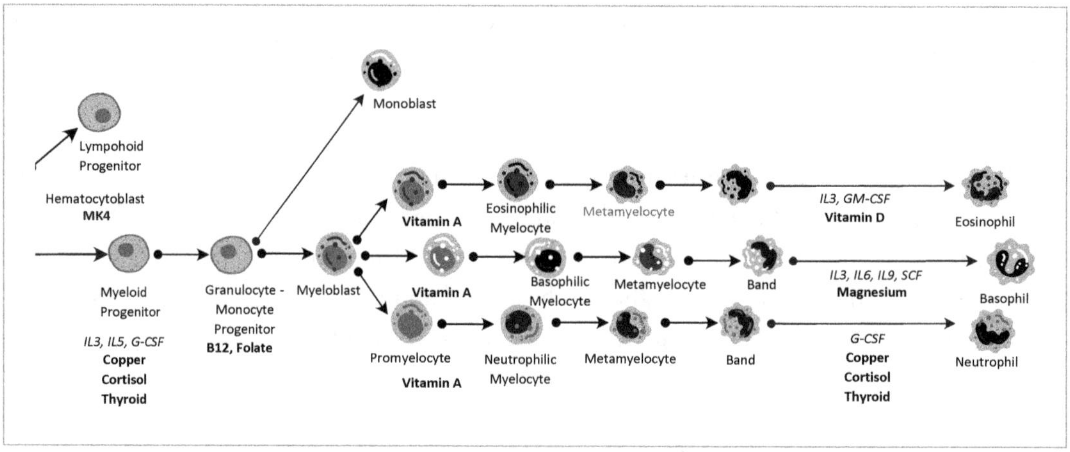

Figure 4: Granulocytes Maturation

Causes of Elevated Immature Granulocytes

See the following sections: Basophils, Eosinophils, Neutrophils, and White Blood Cell (WBC) Count.

When assessing the cause of abnormally high or low values of immature granulocytes, it is important to consider the entire differential. Because the immature granulocyte test is a combination of all young granulocytes, determining the cause requires assessing which granulocytes are elevated.

Other Possible Causes: infection, autoimmune disease, acute physical trauma, hyperthyroidism

Treatment Strategies for Elevated Immature Granulocytes

See the following sections: Basophil, Eosinophil, Neutrophil, and White Blood Cell (WBC) Count.

Causes of Low Immature Granulocytes

See the following sections: Basophils, Eosinophils, Neutrophils, and White Blood Cell (WBC) Count.

Other Possible Causes: aplastic anemia, hypothyroidism, autoimmune disease, chronic inflammatory conditions (inflammatory bowel disease), certain medications (antibiotics, antivirals), malnutrition, mycotoxin exposure

Treatment Strategies for Low Immature Granulocytes

See the following sections: Basophil, Eosinophil, Neutrophil, and White Blood Cell (WBC) Count.

References

1. Yu, L.-L & Jin, Y.-M & Li, M.-M & Chen, X.-J & Zheng, Xiangkuo. (2016). Changes and reference intervals of immature granulocytes in the peripheral blood of women according to pregnancy trimester. 9. 8169–8175

Platelet Count (PLT)

The platelet count (PLT) measures the total number of platelets in a sample. This is found in the complete blood count (CBC) panel.

Platelets are also called thrombocytes. *Thrombo* is Greek for "clump." The production of platelets is regulated by thrombopoietin. Platelets have a circadian rhythm, and the highest counts are found at midday. They make up less than 1% of blood cells.

Platelets are formed from myeloid progenitors. The production of platelets is regulated by thrombopoietin interleukins IL-3, IL-6, and IL-11. Vitamin A directly upregulates the genetic expression of thrombopoeitin, while both vitamin A and thyroid hormones upregulate the expression of erythropoietin (EPO). EPO also contributes to platelet formation, specifically the maturation of megakaryoblasts to megakaryocytes. Each megakaryocyte produces thousands of platelets.

Platelets function through adhesion and aggregation. Adhesion is the sticking of platelets to affected tissues, and aggregation is the sticking of platelets to each other. Blood-clotting disorders may affect the normal function of platelets regardless of counts. Platelets also play a role in innate immunity, binding to pathogens and killing them.

Pregnancy

Platelet counts drop between 15% and 20% throughout the course of gestation; this is why it is important that the platelet levels in the first trimester are addressed if low. In the first trimester, platelet reactivity decreases to allow for less clotting and easier blood flow. In the third trimester, platelet reactivity increases to prepare for childbirth.[1]

Postpartum

Within 14 days postpartum, platelet counts increase, regardless of birth type. There can be an increase of two- or threefold in preeclamptic births.[2] This rise will stay elevated until approximately eight weeks postpartum.

> Platelet activity fluctuates throughout pregnancy and is a normal feature of pregnancy due to the complex and changing ratios of coagulation factors, collagen changes, hormones, and other physiological factors. There is a high turnover of platelets throughout pregnancy based on these features. Platelets live in circulation for approximately eight or nine days, so changes can be seen almost weekly.

When analyzing and comparing platelet counts from different pregnancy periods, you should consider large jumps up or down as potentially pathogenic.

STANDARD LAB RANGE: 150 – 450 × 10^9/L

Trimester	Standard Pregnancy Ranges	**Functional Pregnancy Ranges**
Preconception	150–450	**150 – 450**
First Trimester	150–350	**150 – 250**
Second Trimester	135–350	**150 – 350**
Third Trimester	121–350	**150 – 350**
Postpartum	150–450	**150 – 450**

It is important to consider other lab parameters. Some women have platelet counts less than 150 × 10^3/μL without complication.[3]

Causes of Elevated Platelet Count (PLT)

Elevated platelets (>350 × 10^9/L) are a sign of serious disease and should be assessed by a maternal-fetal medicine physician or other specialized medical provider. Between 30% and 50% of patients with elevated platelets, known as thrombocytosis, will not successfully deliver a healthy baby.[4]

Myeloproliferative Diseases: Myeloproliferative disorders (MPDs) are blood cancers caused by changes in the stem cells inside bone marrow. Polycythemia vera (PV) and thrombocythemia fall into this category.

Autoimmune Joint Inflammation: It is common to see elevated platelets in patients with rheumatoid arthritis (RA). Generally, those with RA and other autoimmune joint diseases do well in pregnancy. Approximately 50% of women will have lower disease activity in pregnancy; between 20% and 40% will have remission of symptoms in the third trimester; and 20% will have a worsening of symptoms, including elevated platelets, during pregnancy.[7] Between 39% and 90% of women will have an RA flare during the first four months postpartum.[8] Autoimmune responses seem dependent on fetal-placental genetics. Fetuses with genetic material more like the mother will

Some studies have linked slightly elevated first-trimester platelets (>250 × 10^9/L) between weeks 8 to 10 with miscarriage; less than 250 × 10^9/L seems protective for early fetal growth.[5] As always, this measure should not be taken on its own and should be assessed with other blood parameters to determine risk factors.

Elevated first-trimester platelets, mean platelet volume (MPV), and red blood cell (RBC) counts in the first trimester increase the risk of postpartum hemorrhage.[6]

elicit a greater response, causing more inflammation. The less similar the genetic material, the more likely there is to be remission of symptoms in pregnancy.[9]

Oral Contraceptive Use: It has been well established that women on combination oral contraceptives have elevated platelet counts. Estrogen increases platelet count and plasma concentrations of clotting factors by increasing gene transcription. In the third trimester, when estrogen levels are their highest, this action helps prepare for the required increase in clotting needed for childbirth. This may be observed in the preconception phase and may contribute to implantation failure due to changes in blood-clotting factor expression and regulation. This risk is more likely in those with preexisting blood-clotting disorders.

Iron Deficiency: Iron is a regulator of both thrombopoietin and EPO, yet most patients with iron deficiency will have normal elevated platelet counts.[10] A classic pattern seen in iron deficiency would be normal-to-elevated platelet counts, low serum total iron, low ferritin, low transferrin saturation, and low mean platelet volume (MPV).

Hyperthyroid Disorders/Autoimmune Thyroid Disorders: Excess thyroid hormones can cause an increase in the production of thrombopoietin and EPO. Both are needed for the maturation of megakaryoblasts to megakaryocytes and, eventually, platelets. Immune thrombocytopenia can be seen with several different autoimmune diseases, such as Hashimoto's and Graves'. Inflammation triggers an increase in platelet production, and then autoimmune responses shorten the lifespan of the platelets themselves. Unmanaged Hashimoto's is associated with higher platelet counts, while Graves' is associated with higher mean platelet volume (MPV).[11] With abnormal platelet counts, additional thyroid testing should be run. (See Thyroid-Stimulating Hormone (TSH) Section.)

Vitamin D Deficiency: Several studies have shown that low vitamin D is associated with higher platelet counts as well as higher MPV levels. This seems to be highly associated with autoimmune disease as well. Testing for vitamin D should be standard in pregnancy, but if elevated platelet counts and MPV are observed, additional vitamin D testing is warranted. (See Vitamin D, 25-Hydroxy (25-Hydroxycalciferol, 25OH-D) Section.)

Other Possible Causes: pesticide exposure, sickle cell anemia

Treatment Strategies for Elevated Platelet Count (PLT)

Diet

Diet plays an important role in the regulation of platelet activity. When platelets are elevated, you must regulate function to reduce the risk of excess clotting disease risk. Diets that are high in omega-3 fatty acids and foods high in anti-inflammatories are important. Mediterranean dietary patterns have been shown to help reduce the inflammation of underlying elevated platelets and help control clotting. Reducing caffeine intake can also help regulate clotting activity. Caffeine has been shown to increase platelet aggregation, specifically energy drinks. Dark chocolate, foods with low glycemic index, garlic, ginger, omega-3 fatty acids, onion, purple grape juice, tomatoes, and wine (red grapes during pregnancy) all reduce platelet aggregation.[12]

Allicin, found in garlic, is also effective at regulating platelet formation. Allicin inhibits human platelet aggregation in vitro without affecting cyclooxygenase or thromboxane synthase activity, which is the primary clotting factor of childbirth.[13] Raw garlic is best, as the allicin is partially destroyed in cooking. Polyphenol-rich foods such as pomegranates have been shown to reduce platelet production and regulate platelet aggregation.[14]

Lifestyle

Light activity is important. A sedentary lifestyle can increase the risk of complications associated with elevated platelets. Yoga and walking are two beneficial activities. Smoking and vaping can increase the risk of clotting and should be discontinued in all pregnancies, but especially in those with elevated platelet counts. Sleep is also important because that is when the body heals any damage. Sleep deprivation, such as sleep apnea in pregnancy, can worsen inflammation and trigger increased platelet counts.

Supplements

Vitamin D3 supplementation has been shown to decrease platelet counts.[15] Correct dosing would vary based on serum vitamin D testing. Generally, the average dosage used in studies was 50,000 IU weekly for six weeks orally followed by 1,800 IU/day vitamin D (nonpregnant). (See Vitamin D Section.) Fish oil supplements of between 2,000 and 3,000 mg total omega can also be useful in regulating clotting factors. Caution should be taken with DHA-only (docosahexaenoic acid) supplements, as they could increase bleeding risk. Fish oil supplements that contain both EPA (eicosapentaenoic acid) and DHA do not show a correlation to an increased risk in hemorrhage and bleeding incidence.[16]

Supplementing with iron can be beneficial if increased platelets are associated with a deficiency in iron. (See Iron Section.)

Alpha-lipoic acid (ALA) is an antioxidant supplement that has increasing uses in pregnancy-complication prevention. ALA has been shown to decrease platelet counts.[17] Vitamin C in doses between 250 mg and 1,000 mg per day over the course of a week has been shown to reduce the expression of IL-6 and thus decrease thrombopoiesis.[18]

Additional Testing

prothrombin time (PT); activated partial thromboplastin time (aPTT); antinuclear antibodies (ANA); iron and TIBC; ferritin; comprehensive thyroid profile II; thyroid peroxidase antibodies (TPOAb); thyroglobulin antibody (TgAb); thyroid receptor antibodies; vitamin D, 25-hydroxy (25-hydroxycalciferol, 25OH-D)

Causes of Low Platelet Count (PLT)

Thrombocytopenia in pregnancy, defined as a platelet count of under 150 × 10^9/L, is the second most common hematological abnormality in pregnancy.[19]

Significant drops in platelets can happen early in preeclampsia before hypertension and renal disease appear.[20]

Most guidelines raise concern at platelet count <100 × 10^9/L, which occurs in <1% of all term deliveries.[21] Less than 150 × 10^9/L is associated with a twofold increased risk of postpartum hemorrhage.

If platelet counts are low in the first trimester, the most likely

Gestational Thrombocytopenia (GT): It is important to know the platelet counts before pregnancy and into the first trimester to assess for a normal drop. Typically, in GT, platelet levels do not drop below 130 × 10^9/L. GT is associated with hemodilution. There is a 50% increase in the plasma of the blood during pregnancy, and hemodilution can change many parameters of the CBC. GT is diagnosed when all other causes have been ruled out.

Lupus: Thrombocytopenia is found in approximately 40% of patients with systemic lupus erythematosus (SLE). Testing antinuclear antibodies (ANA), if not diagnosed previously, may help identify etiology.[22]

Selenium Deficiency: Though selenium doesn't play a direct role in the formation of platelets, it is needed to produce the antioxidant glutathione. Glutathione is important for reducing the reactive oxygen species (ROS) and oxidative stress in platelet cells, keeping them alive longer.

Vitamin B9 (Folate) and Vitamin B12 (Cobalamin) Deficiency: Blast cells require vitamin B12 and vitamin B9 for proliferation during their differentiation phase, via methylation and mitosis support. Megakaryoblast-to-megakaryocyte production and the transcription of platelets require methylation nutrients. There is an interesting connection between low platelets and elevated homocysteine. A higher homocysteine level with lower platelets is associated with higher diastolic blood pressure. If platelets are low, testing homocysteine may

factors are immune thrombocytopenia, genetics, and nutritional deficiencies. If thrombocytopenia presents in the second or third trimesters, you should rule out preeclampsia and HELLP syndrome, as well as nutritional deficiencies, before diagnosing as idiopathic gestational thrombocytopenia.

be a useful tool to assess methylation and the need for homocysteine support. (See Homocysteine Section.)

Zinc Deficiency: Zinc deficiency is found in those with immune thrombocytopenia. Zinc helps to regulate immune responses that can cause cell death. It also helps to decrease the expression of c-reactive protein (CRP) on platelet cells and regulates blood-clotting factors. Zinc deficiency is associated with prolonged bleeding times.

Protein-Deficient Diet

Protein-deficient diets have been associated with lower platelet counts.[23] The pattern seen in low-protein diets is low platelets and low mean platelet volume (MPV), but normal platelet distribution width (PDW).

Vitamin A Deficiency: Vitamin A is required for the genetic expression of thrombopoietin. A study from 1923 used vitamin A-deficient diets to elicit thrombocytopenia and then corrected with vitamin A supplementation. Vitamin A needs go up sixfold in the third trimester in preparation for childbirth, a portion of which is used in platelet expression.[24] This may also be caused by over-supplementing with vitamin D, as vitamin D and vitamin A have counteractive properties.

HELLP Syndrome: Lower platelet counts in HELLP syndrome are associated with hemolysis, or the destruction of blood cells. This is often the first marker, before hypertension and elevated liver enzymes present. A significant and rapid drop in platelets should be investigated. A comprehensive metabolic panel (CMP) should be run in cases of rapid platelet drops.

Stress: There is a negative association between cortisol and platelets. Studies link a decrease in platelets with physical and emotional stress.[25] This can be characterized by easy bruising.

Hypothyroidism: Thyroid hormones stimulate the genetic expression of thrombopoietin and EPO. Both are needed for the maturation of megakaryoblasts to immature megakaryocytes.[26]

Other Possible Causes: medications (nonsteroidal anti-inflammatories), viral infections, genetic disorders, hemolysis, vitamin B12 (cobalamin) deficiency, liver disease, alcohol use, bone-marrow disorders, environmental toxin exposure, mycotoxin exposure

Treatment Strategies for Low Platelet Count (PLT)

Diet

Coconut water has been shown to help increase platelet counts as well as improve clotting time. The younger the coconut, the better the outcomes. The mechanism of action is currently unknown. Flavonoids and polyphenols found in a variety of fruits and vegetables can help to increase platelet counts by reducing platelet loss via oxidative stress. Focusing on the nutrients that go into proper platelet differentiation and formation is key to increasing platelets through diet. Focus must also be on causes of cell death. Nutrient focus is on vitamin B12 (cobalamin), vitamin B9 (folate), zinc, and vitamin A. Again, studies show that adhering to a Mediterranean-style diet that is high in fat and antioxidants helps increase platelets as much as it helps to reduce excess counts.[27] The Brewer Diet would also be of benefit in these scenarios, as would the New Nordic Diet.

Lifestyle

Decrease toxin exposure. When platelets are low, we think of two things: issues in their production or a decrease in cell life. Pesticides on produce, specifically glyphosates, are associated with thrombocytopenia as these pesticides decrease cell lifespan and cause apoptosis of platelet cells.[28] Choosing local produce free of glyphosates can reduce exposure. In areas where local and pesticide-free produce is not available, patients should be instructed to thoroughly wash their produce with soap and water or do a vinegar soak.

Supplements

N-acetyl cysteine (NAC) is an antioxidant supplement used in the treatment of thrombocytopenia. A few case studies have shown a positive increase in platelet counts with supplementation. NAC has a long safety record in pregnancy care, mostly in the treatment of acetaminophen overdose. Research is pointing to the use of NAC in a variety of other pregnancy complications as well.[29] Additional vitamin B12 (cobalamin), in the form of injection therapy, may be useful to help increase platelet levels in the presence of both poor formation and toxin exposure. Studies show that vitamin B12 supplementation may help protect against the damage associated with glyphosate exposure.[30] Overdosing on vitamin B12 is possible, so make sure to assess its function before administering injection therapy, by looking at other CBC values as well as possibly homocysteine, methylmalonic acid, and serum B12.

Caution

High-dose alpha-lipoic acid supplementation of 80 mg/kg/d was associated with a severe drop in platelet counts.[31] When using this supplementation in the prevention of pregnancy complications, be sure to assess platelet counts during use.

Additional Testing

antinuclear antibodies (ANA); homocysteine; vitamin B12 (cobalamin); comprehensive metabolic panel (CMP); vitamin D, 25-hydroxy (25-hydroxycalciferol, 25OH-D); lactate dehydrogenase (LDH); oral zinc tolerance test

References

1. Burke, N, Flood, K, Murray, A, Cotter, B, Dempsey, M, Fay, L, Dicker, P, Geary, MP, Kenny, D, Malone, FD. Platelet reactivity changes significantly throughout all trimesters of pregnancy compared with the nonpregnant state: a prospective study. BJOG 2013; DOI: 10.1111/1471–0528.12394

2. Reese JA, Peck JD, Deschamps DR, et al. Platelet Counts during Pregnancy. N Engl J Med. 2018;379(1):32–43. doi:10.1056/NEJMoa1802897

3. Aune B, Gjesdal K, Oian P. Late-onset postpartum thrombocytosis in preeclampsia. Acta Obstet Gynecol Scand. 1999;78(10):866–870

4. Jønsson V, Bock JE, Mortensen TH, Staun M, Thorsen S. Svangerskabsrelateret trombocytose [Pregnancy-related thrombocytosis]. Ugeskr Laeger. 2002;164(34):3946–3949

5. Shao X, Wang D, Xu Y, et al. The high platelet counts as predictor for early foetal demise. Ann Med. 2021;53(1):1502–1508. doi:10.1080/07853890.2021.1968027

6. Robinson, M.R., Patxot, M., Stojanov, M. et al. Postpartum hemorrhage risk is driven by changes in blood composition through pregnancy. Sci Rep 11, 19238 (2021). doi.org/10.1038/s41598–021-98411-z

7. Krause ML, Makol A. Management of rheumatoid arthritis during pregnancy: challenges and solutions. Open Access Rheumatol. 2016. 8:23–36

8. Van der Horst-Bruinsma IE, de Vries RR, de Buck PD, van Schendel PW, Breedveld FC, Schreuder GM, et al. Influence of the HLA-class II incompatibility between mother and fetus on the development and course of rheumatoid arthritis of the mother. Ann Rheum Dis. 1998 May. 57(5):286–90

9. Dissanayake TD, Maksymowych WP, Keeling SO. Peripartum issues in the inflammatory arthritis patient: A survey of the RAPPORT registry. Sci Rep. 2020 Feb 28. 10(1):3733

10. Kadikoylu G, Yavasoglu I, Bolaman Z, Senturk T. Platelet parameters in women with iron-deficiency anemia. J Natl Med Assoc. 2006;98(3):398–402

11. Cao YT, Zhang KY, Sun J, et al. Platelet abnormalities in autoimmune thyroid diseases: A systematic review and meta-analysis [published correction appears in Front Immunol. 2023 Feb 21;14:1166711]. Front Immunol. 2022;13:1089469. Published 2022 Dec 22. doi:10.3389/fimmu.2022.1089469

12. McEwen BJ. The influence of diet and nutrients on platelet function. Semin Thromb Hemost. 2014;40(2):214–226. doi:10.1055/s-0034–1365839

13. Mayeux, P.R., Agrawal, K.C., Tou, J.S.H. et al. The pharmacological effects of allicin, a constituent of garlic oil. Agents and Actions 25, 182–190 (1988). doi.org/10.1007/BF01969110

14. Mattiello T, Trifirò E, Jotti GS, Pulcinelli FM. Effects of pomegranate juice and extract polyphenols on platelet function. J Med Food. 2009;12(2):334–339. doi:10.1089/jmf.2007.0640

15. Kucukay MB, Alanli R. Vitamin D Replacement Effect on Platelet Counts. J Coll Physicians Surg Pak. 2021;31(9):1064–1068. doi:10.29271/jcpsp.2021.09.1064

16. Begtrup KM, Krag AE, Hvas AM. No impact of fish oil supplements on bleeding risk: a systematic review. Dan Med J. 2017;64(5):A5366

17. Petca A, Bot M, Maru N, et al. Benefits of α-lipoic acid in high-risk pregnancies (Review). Exp Ther Med. 2021;22(5):1232. doi:10.3892/etm.2021.10666

18. Gholizadeh M, Ghafour Saeedy SA, Abdi A, Khademi F, Lorian K, Clark CCT, Djafarian K. Vitamin C reduces interleukin-6 plasma concentration: a systematic review and meta-analysis of randomized clinical trials. Clinical Nutrition Open Science. 2021;40:1–14. ISSN 2667–2685. doi.org/10.1016/j.nutos.2021.09.003. (www.sciencedirect.com/science/article/pii/S2667268521000358)

19. Mangla A, Hamad H. Thrombocytopenia in Pregnancy. [Updated 2022 Nov 30]. In: StatPearls [Internet]. Treasure Island (FL): StatPearls Publishing; Jan 2023. www.ncbi.nlm.nih.gov/books/NBK547705

20. Ciobanu AM, Colibaba S, Cimpoca B, Peltecu G, Panaitescu AM. Thrombocytopenia in Pregnancy. Maedica (Bucur). 2016;11(1):55–60

21. Govindappagari S, Moyle K, Burwick RM. Mild Thrombocytopenia and Postpartum Hemorrhage in Nulliparous Women With Term, Singleton, Vertex Deliveries. Obstet Gynecol. 2020;135(6):1338–1344. doi:10.1097/AOG.0000000000003861

22. Galanopoulos N, Christoforidou A, Bezirgiannidou Z. Lupus thrombocytopenia: pathogenesis and therapeutic implications. Mediterr J Rheumatol. 2017;28(1):20–26. Published 2017 Mar 28. doi:10.31138/mjr.28.1.20

23. Olayanju AO, Ukaejiofo EO, Sulaiman HA, et al. Impact of hypoproteic diet on liver function and thrombopoiesis in New Zealand white rabbits. Hematol Transfus Int J. 2016;3(1):147–152. DOI: 10.15406/htij.2016.03.00060

24. Bedson SP, Zilva SS. The Influence of Vitamin A on the Blood-Platelets of the Rat. Br J Exp Pathol. 1923;4(1):5–12

25. Hemati Z, Kiani D. The comparison of perceived stress in idiopathic thrombocytopenic purpura patients referred to Seyed Al-Shohada Hospital with healthy people in Isfahan, Iran, 2013. Int J Hematol Oncol Stem Cell Res. 2015;9(2):67–71

26. Ma Y, Freitag P, Zhou J, Brüne B, Frede S, Fandrey J. Thyroid hormone induces erythropoietin gene expression through augmented accumulation of hypoxia-inducible factor-1. Am J Physiol Regul Integr Comp Physiol. 2004;287(3):R600-R607. doi:10.1152/ajpregu.00115.2004

27. Hernáez Á, Lassale C, Castro-Barquero S, et al. Mediterranean Diet Maintained Platelet Count within a Healthy Range and Decreased Thrombocytopenia-Related Mortality Risk: A Randomized Controlled Trial. Nutrients. 2021;13(2):559. Published 2021 Feb 8. doi:10.3390/nu13020559

28. Varol E, Ogut S, Gultekin F. Effect of pesticide exposure on platelet indices in farm workers. Toxicol Ind Health. 2014;30(7):630–634. doi:10.1177/0748233712462477

29. Español, I., Leal, J.D., Blanquer, M. et al. N-Acetylcistein for thrombotic thrombocytopenic purpura: an observational case series study. Ann Hematol 102, 2069–2075 (2023). doi.org/10.1007/s00277–023-05248–9

30. Ngatuni D, Wairagu P, Jillani N, Isaac AO, Nyariki JN. A glyphosate-based herbicide disrupted hematopoiesis and induced organ toxicities, ameliorated by vitamin B12 in a mouse model. Saudi J Biol Sci. 2022;29(6):103278. doi:10.1016/j.sjbs.2022.03.028

31. Liu J, Song Q, Huang Y, Sun W, Lu D, Zhou B. R-lipoic acid overdosing affects platelet life span via ROS mediated autophagy. Platelets. 2018;29(7):695–701. doi:10.1080/09537104.2017.1356450

Mean Platelet Volume (MPV)

Mean platelet volume (MPV) is a measure of the average platelet size. It is usually found on the complete blood count (CBC) but not always. It is used to assess platelet function.

Immature platelets are larger than more mature platelets. When the MPV is elevated, it can mean that there are more immature platelets in the bloodstream. This measure can help in determining the cause of changes in total platelet counts.

Pregnancy

MPV values do not change much in pregnancy. There is only a slight increase in the first trimester that remains stable through the second trimester. Another slight increase can be seen in the third trimester with increased cell turnover before delivery.

Postpartum

A slight increase in MPV may be seen postpartum. Large increases can be seen post-cesarean delivery. This should be resolved quickly. There is limited information on normal postpartum changes in MPV.

STANDARD LAB RANGE: 6.4 – 11 fL

Trimester	Standard Pregnancy Ranges	**Functional Pregnancy Ranges**
Preconception	6.4 – 11	**6.4 – 11**
First Trimester	7.7 – 10.3	**7.7 – 10.1**
Second Trimester	7.8 – 10.2	**7.7 – 10.3**
Third Trimester	8.2 – 10.4	**8.2 – 10.4**
Postpartum	6.4 – 11	**6.4 – 11**

Causes of Elevated Mean Platelet Volume (MPV)

See Platelet Count (PLT) Section.

Elevated MPV >10.1 fL in the first trimester is a predictive biomarker

Impairment of Uteroplacental Circulation: Changes in the production of platelets can indicate disease in early pregnancy. During the first months of pregnancy, when the uteroplacental spiraling is

for preeclampsia and IUGR risk.[1]

MPV is significantly higher in the third trimester of patients with cholestasis.[2]

forming. This process requires adequate regulation of platelets and aggregation. Abnormal changes in this process can lead to issues with the structure of the arterial spirals and with placental function that leads to IUGR or placental presentations.

Hyperthyroidism: A high MPV with normal platelet counts may indicate hyperthyroidism. In the first trimester, a condition called gestational transient thyrotoxicosis can be a cause of this pattern. This is a transient condition that corrects itself within the first few months of pregnancy. (See Thyroid-Stimulating Hormone (TSH) Section.)

Hemolysis: A high MPV with low platelet counts means platelets are being destroyed via hemolytic mechanisms, toxic exposure, or autoimmune responses.

Overexercising: A high MPV can also be seen in professional athletes and those who participate in vigorous physical activity, such as CrossFit and long-distance running. This is due to muscle damage that occurs during strenuous exercise and the need for repair.

Vitamin D Deficiency: Several studies have shown that low vitamin D is associated with higher platelet counts, as well as higher MPV levels. This seems to be highly associated with autoimmune disease as well. Testing for vitamin D should be standard in pregnancy, but if elevated platelet counts and MPV are observed, additional vitamin D testing is warranted.[3]

Polycythemia: A high MPV with high platelet counts may indicate excess production in the bone marrow.

Other Possible Causes: cancer, chronic inflammatory diseases (inflammatory bowel disease), smoking/vaping

Treatment Strategies for Elevated Mean Platelet Volume (MPV)

See Platelet Count (PLT) Section.

Additional Testing

vitamin D, 25-hydroxy (25-hydroxycalciferol, 25OH-D); lactate dehydrogenase (LDH); bile acid, serum; comprehensive metabolic panel (CMP); c-reactive protein (CRP); comprehensive thyroid profile II; reverse T3 (rT3); thyroid peroxidase antibodies (TPOAb); thyroglobulin antibody (TgAb); thyroid receptor antibodies (TRAb); comprehensive stool testing

Causes of Low Mean Platelet Volume (MPV)

See Platelet Count (PLT) Section.

A low MPV with low platelet counts can indicate a disruption in platelet production, reducing the number of young platelets.

Treatment Strategies for Low Mean Platelet Volume (MPV)

See Platelet Count (PLT) Section.

References

1. Kanat-Pektas, M., Yesildager, U., Tuncer, N., Arioz, D.T., Nadirgil-Koken, G. and Yilmazer, M. (2014), MPV and adverse perinatal outcome. J Obstet Gynaecol Res, 40: 1840–1845. doi.org/10.1111/jog.12433

2. Silva J, Magenta M, Sisti G, Serventi L, Gaither K. Association Between Complete Blood Count Components and Intrahepatic Cholestasis of Pregnancy. Cureus. 2020;12(12):e12381. Published 2020 Dec 30. doi:10.7759/cureus.12381

3. Feketea G, Vlacha V, Pop RM, Bocsan IC, Stanciu LA, Buzoianu AD and Zdrenghea M (2022) Relationship Between Vitamin D Level and Platelet Parameters in Children With Viral Respiratory Infections. Front. Pediatr. 10:824959. doi: 10.3389/fped.2022.824959

Prothrombin Time (PT)

The prothrombin time (PT) test is used to assess the clotting ability of blood. It measures the time it takes for blood to clot after certain clotting factors are activated with the addition of thromboplastin (a mixture of tissue factor, calcium, and phospholipid). It is a separate indice.

The coagulation cascade is a series of interconnected enzymatic reactions that culminate in the formation of a blood clot. It is divided into three main pathways: the extrinsic pathway, the intrinsic pathway, and the common pathway. The extrinsic and intrinsic pathways each have an amplification phase and converge to form the common pathway.

The extrinsic pathway is triggered when tissue damage exposes tissue factor (Factor III) to the blood. Tissue factor forms a complex with Factor VII, activating it. Activated Factor VII (Factor VIIa) and calcium then convert Factor X to its active form, Factor Xa, initiating the common pathway.

The intrinsic pathway is triggered when exposed collagen activates Factor XII. Factor XIIa activates Factor XI, which then activates Factor IX in the presence of Factor VIII and calcium. Then Factor IXa, Factor VIIIa, and calcium form a complex to activate Factor X to Factor Xa, initiating the common pathway.

The common pathway may result after the activation of Factor X at the end of either the intrinsic or extrinsic pathways. Factor X, Factor Va, and calcium bind together to form prothrombinase. This activates prothrombin (Factor II) into thrombin (Factor IIa). Thrombin then cleaves fibrinogen (Factor I) into fibrin (Factor Ia). Then, thrombin cleaves Factor XIII into Factor XIIIa, which binds with calcium to create fibrin cross-links to stabilize the clot.

The prothrombin time (PT) test specifically evaluates the extrinsic pathway of the coagulation cascade. The test measures the activity of Factor I, Factor II, Factor V, Factor VII, and Factor X. It is also the only vitamin K biomarker.

Factor I: Factor I is also known as fibrinogen. Fibrinogen is a glycoprotein that is converted to fibrin, a fibrous protein that forms the base of blood clots.

Factor II: Factor II is also known as prothrombin. Prothrombin is a glycoprotein that is activated into Factor IIa (thrombin). Factor II is vitamin K-dependent.

Factor V: Factor V is also known as proaccelerin or labile factor. It is a large glycoprotein that is activated by thrombin. Thrombin cleaves off a small peptide from Factor V to make Factor Va, which is the active form needed for pro-coagulation actions. Factor V affects the amplification phase of the coagulation cascade. It acts as a cofactor for Factor X, which enhances the conversion of prothrombin to thrombin.

Factor VII: Factor VII is also known as proconvertin or stable factor. Factor VII is vitamin K-dependent.

Factor X: Factor X is also known as Stuart-Prower Factor. Factor X is vitamin K-dependent.

A decreased production of coagulation factors leads to prolonged prothrombin time. The prothrombin time is better at assessing causes of bleeding versus causes of clotting.

Pregnancy

During pregnancy, there is increased production of clotting factors, specifically Factor I, Factor II, Factor VII, Factor VIII, Factor IX, and Factor XII, as well as a decrease in protein S levels and an inhibition of fibrinolysis. Toward the end of pregnancy, there is also a significant fall in the activity of protein C.[1] These changes are important for balancing clotting in the prevention of bleeding but may also increase the risk of thromboembolism during pregnancy and postpartum. Around 50% of women have elevated thrombin-antithrombin complexes in the first trimester, with 100% having elevated levels in the second and third trimesters. This increase in antithrombin helps to regulate clotting and reduces the risk of thromboembolism. Thus, these mechanisms help to balance clotting activities in pregnancy. This causes a relatively small shift in prothrombin time in pregnancy, with only a slight shortening of clotting time.[2]

Postpartum

Blood loss in pregnancy can have an impact on postpartum prothrombin time. There is a slight increase in PT with increasing volumes of blood loss.[3]

> Activated partial thromboplastin time (aPTT) is often used with PT to differentiate causes.

Prothrombin Time (PT)

STANDARD LAB RANGE: 9.1 – 12 SECONDS

Trimester	Standard Pregnancy Ranges	**Functional Pregnancy Ranges**
Preconception	9.1 – 12	**9.1 – 12**
First Trimester	9.7 – 13.5	**8.9 – 12.2**
Second Trimester	9.5 – 13.4	**8.6 – 12.1**
Third Trimester	9.6 – 12.9	**8.7 – 12.1**
Postpartum	9.1 – 12	**9.1 – 12**

Different preparations of thromboplastin reagents are available and give different prothrombin time results, even when using the same blood sample. Because of this, the World Health Organization (WHO) introduced the international normalized ratio (INR), which is now becoming the standard format for prothrombin time results and is available with the LabCorp prothrombin (PT) test.

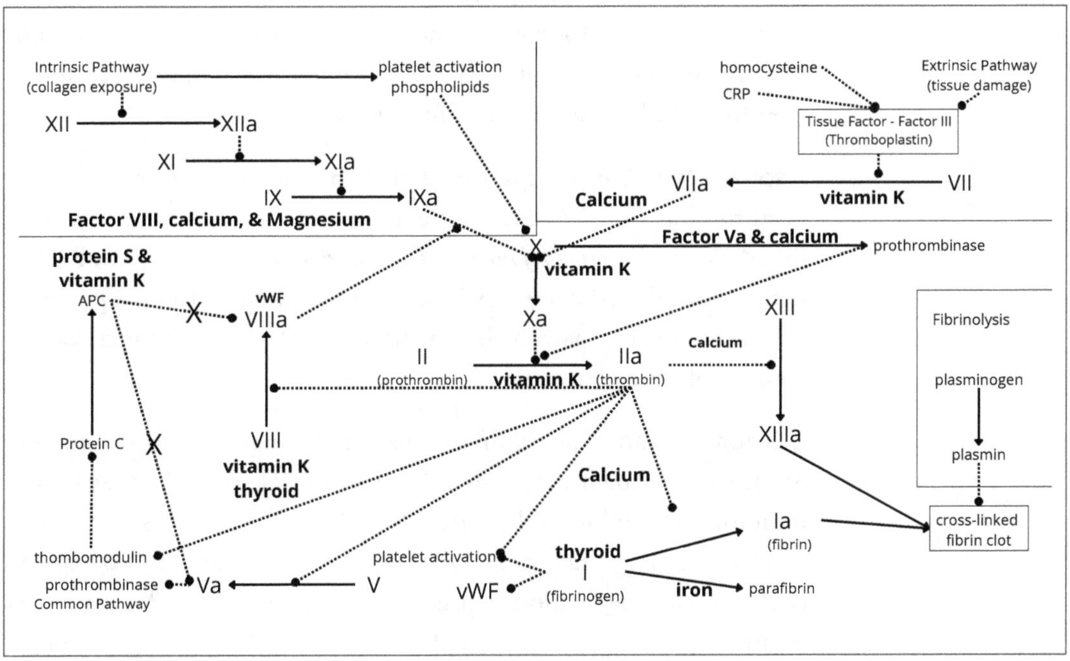

Figure 5: Coagulation Cascade

Causes of Prolonged Prothrombin Time (PT)

Liver Disease: The liver synthesizes many of the coagulation factors, including prothrombin, Factor VII, Factor IX, and Factor X, as well as proteins C and S. Liver disease can impair the synthesis of these factors, leading to prolonged clotting time. In liver disease, PT will be prolonged with normal partial thromboplastin time (PTT).

Vitamin K Deficiency: Prolonged prothrombin time is considered the most sensitive screening test for detecting early and/or mild vitamin K deficiency. Yet studies have shown that it is more of an indicator of late-stage vitamin K deficiency, particularly in pregnancy. A 2022 study on critical illness polyneuropathy (CIP) and vitamin K found that 59.2% of women with intrahepatic cholestasis of pregnancy (ICP) were diagnosed with vitamin K deficiency, yet 98.6% of women had normal coagulation indices.[4] Vitamin K deficiency is usually shown as prolonged PT and aPTT with normal fibrinogen. Vitamin K plays a role in the post-translational modification of glutamic residues on clotting factors. This process is known as gamma-carboxylation and helps to convert inactive precursor proteins to their active forms. This includes Factor II, Factor VII, Factor IX, and Factor X, as well as protein C, protein S, and protein Z. Vitamin K deficiency can be found in even slight increases in prothrombin time.

Aspirin Use: Aspirin doses of 2 to 3 mg/day can cause prolonged prothrombin time.[5] A 2023 systemic review and meta-analysis published in the *American Journal of Obstetrics & Gynecology MFM* (for maternal-fetal medicine) concluded that low-dose aspirin is a potential risk factor for postpartum hemorrhage and does slightly increase the amount of postpartum blood loss.[6]

Curcumin Use: Curcumin is the active ingredient in turmeric. Studies have shown that curcumin prolongs PT and aPTT, as well as inhibiting thrombin and Factor Xa activity, thus increasing the risk of bleeding. Moderate doses of between 500 mg and 1,000 mg/day could impact coagulation, but generally anticoagulant effects are seen at doses closer to between 2,000 mg and 3,000 mg/day when taken over an extended period of time. This is unlikely to be seen in turmeric supplementation or dietary intake, as the concentration of curcumin and other active ingredients is only between 2% and 5% by weight.

So the typical dietary use doesn't deliver the high doses of curcumin needed to affect clotting time.

Antiphospholipid Antibodies: Antiphospholipid antibody syndrome is characterized by recurrent thromboembolic events or pregnancy loss with detectable antiphospholipid antibodies. These antibodies can cause an increased conversion of prothrombin to thrombin, leading to an overall decrease in prothrombin levels. Decreased prothrombin levels can lead to a prolonged prothrombin time.[7]

Genetic Deficiencies in Clotting Factors: Running the thromboplastin time (PTT) test may help with differentiation. Prolonged PT with prolonged PTT may indicate a decrease or defect in Factor I, Factor II, Factor V, or Factor X. A prolonged PT with a normal PTT may indicate a decrease or defect in Factor VII, as well as vitamin K deficiency.

Other Possible Causes: vitamin C deficiency, certain medications (anticoagulants), genetics

Treatment Strategies for Prolonged Prothrombin Time (PT)

Diet

Consuming vitamin K-rich foods may become a focus. This includes cooked green leafy vegetables (kale, spinach, mustard greens, collard greens, turnip greens, and beet greens), parsley, fruits such as kiwi and avocado, as well as fermented soy (natto, miso, tofu, and tempeh). Avoiding foods known to be blood thinners is also important when PT is prolonged. Alcohol can impair liver function and has been known to thin the blood. It impairs the synthesis of clotting factors, which can exacerbate prolonged PT. Sodium dehydroacetate is a food additive, preservative, and antimicrobial agent. It has been shown to cause a depletion of vitamin K and is associated with increased bleeding risk. It is commonly found in the preservation of dairy products such as cheese, butter, and margarine, as well as starchy products such as breads and cakes.

Much more is known about the absorption and metabolism of vitamin K1 than there is known about vitamin K2, mostly because vitamin K1 is the most common form routinely measured in blood work. Concentrations of vitamin K2 in the plasma are very low or undetectable. Blood levels of vitamin K peak approximately 12 to 24 hours after consumption or supplementation. Although vitamin K is stored in the liver, it has a rapid turnover and a short half-life. Each form of vitamin K has a different half-life. Vitamin K1 has a half-life of approximately one and a half to two hours. Vitamin K2's half-life varies, based on the form, from 3 to 60 hours. The body retains only between 30% and 40% of any oral consumption or dosage of vitamin K, with 70% cleared within a few hours. Currently, there is no established upper limit for vitamin K consumption, due to a lack of known side effects with excess consumption of natural forms. The current recommended dietary allowance (RDA) for pregnancy is 90 µg.

Supplements

Omega-3 fatty acids in high amounts, particularly isolated DHA supplements, have been shown to impair blood-clotting ability, increasing bleeding risk. Consuming omega-3 fatty acids should not have this same effect, but it seems to be variable by patient.[8] Certain herbs and other dietary supplements may have anticoagulation properties and may lead to potentially longer prothrombin times. These include garlic supplements, ginkgo biloba, ginger supplements, vitamin E, bromelain, and curcumin.

Vitamin K supplements have not been shown to cause birth defects or other problems in pregnancy. The only form with consistent toxic side effects is the synthetic water-soluble form called menadione, also known as vitamin K3. Because of its water-soluble instead of a fat-soluble structure, the body doesn't recognize it as elevated and fails to excrete the excess. This form has been associated with hemolytic anemia and hyperbilirubinemia. According to some sources, dosages of 10 mg per day starting at 36 weeks gestation are safe and recommended in those at a higher risk of vitamin K deficiency.

Additional Testing

complete blood count (CBC); comprehensive metabolic panel (CMP); activated partial thromboplastin time (aPTT); antiphospholipid antibodies; thrombin time (TT); specific factor assays; fibrinogen

Causes of Shortened Prothrombin Time (PT)

This is less common; other tests are better at assessing increased clotting. Prothrombin time is rarely shortened in blood-clotting disorders. Other tests are more accurate in identifying increased clotting risk. Prothrombin time is more accurate in assessing the risk of bleeding and less

Factor V Leiden: This condition is caused by a mutation in the F5 gene, which provides the instructions for making Factor V. Women with this genetic mutation have a higher risk of increased clotting, specifically deep vein thrombosis (DVT) and venous thromboembolism (VTE), as well as a pulmonary embolism. Normally, activated protein C works as a natural anticoagulant that inactivates Factor V and Factor VIII, regulating clotting. However, in Factor V Leiden, the mutated factor is resistant to inactivation by protein C. Those with Factor V Leiden may have a history of increased menstrual clotting with a lighter flow, DVT, history of miscarriage, and/or higher hemoglobin levels.[9] Prothrombin time may not be affected in all cases.

effective in assessing the risk of clotting.

Advanced Maternal Age: Studies show that PT and INR are shorter in women who are of advanced maternal age.[10]

Other Possible Causes: thrombophilia conditions, inflammation with high fibrinogen, genetics

Treatment Strategies for Shortened Prothrombin Time (PT)

Diet

Minimizing the risk of blood clots may lean on increasing foods that have blood-thinning as well as antioxidant effects.

Supplements

Certain herbs and other dietary supplements may have anticoagulation properties and may lead to potentially longer prothrombin times. These include garlic supplements, ginkgo biloba, ginger supplements, vitamin E, bromelain, and curcumin. Conditions that result in a shortened prothrombin time should be treated by medical professionals.

Additional Testing

complete blood count (CBC); d-dimer; activated partial thromboplastin time (aPTT); dilute Russell's Viper Venom Time (dRVVT); specific factor assays; antiphospholipid antibody testing; thrombin time (TT); fibrinogen

References

1. Bremme KA. Haemostatic changes in pregnancy. Best Pract Res Clin Haematol. 2003;16(2):153–168. doi:10.1016/s1521–6926(03)00021–5

2. Covali R, Socolov D, Socolov R. Coagulation tests and blood glucose before vaginal delivery in healthy teenage pregnant women compared with healthy adult pregnant women. Medicine (Baltimore). 2019;98(5):e14360. doi:10.1097/MD.0000000000014360

3. Gillissen A, van den Akker T, Caram-Deelder C, et al. Coagulation parameters during the course of severe postpartum hemorrhage: a nationwide retrospective cohort study. Blood Adv. 2018;2(19):2433–2442. doi:10.1182/bloodadvances.2018022632

4. Cemortan M, Sagaidac I, Cernetchi O. Assessment of vitamin K levels in women with intrahepatic cholestasis of pregnancy. BMC Pregnancy Childbirth. 2022;22(1):534. Published 2022 Jul 1. doi:10.1186/s12884–022-04875-w

5. QUICK AJ, CLESCERI L. Influence of acetylsalicylic acid and salicylaide on the coagulation of blood. J Pharmacol Exp Ther. 1960;128:95–98

6. Jiang Y, Chen Z, Chen Y, et al. Low-dose aspirin use during pregnancy may be a potential risk for postpartum hemorrhage and increased blood loss: a systematic review and meta-analysis. Am J Obstet Gynecol MFM. 2023;5(4):100878. doi:10.1016/j.ajogmf.2023.100878

7. Ortel TL. Antiphospholipid syndrome: laboratory testing and diagnostic strategies. Am J Hematol. 2012;87 Suppl 1(Suppl 1):S75-S81. doi:10.1002/ajh.23196

8. Vanschoonbeek K, Feijge MA, Paquay M, et al. Variable hypocoagulant effect of fish oil intake in humans: modulation of fibrinogen level and thrombin generation. Arterioscler Thromb Vasc Biol. 2004;24(9):1734–1740. doi:10.1161/01.ATV.0000137119.28893.0b

9. van Dunné FM, Doggen CJ, Heemskerk M, Rosendaal FR, Helmerhorst FM. Factor V Leiden mutation in relation to fecundity and miscarriage in women with venous thrombosis. Hum Reprod. 2005;20(3):802–806. doi:10.1093/humrep/deh640

10. Dai J, Mao P, Pu C, Wang X, Liu X. Trimester-specific reference intervals and profile of coagulation parameters for Chinese pregnant women with diverse demographics and obstetric history: a cross-sectional study. BMC Pregnancy Childbirth. 2023;23(1):421. Published 2023 Jun 6. doi:10.1186/s12884–023-05571-z

Activated Partial Thromboplastin Time (aPTT)

The activated partial thromboplastin time (aPTT) test is used to assess the clotting ability of blood. It measures the time it takes for blood to clot after certain clotting factors are activated with the addition of various reagents that activate Factor XII.

Partial thromboplastin time (PTT) and aPTT are similar and are often used interchangeably but vary slightly based on the activator. aPTT is tested by adding an activator that speeds up the clotting time and results in a narrower reference range.

The intrinsic pathway is triggered when exposed collagen activates Factor XII. Factor XIIa activates Factor XI, which then activates Factor IX in the presence of Factor VIII and calcium. Then Factor IXa, Factor VIIIa, and calcium form a complex to activate Factor X to Factor Xa, initiating the common pathway.

The activated partial thromboplastin time (aPTT) test specifically evaluates the intrinsic pathway of the coagulation cascade.

Factor VIII: Also known as antihemophilic factor A. Factor VIII is needed for the formation of tenase complex, which activates Factor X. Deficiencies lead to hemophilia A.

Factor IX: Also known as Christmas factor. Factor IX is a component of the tenase complex, along with Factor VIII and calcium. It activates Factor X. Deficiencies lead to hemophilia B.

Factor XI: Also known as plasma thromboplastin antecedent (PTA). Factor XI is part of the amplification of the coagulation cascade. It activates Factor IX. Deficiencies lead to hemophilia C.

Factor XII: Also known as Hageman factor. Foreign substances activate Factor XII. Factor XII activates Factor XI.

Prekallikrein: Also known as Fletcher factor. Prekallikrein is activated by foreign substances, which leads to the activation of Factor XII.

High Molecular Weight Kininogen (KNG): Cofactor of prekallikrein.

Pregnancy

During pregnancy, there is increased production of clotting factors, specifically Factor I, Factor II, Factor VII, Factor VIII, Factor IX, and Factor XII, as well as a decrease in protein S levels and an inhibition of fibrinolysis. Toward the end of pregnancy, there is also a significant fall in the activity of protein C.[1] These changes are important for balancing clotting in the prevention of bleeding but may also increase the risk of thromboembolism during pregnancy and postpartum. Approximately 50% of women have elevated thrombin-antithrombin complexes in the first trimester, with 100% having elevated levels in the second and third trimesters. This increase in antithrombin helps to regulate clotting and reduces the risk of thromboembolism. Thus, these mechanisms help to balance clotting activities in pregnancy. aPTT and PTT ranges decrease slightly in pregnancy, with the increased hypercoagulative state of pregnancy. There is a measurable decrease in aPTT between the first and third trimester in preparation for childbirth.

Postpartum

Life-threatening hemorrhage during childbirth is preceded by low fibrinogen and prolonged aPTT soon after its onset.[2]

STANDARD LAB RANGE: 24 – 33 SECONDS

Trimester	Standard Pregnancy Ranges	**Functional Pregnancy Ranges**
Preconception	26.3 - 39.4	**24 - 33**
First Trimester	24.3 - 38.9	**24 - 33**
Second Trimester	24.2 - 38.1	**24 - 33**
Third Trimester	24.7 - 35	**24 - 33**
Postpartum	26.3 - 39.4	**24 - 33**

Causes of Prolonged Activated Partial Thromboplastin Time (aPTT)

Lupus Anticoagulant Syndrome: Lupus anticoagulant (LA) is an autoimmune antibody that is associated with antiphospholipid antibody syndrome. Lupus anticoagulants target phospholipid-binding proteins of cell membranes, prothrombin, and beta2-glycoprotein. This inhibits phospholipid-dependent coagulation, which increases the formation of small clots. It is more common in people with lupus, so it is called the lupus anticoagulant syndrome. Because lupus anticoagulant is an attack on the phospholipids, it interferes with the mechanisms of action of the test, causing a prolonged clotting time, even though the disease itself causes increased clotting. Often a more specific lupus anticoagulant test, the aPTT-LA is used to differentiate lupus anticoagulant as a cause of prolonged aPTT. The Russell's Viper Venom Time (dRVVT) test is more accurate at detecting LA.

Antiphospholipid Antibody Syndrome: Antiphospholipid antibodies target phospholipid-binding proteins and complexes. These antibodies increase thrombosis but cause prolonged aPTT. This includes lupus anticoagulant, anticardiolipin antibodies, anti-β2 glycoprotein I antibodies, and antiphosphatidylserine antibodies. These antibodies are associated with increased placental dysfunction and increased risk of pregnancy complications that include miscarriage, intrauterine growth restriction, and preeclampsia.

Hypothyroidism: Hypothyroidism has been shown to have a pronounced effect on aPTT testing. This is most likely associated with a decrease in coagulation Factor VIII and/or von Willebrand factor. Thyroid hormones are required for their expression. This has been found with subclinical hypothyroidism as well as overt hypothyroidism. This may be why there is also a connection between subclinical hypothyroidism in the third trimester and an increased risk of postpartum hemorrhage.[3 4]

Von Willebrand Disease (vWD): Von Willebrand disease (vWD) is the most common inherited bleeding disorder characterized by a defect in von Willebrand factor needed for proper clotting. vWF is a carrier protein for VIII, protecting it from degradation. It also mediates platelet adhesion and aggregation. There are several types of vWD. Prolonged aPTT may present with vWD but not always.

Genetic Deficiencies in Clotting Factors: Running the prothrombin time (PT) test may help with differentiation. Prolonged PTT/aPTT with normal PT may indicate a decrease or defect in Factor VIII, Factor IX, Factor XI, Factor XII, von Willebrand disease, lupus anticoagulant, or factor autoantibodies. A prolonged PTT/aPTT with prolonged PT may indicate a decrease or defect in Factor I, Factor II, Factor V, or Factor X. A slightly prolonged PTT/aPTT with a normal PT may indicate normal clotting; however, a slight increase in PTT/aPTT may show mild issues with von Willebrand disease or lupus anticoagulant. There is more often a prolonged time of double the standard range in factor disease.

Other Possible Causes: vitamin K deficiency, liver disease, disseminated intravascular coagulation, hemophilia A, hemophilia B, von Willebrand factor disease, anticoagulant therapy, rheumatoid arthritis, herbal medications (curcumin)

Treatment Strategies for Prolonged Activated Partial Thromboplastin Time (aPTT)

See Prothrombin Time (PT) Section.

Diet

In cases of mild prolonged clotting time, addressing vitamin K deficiency may be beneficial.

Additional Testing

complete blood count (CBC); comprehensive thyroid profile II; comprehensive metabolic panel (CMP); reverse T3 (rT3); prothrombin time (PT); thrombin time (TT); von Willebrand factor (vWF); dilute Russell's Viper Venom Time (dRVVT); antiphospholipid antibody testing; antinuclear antibodies (ANA); specific factor assays; fibrinogen

Causes of Shortened Activated Partial Thromboplastin Time (aPTT)

Hyperthyroidism: Hyperthyroidism has been associated with shortened aPTT and increased fibrinogen.[5]

Other Possible Causes: issues with collection, initial disseminated intravascular coagulation, acute internal bleeding, cancer

Treatment Strategies for Shortened Activated Partial Thromboplastin Time (aPTT)

See Prothrombin Time (PT) Section.

Diet

Minimizing the risk of blood clots may lean on increasing foods that have blood-thinning effects as well as antioxidant effects.

Additional Testing

complete blood count (CBC); d-dimer; prothrombin time (PT); thrombin time (TT); fibrinogen, comprehensive thyroid profile II; reverse T3 (rT3); thyroid peroxidase antibodies (TPOAb); thyroglobulin antibody (TgAb); thyroid receptor antibodies (TRAb)

References

1. Bremme KA. Haemostatic changes in pregnancy. Best Pract Res Clin Haematol. 2003;16(2):153–168. doi:10.1016/s1521–6926(03)00021–5

2. Gillissen A, van den Akker T, Caram-Deelder C, et al. Coagulation parameters during the course of severe postpartum hemorrhage: a nationwide retrospective cohort study. Blood Adv. 2018;2(19):2433–2442. doi:10.1182/bloodadvances.2018022632

3. Hjelm Lundgaard M, Carlé A, Birgitte Christiansen U, Sørensen A, Risom Kristensen S, Andersen SL. Prolonged APTT and autoimmune overt hypothyroidism identified postpartum: a case report. Eur Thyroid J. 2022;11(4):e220109. Published 2022 Jul 15. doi:10.1530/ETJ-22–0109

4. Hizkiyahu R, Badeghiesh A, Baghlaf H, Dahan MH. Associations between hypothyroidism and adverse obstetric and neonatal outcomes: a study of a population database including over 184,000 women with hypothyroidism. J Matern Fetal Neonatal Med. 2023;36(2):2278027. doi:10.1080/14767058.2023.22780 27

5. Lippi G, Franchini M, Targher G, et al. Hyperthyroidism is associated with shortened APTT and increased fibrinogen values in a general population of unselected outpatients. J Thromb Thrombolysis. 2009;28(3):362–365. doi:10.1007/s11239–008-0269-z

Fibrinogen

The fibrinogen test measures the amount of fibrinogen in a blood sample. It is a single analyte.

Fibrinogen, also known as Factor I, is a glycoprotein. It is the precursor for fibrin, the insoluble protein that forms the structure of blood clots.

During the coagulation cascade, thrombin cleaves fibrinogen into fibrin monomers. These monomers are polymerized to form insoluble fibrin strands. This forms a mesh of fibrin strands that trap platelets and other blood components to form a stable clot at the site of injury. Once formed, fibrin strands are cross-linked by activated Factor XIII.

Fibrinogen also plays a role in platelet activation and aggregation and interacts with von Willebrand factor.

The production and function of fibrinogen are tightly controlled. The conversion of fibrinogen to fibrin is a critical and rate-limiting step in clot formation. This step is regulated by thrombin. The function of fibrinogen and the conversion of fibrinogen to fibrin is measured with the thrombin time (TT) test.

Pregnancy

The overall production of fibrinogen and thrombin increases in pregnancy. There is also a decrease in overall thrombin time progressively throughout pregnancy.[1 2] This is representative of the hypercoagulation state that exists starting in early pregnancy. Throughout pregnancy, and especially toward the end, fibrinogen levels can increase nearly double preconception ranges.

Postpartum

Fibrinogen levels decrease postpartum. The severity of the decrease may depend on birth method and outcomes. Excess bleeding during delivery, either via increased blood loss in surgical delivery or after hemorrhage, can cause a sharp drop in fibrinogen levels. The amount of fibrinogen polymerized into fibrin to aid in clotting exceeds production.

STANDARD LAB RANGE: 193 – 507 mg/dL

Trimester	Standard Pregnancy Ranges	**Functional Pregnancy Ranges**
Preconception	193 – 507	**200 – 500**
First Trimester	244 – 510	**300 – 500**
Second Trimester	291 – 538	**300 – 500**
Third Trimester	373 – 619	**300 – 500**
Postpartum	233 – 496	**200 – 500**

Causes of Elevated Fibrinogen

There is more literature on the effects of low fibrinogen in pregnancy than on the effects of elevated fibrinogen in pregnancy.

Acute Inflammation: Fibrinogen synthesis is stimulated by inflammatory cytokines, particularly interleukin-6 (IL-6), and thus can be seen in acute inflammatory reactions.

Nutritional Deficiencies: Elevated fibrinogen levels have been associated with lower iron, vitamin E, and vitamin B6 (pyridoxine) levels, particularly in women.[3] Fibrinogen activity is inversely related to iron levels, as ferric iron (Fe^{3+}) initiates the hydroxyl radical-catalyzed conversion of fibrinogen to parafibrin.

Other Possible Causes: hyperthyroidism, rheumatoid arthritis, autoimmune disease, inflammatory bowel disease, kidney inflammation/infection, cardiovascular inflammation, lipid peroxidation, gallbladder obstruction, adrenal hyperfunction, acute stress, genetics, cancer

Treatment Strategies for Elevated Fibrinogen

Diet

Minimizing the risk of blood clots may require increasing foods that have blood-thinning effects as well as antioxidant effects. Lipid peroxidation may be affected by dietary intake of fatty acids and antioxidants. Balance between omega-6, omega-3, and omega-9 fatty acids is key. High dietary intake of long-chain fatty acids, trans-fatty acids, and even excess polyunsaturated fatty acid intake can increase the susceptibility of lipoprotein oxidation. Those with excessively elevated fibrinogen may benefit from changes in the composition of their fatty acid intake. They should focus on reducing trans and processed fats in their diet, increasing a mix of healthy fats that come from whole animal products (whole fish, bone-in and skin-on chicken), nuts, and seeds. Cooking with tallow, lard, and butter and avoiding heat-sensitive seed oils can also be beneficial in balancing fatty-acid levels to reduce lipid peroxidation. Antioxidants such as vitamin E help to stabilize polyunsaturated fats and reduce oxidative stress in lipid membranes. Vitamin E-rich foods such as sunflower seeds (fresh), cooked spinach, raab, avocado, sardines, and salmon should be prioritized.

Supplements

Vitamin D supplements have been shown to lower fibrinogen levels. So far, there has not been a direct link. Indirectly, vitamin D supplements downregulate interleukin production and may affect fibrinogen synthesis by decreasing cytokine production.[4] Alpha-lipoic acid is an antioxidant that has shown promise in the prevention and treatment of pregnancy complications. It helps modify coagulation by inhibiting platelet activation, affecting the intrinsic coagulation pathway, and reducing fibrinogen. Dosage is approximately 600 mg per day.

Additional Testing

complete blood count (CBC); iron and TIBC; ferritin; comprehensive metabolic panel (CMP); comprehensive thyroid profile II; reverse T3 (rT3); thyroid peroxidase antibodies (TPOAb); thyroglobulin antibody (TgAb); thyroid receptor antibodies (TRAb); c-reactive protein (CRP); antinuclear antibodies (ANA); prothrombin time (PT)

Causes of Low Fibrinogen

Levels <3 g/L (300 mg/dL) in pregnancy are a sign of coagulation abnormalities.[5] Low fibrinogen is a reliable biomarker to predict postpartum hemorrhage in pregnant women presenting with HELLP syndrome.

Low fibrinogen levels prior to delivery can be a predictive biomarker for postpartum hemorrhage.[6] It may also be an independent marker of hemorrhage

Hypothyroidism: Thyroid hormones are responsible for the synthesis of several hepatic proteins and clotting factors, including fibrinogen. Studies show an inverse relationship between TSH and fibrinogen levels. Low TSH is associated with elevated fibrinogen levels, and elevated TSH is associated with lower fibrinogen levels.[9] [10]

Iron Overload/Hemochromatosis: There is an inverse relationship between iron and serum fibrinogen levels. The polymerization of fibrinogen is elevated in iron saturation conditions. This rapidly degrades fibrinogen to fibrin strands, decreasing serum fibrinogen levels while increasing clot formation.[11] [12] It is well documented that iron excess increases thrombosis and, in pregnancy, is associated with placental dysfunction and pregnancy complications.[13]

Other Possible Causes: liver disease, internal bleeding (placental abruption, Crohn's disease digestive bleeding), chronic inflammation

severity.[7] Levels <200 mg/dL are associated with a 100% positive predictive value of developing severe postpartum hemorrhage.[8]	and tissue damage, infection, certain medications (anticoagulants, antiseizure), genetics, cancer

Treatment Strategies for Low Fibrinogen

Diet

Protein is essential to produce fibrinogen. During pregnancy, the need for protein almost doubles by the third trimester. For those struggling to increase protein, please visit my website (www.FunctionalMaternity.com/ebooks.html) and download my *Protein Packed Pregnancy* e-book. One small study found that fibrinogen levels increased between 20% and 40% after patients consumed, in addition to their regular diet, a protein shake each day that contained 15% of the individuals' calculated daily protein needs.[14] Additionally, supporting thyroid hormone production via nutrition may also be important if hypothyroidism is a factor. (See Thyroid-Stimulating Hormone (TSH) Section.)

Additional Testing

complete blood count (CBC); iron and TIBC; ferritin; comprehensive metabolic panel (CMP); comprehensive thyroid profile II; c-reactive protein (CRP); vitamin D, 25-hydroxy (25-hycroxycalciferol, 25OH vitamin D); prothrombin time (PT)

References

1. Gong JM, Shen Y, He YX. Reference Intervals of Routine Coagulation Assays During the Pregnancy and Puerperium Period. J Clin Lab Anal. 2016;30(6):912–917. doi:10.1002/jcla.21956

2. Bagot CN, Leishman E, Onyiaodike CC, Jordan F, Freeman DJ. Normal pregnancy is associated with an increase in thrombin generation from the very early stages of the first trimester. Thromb Res. 2017;157:49–54. doi:10.1016/j.thromres.2017.06.027

3. James S, Vorster HH, Venter CS, et al. Nutritional status influences plasma fibrinogen concentration: evidence from the THUSA survey. Thromb Res. 2000;98(5):383–394. doi:10.1016/s0049–3848(00)00197–3

4. Rautenbach PH, Nienaber-Rousseau C, de Lange-Loots Z, Kruger IM, Pieters M. Associations Between 25-Hydroxyvitamin D and Total and γ' Fibrinogen and Plasma Clot Properties and Gene Interactions in a Group of Healthy Black South African Women. Front Cardiovasc Med. 2022;9:868542. Published 2022 Jul 12. doi:10.3389/fcvm.2022.868542

5. Cui C, Ma S, Qiao R. Prenatal Plasma Fibrinogen Level Predicts Postpartum Hemorrhage of Patients With HELLP Syndrome. Clin Appl Thromb Hemost. 2020;26:1076029619894057. doi:10.1177/1076029619894057

6. Vermeulen T, Van de Velde M. The role of fibrinogen in postpartum hemorrhage. Best Pract Res Clin Anaesthesiol. 2022;36(3–4):399–410. doi:10.1016/j.bpa.2022.10.002

7. Cortet M, Deneux-Tharaux C, Dupont C, et al. Association between fibrinogen level and severity of postpartum haemorrhage: secondary analysis of a prospective trial. Br J Anaesth. 2012;108(6):984–989. doi:10.1093/bja/aes096

8. Matsunaga S, Takai Y, Seki H. Fibrinogen for the management of critical obstetric hemorrhage. J Obstet Gynaecol Res. 2019;45(1):13–21. doi:10.1111/jog.13788

9. Hertzberg KM, Pindyck J, Mosesson MW, Grieninger G. Thyroid hormone stimulation of plasma protein synthesis in cultured hepatocytes. J Biol Chem. 1981;256(2):563–566

10. Ma J, Liu R, Wu D, et al. Utility of plasma fibrinogen in the differential diagnosis of thyrotoxicosis. Int J Clin Exp Med. 2015;8(1):1220–1226. Published Jan 15, 2015.

11. Padron-Monedero A, Rodríguez-Artalejo F, Lopez-Garcia E. Dietary micronutrients intake and plasma fibrinogen levels in the general adult population. Sci Rep. 2021;11(1):3843. Published 2021 Feb 15. doi:10.1038/s41598–021-83217-w

12. Rautenbach PH, Nienaber-Rousseau C, de Lange-Loots Z, Pieters M. Certain Associations Between Iron Biomarkers and Total and γ' Fibrinogen and Plasma Clot Properties Are Mediated by Fibrinogen Genotypes. Front Nutr. 2021;8:720048. Published 2021 Aug 10. doi:10.3389/fnut.2021.720048

13. Ng SW, Norwitz SG, Norwitz ER. The Impact of Iron Overload and Ferroptosis on Reproductive Disorders in Humans: Implications for Preeclampsia. Int J Mol Sci. 2019;20(13):3283. Published 2019 Jul 4. doi:10.3390/ijms20133283

14. Caso G, Mileva I, Kelly P, Ahn H, Gelato MC, McNurlan MA. Feeding acutely stimulates fibrinogen synthesis in healthy young and elderly adults. J Nutr. 2009;139(11):2032–2036. doi:10.3945/jn.109.107532

Red Blood Cell (RBC) Count

The red blood cell (RBC) count measures the total number of red blood cells in a blood sample. It is part of the complete blood count (CBC).

The production of red blood cells happens in the marrow of the bones and is triggered by the hormone erythropoietin (EPO), which, in turn, is stimulated by hypoxia in cells and iron concentrations. RBCs are formed from myeloid progenitors.

Erythropoiesis (red blood cell formation) takes about one week to complete. There are multiple steps in the formation of red blood cells, and each step is influenced by or governed by hormones and nutrients. In the first phases of RBC production, erythroblast cells look like all other cells in the body, each with a nucleus and organelles. During this phase of development, iron is accumulated as ferritin, and the other components of hemoglobin are synthesized. Most of the hemoglobin production occurs in the early phases of RBC development, with 35% of hemoglobin synthesis occurring in young RBCs called reticulocytes.

Pregnancy

Red blood cell production increases by 35% starting at 20 weeks gestation. Due to changes in hemodilution, total RBC counts do not increase and may show a decrease in blood work.

Postpartum

Changes may depend on birth experience. There is a slight decrease in counts due to the normal blood loss of pregnancy. Immediately after delivery, plasma volume decreases due to increased diuresis, and the blood volume returns to nonpregnant values. Hemoglobin and hematocrit increase consequently. Plasma volume increases again two to five days postpartum.

> RBC values are used to assess different types of anemia. Anemia is complicated, and most of the concentration of diagnosis and treatment is centered around iron deficiency and iron supplementation. Several nutrients and hormones play into the production and function of RBCs. Make sure not to narrow the focus of treatment to isolated iron supplementation. There are cases and presentations of anemia without iron deficiency, and supplementation with iron may cause a more severe presentation of anemia or other complications in pregnancy. Correct differentiation and treatment are crucial to pregnancy and childbirth success. Certain patterns in the CBC will give you clues to underlying etiology of anemia or other complications.

For more information on anemia in pregnancy, please refer to chapter 9 of my book *Functional Maternity: Using Functional Medicine and Nutrition to Improve Pregnancy and Childbirth Outcomes.*

STANDARD LAB RANGE: 3.77 – 5.28 × 10^6/µL

Trimester	Standard Pregnancy Ranges	**Functional Pregnancy Ranges**
Preconception	3.77 - 5.28	**3.9 - 5.28**
First Trimester	3.42 - 4.55	**4.3 - 4.6**
Second Trimester	2.81 - 4.49	**4.0 - 4.2**
Third Trimester	2.72 - 4.43	**3.9 - 4.4**
Postpartum	3.77 - 5.28	**3.9 - 5.28**

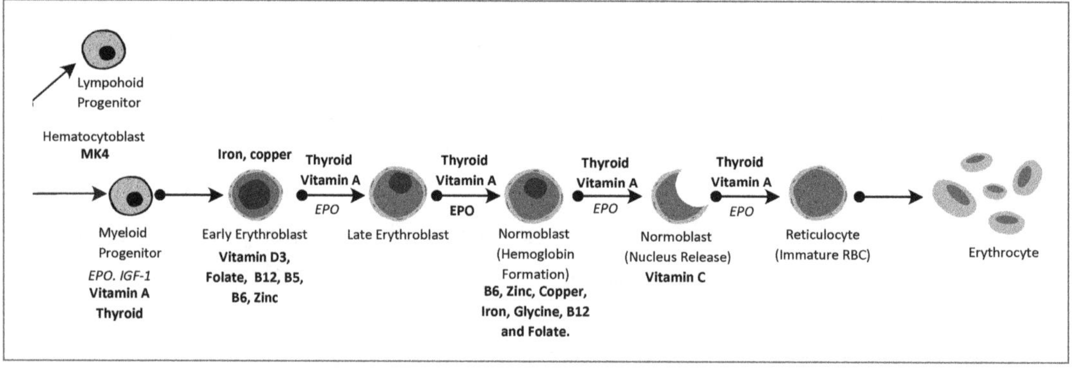

Figure 6: Erythrocyte Maturation

Erythropoiesis is stimulated by EPO. EPO requires Vitamin A and thyroid hormones for genetic expression. Iron is the structural component of heme and is accumulated in the cells in the early erythroblast phase. Copper regulates iron transport to the cells. Iron begins to accumulate in the early erythroblast phase as ferritin. Mitosis is dependent on vitamin D, iron, folic acid, vitamins B5, B6, and B12 (pantothenic acid, pyridoxine, and cobalamin), zinc, and glucose. Hemoglobin formation is dependent on vitamin B6 (pyridoxine), zinc, copper, iron, glycine, vitamin B12 (cobalamin), and vitamin B9 (folate). Vitamin C is required for demethylation after hemoglobin formation for the release of the nucleus.

RBC count value is not useful on its own and must be used in conjunction with the other CBC values.

Causes of Elevated Red Blood Cell (RBC) Count

There may be a slight increase of RBC count in those living at altitudes above 5,000 feet.

Dehydration: Dehydration can skew CBC results with either higher than reference range RBC counts or falsely normal RBC counts. Hematocrit can also be skewed in dehydration patterns. If dehydration is suspected, have patients hydrate for several days then retest for accuracy.

Polycythemia: Polycythemia is a rare blood disorder that is characterized by an abnormal increase in the total number of red blood cells. There are two main types: primary polycythemia (polycythemia vera, or PV) and secondary polycythemia. The increase in red blood cells in PV is primarily due to a bone-marrow disorder, while secondary polycythemia results from conditions leading to increased EPO production, such as chronic hypoxia or kidney cysts and tumors. Typically, this would present with elevated RBCs as well as elevated platelets but not always.

PV in pregnancy is very rare but does occur. This is a condition that needs proper medical management. Typically, you will see an additional increase in white blood cell (WBC) counts, platelet counts, hematocrit, total bilirubin, and alkaline phosphatase (ALP) and a decrease in mean corpuscular volume (MCV), mean corpuscular hemoglobin (MCH), and serum iron. It is well documented that elevated cortisol can be a cause of polycythemia conditions (both WBC and RBC) because it stimulates all progenitor cells and extends their life, increasing overall cell production. PV is often seen in early Cushing's syndrome.[1]

Hypoxia: Low oxygen can cause the body to increase RBC production by increasing EPO production. Causes of hypoxia could be a lung disease (such as asthma), sleep apnea, or issues with the transport of oxygen across cell membranes due to lipid peroxidation. Carbon dioxide (CO_2) levels often increase in those who are smoking or vaping, as well as those with apnea. Hemoglobin binds to CO_2 more readily than oxygen. CO_2-bound hemoglobin is nonfunctional. This creates cellular hypoxia, which increases EPO production and, in turn, more RBCs and hemoglobin. This can also be seen in certain types of anemia such as thalassemia, in which the blood cells do not function correctly and do not transport oxygen effectively to the cells. This hypoxic pattern increases EPO and RBC production.

Iron Overload/Hemochromatosis: Hemochromatosis can present with or without elevated RBC counts. Looking at other CBC values can help you identify this pattern. Additionally, testing an iron and TIBC panel and ferritin can help differentiate this pattern.

Other Possible Causes: asthma, sleep apnea, adrenal hyperfunction, hyperthyroidism, cystic fibrosis, altitude, excess erythropoietin (EPO) production

Treatment Strategies for Elevated Red Blood Cell (RBC) Count

The key to treatment is identifying the underlying cause of elevation.

Diet

In pregnancy, hydration becomes problematic as the need for fluids increases. The increase in plasma begins in the first trimester. As amniotic fluid levels increase, fluid needs peak at the end of the second trimester through 34 weeks. Eating hydrating foods can increase fluid consumption without increasing water intake. This can be done through consuming foods such as watermelon, cucumber, cantaloupe, fresh fruits, and vegetables, and by increasing the consumption of soups and stews, smoothies, or coconut water. If iron overload is identified, decreasing red meat intake and focusing on plant-based iron are important steps to prevent excess iron accumulation. One of the active ingredients of green tea, catechin, can help reduce the damage associated with excess iron accumulation and may be an iron chelator.[2] (See Iron Section.) Reducing trans fats and processed foods in the diet can also be helpful in reducing lipid peroxidation that may interfere with oxygen transfer to the cells.

Lifestyle

A sleep study may be used to assess sleep apnea, and a CPAP (continuous positive airway pressure) machine may be a useful tool to increase oxygenation. Exposure to lung irritants such as cleaning chemicals, smoking, vaping, and other inhaled toxins should be addressed if necessary. If PV is suspected, they should be treated by medical specialists.

Supplements

Electrolyte supplements may help increase hydration. If iron overload is present, turmeric supplements may be useful. Turmeric has been shown to bind to excess iron in cells and help the body excrete it. Use caution with turmeric supplements, as high amounts of curcuminoids may affect blood clotting.

Additional Testing
ferritin; iron and TIBC; comprehensive metabolic panel (CMP)

Causes of Low Blood Cell (RBC) Count

Due to hemodilution, a lower RBC count may be a normal presentation. It is important to look at all CBC values, not just the RBC count.

Iron Deficiency: Iron is part of the structural component of hemoglobin, and a deficiency of iron can cause low RBC formation. Iron is also needed to stimulate the synthesis of EPO. Iron deficiency is rarely a solo nutritional deficiency. It is more common in certain underlying medical conditions, such as inflammatory bowel disease (IBD). In all cases of low RBC, additional testing should be done to assess iron levels. According to the American Pregnancy Association, only between 15% and 25% of pregnancies in America experience iron deficiency.

A study of young pregnant women found that 25% were anemic in the third trimester, and of those women, only 6.1% had iron-deficiency anemia.[3] This means our focus needs to shift from iron supplementation without testing in cases of low RBC, hemoglobin, and anemia in pregnancy. If both the mean corpuscular hemoglobin (MCH) and mean corpuscular hemoglobin concentration (MCHC) are low in conjunction with low RBC, it is important to rule out iron-deficiency anemia. (See Iron Section.)

Copper Deficiency: Copper deficiency can cause iron deficiency or issues in iron utilization. Copper is a structural element of ceruloplasmin, which converts ferrous iron (Fe^{2+}) to ferric iron (Fe^{3+}) so it can bind to transferrin. Copper also activates hepcidin, a hormone that regulates iron absorption and release. If the MCHC is elevated, it is important to rule out copper deficiency. (See Mean Corpuscular Hemoglobin Concentration (MCHC) Section.)

Zinc Deficiency: Zinc is a key modulator of intestinal iron absorption and tissue iron distribution via ferroportin, a transmembrane protein that exports iron from cells. Zinc is essential to enzyme systems that influence cell division and proliferation in mitosis, aid in the formation of the pyrroles, and increase oxygen affinity of hemoglobin. Zinc, copper, and iron deficiencies often go hand in hand. Over-supplementation with zinc can cause copper deficiency. There is a normal decrease in zinc levels through pregnancy.[4]

Vitamin C Deficiency: Ascorbic acid facilitates iron absorption by forming a chelate with ferric iron and also aids in transferrin iron uptake.[5] In patterns of vitamin C deficiency, you will see normal or higher serum iron levels, where the iron is struggling to be pulled into the cells. Vitamin C deficiency can also cause a functional vitamin B9 (folate) deficiency and is associated with macrocytic anemia patterns. (See Mean Corpuscular Volume (MCV) Section.)

Vitamin A Deficiency: Vitamin A is required for the genetic expression of EPO, and a low production of EPO causes a decrease in the production of total RBC.[6] You may see this when all parameters of RBC are low-normal. It is a decrease in overall production versus a dysfunction in the steps of production.

Vitamin D Deficiency: Early erythrocyte progenitor cells express receptors for calcitriol, the active form of vitamin D. Vitamin D induces proliferation and maturation of these early cells. Low vitamin D may also cause a lower production of EPO.

Vitamin B2 (Riboflavin) Deficiency: Riboflavin is a cofactor for many of the enzymes needed for iron uptake.

Vitamin B6 (Pyridoxine) Deficiency: Pyridoxine is needed to incorporate iron into the protoporphyrin groups in hemoglobin, the last step in hemoglobin formation. Assessing other values in the CBC can help identify a vitamin B6 component. Additionally, looking at the alanine aminotransferase (ALT)(SGPT) in the comprehensive metabolic panel (CMP) can also help diagnose vitamin B6 deficiency. If the red blood cell distribution width (RDW) is low, this may indicate a vitamin B6 deficiency.

Vitamin B12 (Cobalamin) and Vitamin B9 (Folate) Deficiency: Erythroblasts require vitamin B12 (cobalamin) and vitamin B9 (folate) for proliferation during their differentiation, via methylation and mitosis support. Vitamin B12 also influences EPO responses. Assessing other values in the CBC can help identify a B12 component. If the MCV and MCH are elevated but MCHC is normal, this may indicate a vitamin B12 deficiency. (See Mean Corpuscular Volume (MCV) Section.)

Thyroid Dysfunction: There is a connection between low iron, hypothyroidism, and low RBC.[7] Thyroid hormones are needed for the genetic expression of EPO.[8]

Vegan Diet: Plant-based diets are at a higher risk of nutritional deficiencies such as iron, vitamin B12 (cobalamin), vitamin D, calcium, iodine, and omega-3s in pregnancy.[9] This does not mean a deficiency is inevitable; many women have amazing, nutrient-dense pregnancies on a plant-based diet. In the case of a woman presenting with anemia and a plant-based diet, these areas need to be assessed through additional testing.

Hemolysis: Hemolysis is a condition in which blood cells die faster than they are made. This is caused by toxicity, inflammation, or low antioxidant production. Hemolytic anemia most often presents with low RBC, low or normal hemoglobin, high reticulocytes, high nucleated red blood cells (nRBC), low platelets, low mean platelet volume (MPV), and low neutrophils.

Anemia of Inflammation: Anemia of inflammation is also known as anemia of chronic disease. Although rare, it does happen in pregnancy, especially in older mothers. This is common in women with chronic infections or autoimmune disease. Inflammation reduces iron absorption and erythropoiesis. Anemia of inflammation will also present with low serum iron and transferrin saturation but high ferritin. This is due to tissue damage and the destruction of cells, releasing their stored ferritin into circulation. C-reactive protein (CRP) is a marker used to diagnose anemia of inflammation.[10] Anemia of inflammation typically presents with low RBC counts; low reticulocytes; low monocytes, eosinophils, and basophils; as well as normal hemoglobin, MCV, MCH, and MCHC. (See C-Reactive Protein (CRP) Section.)

Adrenal Hypofunction: Because cortisol plays an overall important role in the stimulation of the progenitor cells, lower levels of cortisol production can decrease overall red blood cell formation. This may be seen when there is overall healthy RBC production but just fewer cells produced. There will also be an overall decrease in lymphocyte production and a two- or threefold increase in the number of white blood cells (WBC) in the peripheral blood.

Environmental Toxin Exposure: Exposure to environmental chemicals poses a multifaceted risk for anemia, disrupting various processes involved in red blood cell production and function. These chemicals can interfere with iron metabolism, leading to iron-deficiency anemia. Some toxins inhibit erythropoiesis in the bone marrow, reducing the overall production of red blood cells. Others may directly affect the structure of hemoglobin, compromising its ability to carry oxygen. Bone-marrow suppression induced by certain toxic substances, including pesticides and benzene, can contribute to anemia.

Additionally, environmental chemicals may induce premature destruction of red blood cells (hemolysis), diminish the function of enzymes involved in hemoglobin synthesis, and disrupt hormonal regulation, affecting EPO levels. The oxidative stress triggered by some toxins can damage red blood cells and contribute to anemia. Nutrient depletion, especially of key vitamins and minerals, may also result from exposure to certain toxins.

Mycotoxin Exposure: Some mycotoxins, such as aflatoxins, can cause bone-marrow suppression and decrease RBC production. Chronic mycotoxin exposure may lead to chronic inflammation and oxidative stress, which can shorten the lifespan of RBCs as well as hemolysis.

Other Possible Causes: molybdenum deficiency, magnesium deficiency, cancer

Treatment Strategies for Low Red Blood Cell (RBC) Count

Diet

A diet rich in nutrients that help to grow red blood cells is important. Liver is a nutrient-dense organ meat that has almost every nutrient needed for erythropoiesis. Clinically, I have not found desiccated liver supplements to be effective. Other foods include legumes and eggs. Identifying the underlying nutritional deficiencies can help with recommendations for foods and individual nutrient focus. For those on vegan diets, adding in nutritional yeast for vitamin B12 (cobalamin), fermented vegetables, and other sources of B12 will be important.

Lifestyle

Women with low RBC counts will most likely be struggling with fatigue. Rest and recuperation are good for them. They should not exert themselves too much until levels have improved.

Supplements

Not everyone needs additional iron supplements when low RBC is present. Differentiation is key to treatment, as too much iron can also cause disease. If iron deficiency is diagnosed, correct supplementation practices are needed. Identification of a pattern is important for correct supplementation. (See Iron Section.)

Additional Testing

ferritin; iron and TIBC; vitamin B12 (cobalamin); comprehensive thyroid profile II; comprehensive metabolic panel (CMP); lactate dehydrogenase (LDH); c-reactive protein (CRP); vitamin D, 25-hydroxy (25-hydroxycalciferol, 25OH-D); copper, total; ceruloplasmin; heavy metal testing; oral zinc tolerance test

References

1. Lodish H, Flygare J, Chou S. From stem cell to erythroblast: regulation of red cell production at multiple levels by multiple hormones. IUBMB Life. 2010;62(7):492–496. doi:10.1002/iub.322

2. Orisakwe OE, Amadi CN, Frazzoli C. Management of Iron Overload in Resource Poor Nations: A Systematic Review of Phlebotomy and Natural Chelators. J Toxicol. 2020;2020:4084538. Published 2020 Jan 27. doi:10.1155/2020/4084538

3. Lee S, Guillet R, Cooper EM, et al. Maternal inflammation at delivery affects assessment of maternal iron status. J Nutr.2014;144(10):1524–1532. doi:10.3945/jn.114.191445

4. Jeng SS, Chen YH. Association of Zinc with Anemia. Nutrients. 2022;14(22):4918. Published 2022 Nov 20. doi:10.3390/nu14224918

5. Lane DJ, Chikhani S, Richardson V, Richardson DR. Transferrin iron uptake is stimulated by ascorbate via an intracellular reductive mechanism. Biochim Biophys Acta. 2013;1833(6):1527–1541. doi:10.1016/j.bbamcr.2013.02.010

6. Zimmermann MB, Biebinger R, Rohner F, et al. Vitamin A supplementation in children with poor vitamin A and iron status increases erythropoietin and hemoglobin concentrations without changing total body iron. Am J Clin Nutr. 2006;84(3):580–586. doi:10.1093/ajcn/84.3.580

7. M'Rabet-Bensalah K et al Thyroid dysfunction and anemia in a large population-based study. Clin Endocrinol (Oxf). 2015 Dec 10. doi: 10.1111/cen.12994. [Epub ahead of print]

8. Ma Y, Freitag P, Zhou J, Brüne B, Frede S, Fandrey J. Thyroid hormone induces erythropoietin gene expression through augmented accumulation of hypoxia-inducible factor-1. Am J Physiol Regul Integr Comp Physiol. 2004;287(3):R600-R607. doi:10.1152/ajpregu.00115.2004

9. Sebastiani G, Herranz Barbero A, Borrás-Novell C, et al. The Effects of Vegetarian and Vegan Diet during Pregnancy on the Health of Mothers and Offspring. Nutrients. 2019;11(3):557. Published 2019 Mar 6. doi:10.3390/nu11030557

10. Finkelstein, J.L., Kurpad, A.V., Thomas, T., Srinivasan, K. and Duggan, C. (2016), Maternal Anemia of Inflammation and Adverse Pregnancy and Neonatal Outcomes in India. The FASEB Journal, 30: 668.3–668.3. doi.org/10.1096/fasebj.30.1_supplement.668.3

Hemoglobin (HB)

The hemoglobin (HB) test measures the total amount of hemoglobin in the blood. This is a part of the complete blood count (CBC) panel.

Serum hemoglobin is a combination of hemoglobin bound to red blood cells (RBCs) and free-floating hemoglobin. There are multiple types of hemoglobin that can be found in circulation and on RBCs; this test counts them all. Hemoglobin subunit beta (HBB), a globin protein, and hemoglobin subunit alpha (HBA) make up the most common form of hemoglobin in RBCs. Other forms include HBF, or fetal hemoglobin, which is found in unborn babies and newborns. HBF is replaced by HBA shortly after birth.

Hemoglobin production is a complex process that involves several steps in the bone marrow. In adults, hemoglobin is composed of four protein chains: two alpha chains and two beta chains. (There are different combinations in fetal hemoglobin.) The synthesis of alpha and beta-globin chains occurs in ribosomes, where amino acids are linked together in a specific sequence to form polypeptide chains. Heme synthesis begins with the formation of a precursor molecule called δ-aminolevulinic acid (δ-ALA) in the mitochondria of the cell. Then δ-ALA is transported into the cytoplasm, where two molecules of δ-ALA combine to form a pyrrole ring in a process called condensation. This step is catalyzed by the enzyme δ-ALA synthase.

Four pyrrole rings are formed through a series of enzymatic reactions, and these rings combine to form a linear tetrapyrrole structure called porphobilinogen. Porphobilinogen undergoes further enzymatic reactions to produce a linear tetrapyrrole structure called porphyrin. The final step in porphyrin synthesis involves the incorporation of iron to produce heme. This step occurs in the mitochondria. The synthesized globin chains and heme molecules come together in the cytoplasm to form hemoglobin.

Hemoglobin is the major carrier of oxygen in RBCs. It is a complex structure that is formed in the early phases of erythropoiesis. Hemoglobin also acts as a buffer for carbon dioxide, formed as a byproduct of cellular metabolism. Not only can low hemoglobin cause hypoxia in the cells, it can also lead to a buildup of "pollution" as the CO_2 fails to be removed correctly.

Pregnancy

During pregnancy, hemoglobin levels vary widely based on gestation and physiology. In the initial few weeks of pregnancy, there is a slight increase in hemoglobin levels as the cessation of the menstrual cycles reserve iron, and hemoglobin production is increased for uteroplacental needs. Later in the first trimester, there can be a slight drop in hemoglobin, as iron absorption decreases significantly during the first trimester, and hemodilution begins. During the second trimester, there is a continued drop in serum hemoglobin due to hemodilution. Hemoglobin concentration physiologically diminishes by approximately 0.5 g/dL during the second trimester.[1] This natural drop in hemoglobin, and subsequent mild hypoxia, triggers an increase in RBC production starting at around 20 weeks gestation. From 20 weeks gestation through approximately 24 weeks, there is a 35% increase in RBC production. This increase in RBC counts also increases hemoglobin counts.

Postpartum

Changes may depend on birth experience. There is a slight decrease due to the normal blood loss of childbirth. Significant elevations have been documented between measurements of hemoglobin taken between six and eight weeks postpartum and those taken between four and six months postpartum, indicating that it takes at least four to six months to restore the physiological dip in hemoglobin to the pre-pregnancy ranges.

Hemoglobin ranges should always be assessed in conjunction with hematocrit, mean corpuscular volume (MCV), mean corpuscular hemoglobin (MCH), mean corpuscular hemoglobin concentration (MCHC), serum ferritin, serum iron, total iron-binding capacity (TIBC), and transferrin saturation (iron saturation) to determine the cause of high or low values. Both high and low hemoglobin concentrations are associated with adverse maternal and infant health outcomes.

According to the *Merck Manual of Diagnosis and Therapy,* pregnancy anemia is defined as hemoglobin <11 g/dL and a hematocrit <33% in the first trimester; hemoglobin <10.5 g/dL and a hematocrit <32% in the second trimester; and hemoglobin <11 g/dL and a hematocrit <33% in the third trimester. It also states that a hemoglobin <10.5 g/dL in the first trimester should be treated prophylactically.

STANDARD LAB RANGE: 11.5 - 15 g/dL

Trimester	Standard Pregnancy Ranges	**Functional Pregnancy Ranges**
Preconception	11.5 - 15	**13.2 - 14.5**
First Trimester	11.6 - 13.9	**11 - 14**
Second Trimester	9.7 - 14.8	**10.5 - 14**
Third Trimester	9.5 - 15	**11 - 14**
Postpartum	11.5 - 15	**11 - 15**

Causes of Elevated Hemoglobin (HB)

See Red Blood Cell (RBC) Count Section.

Hemolysis: In cases of RBC cell death due to oxidative stress, the cells may release hemoglobin. When the RBCs are low and the hemoglobin is elevated, this is a sign of hemolysis.

Fetal Hemoglobin in Maternal Circulation: A hemoglobin level >14.5 g/dL in the second and third trimester can be caused by a leakage of fetal hemoglobin into maternal circulation. Because the hemoglobin value in the CBC is a measure of the total count of all hemoglobin in circulation, it doesn't distinguish between bound, free, or fetal. This is known as fetomaternal hemorrhaging.[4] It is normal for a small amount of this fetal hemoglobin to be found in maternal circulation. In cases of placental dysfunction, this amount increases and causes maternal disease. Preeclamptic placentas accumulate free fetal hemoglobin.[5] Studies on hemolytic changes in pregnancy show that oxidative stress affects the placental functions and increases the release of fetal hemoglobin into maternal circulation.

Unbound hemoglobin is toxic and causes many of the complications seen in the progression of preeclampsia. Iron-rich hemoglobin binds to nitric oxide (NO) and reduces its availability for vasodilation. This causes vasoconstriction and increases the pressure needed to push blood through the system. In addition, hemoglobin spontaneously produces reactive oxygen species (ROS), specifically superoxide, which increases vascular oxidative stress and increases immune inflammatory responses. These inflammatory responses include increased neutrophil and cytokine production. Lastly, iron can affect the action of fer-

---

Elevated hemoglobin >13 g/dL in the first trimester is associated with a higher risk of maternal and fetal complications in pregnancy. This risk increases fourfold if the first-trimester hemoglobin is greater than 14.5 g/dL.[2 3] Levels should decrease throughout pregnancy, not increase, due to hemodilution.

Hemoglobin levels can be slightly higher in those living in altitudes above 5,000 feet.

If hemoglobin in the first trimester is over 13 g/dL in those living below 5,000 feet elevation or over 14 g/dL in those living above 5,000 feet elevation, a repeat of the CBC is warranted, and the woman should be monitored throughout pregnancy for disease.

ro-manganese (Fe-Mn) superoxide dismutase enzymes, neutralizing their functions in reducing oxidative stress.

Progesterone Deficiency: Progesterone has been shown to help reduce hemolysis of RBCs.[6] When elevated hemoglobin is identified, you should test progesterone levels. (See Progesterone Section.)

Hyperthyroidism: Hyperthyroidism can stimulate the production of erythropoietin (EPO), a hormone that promotes the production of red blood cells in the bone marrow. This can lead to an increased production of red blood cells, including hemoglobin. Hemoglobin A2 levels are increased in hyperthyroidism and decreased in hypothyroidism.

Other Possible Causes: dehydration, adrenal dysfunction, asthma and respiratory inflammation, sleep apnea, hypoxia, polycythemia, kidney disease, excess EPO production, iron overload/hemochromatosis

Treatment Strategies for Elevated Hemoglobin (HB)

See Red Blood Cell (RBC) Count Section.

Diet

Manganese-rich foods can help to replace excess iron and increase SOD enzyme activity. Hydration is also key. Eating hydrating food is often more effective than drinking more water. Watermelon, cucumbers, peaches, and coconut water are all good hydrating fruits and vegetables. Omega-3 fatty acids found in fatty fish, flaxseeds, and walnuts have anti-inflammatory properties. Including these foods in the diet may help reduce inflammation and its potential complications. Focus on increasing dietary consumption of copper, zinc, and manganese needed for healthy SOD enzyme formation and function.

Lifestyle

Reducing stress, both emotional and physical, is important for reducing the burden of elevated hemoglobin on the body. This may include working on sleep patterns as well.

Supplements

Antioxidants are important for helping prevent and manage patterns with elevated hemoglobin. Manganese is a trace mineral rarely discussed in nutrition, especially prenatal nutrition. Studies show it has a protective effect against oxidative stress, especially in cases of iron-associated oxidation, such as the release of fetal hemoglobin cardiovascular inflammation. Manganese is a cofactor for an antioxidant called superoxide dismutase (SOD). Manganese and iron can cross-bind to make SOD1. Although the manganese-iron SOD family can use either metal as a cofactor, there are differences in how the enzymes function depending on the cofactor used. Manganese SODs will readily bind to iron, yet iron inactivates the enzyme.[7] These enzymes then increase oxidation in the body. When treating elevated hemoglobin, reducing oxidative stress is a primary goal. There is limited research on the use of SOD supplements in pregnancy, but a few studies are very promising.

Vitamin E can help strengthen RBCs and prevent apoptosis and hemolysis, which releases hemoglobin into circulation.[8] Vitamin E can also be useful for cases of elevated hemoglobin and decreased progesterone. Avoid high-dose vitamin E supplements, keeping dosages below 200 IU. There is limited research on the use of vitamin E supplements in pregnancy. Most studies show benefit in supplementation, with a few showing a slight increased risk in premature rupture of membranes (PROM) in women taking doses of 400 IU of vitamin E in conjunction with 1,000 mg of vitamin C.[9] Other studies show no risk in taking vitamin E doses at or >400 IU in early pregnancy.[10] Additional antioxidants to consider include N-acetyl cysteine (NAC) and alpha-lipoic acid (ALA) depending on presentation and other indices.

Additional Testing

reticulocytes; nucleated red blood cells (nRBC); progesterone; comprehensive metabolic panel (CMP); iron and TIBC; ferritin; comprehensive thyroid profile II; reverse T3 (rT3); thyroid peroxidase antibodies (TPOAb); thyroglobulin antibody (TgAb); thyroid receptor antibodies (TRAb); erythropoietin (EPO); lactate dehydrogenase (LDH)

> Often when elevated hemoglobin levels present in the second and third trimester, this is an "acute crisis management" situation that requires immediate steps in reducing inflammation and damage to the maternal system. Typically, the goal is not treatment but management.

Causes of Low Hemoglobin (HB)

See Red Blood Cell (RBC) Count Section.

Iron Deficiency: Around 30% of anemia cases are caused by iron deficiency. Low hemoglobin can occur when the body doesn't have enough iron to make it. Generally, the body will prioritize hemoglobin synthesis and, in iron deficiency, decreased serum hemoglobin is often the last indice effected. Decreased MCHC may be more sensitive and accurate at identifying iron deficiency. If low hemoglobin is present,

Studies have found that patients with thalassemia and sickle cell anemia have other nutritional deficiencies: between 40% and 75% are deficient in vitamin

A, vitamin C, vitamin D, and/or selenium; between 28% and 38% are deficient in B vitamins.[11]

Hemoglobin levels <10 g/dL in the third trimester are a risk factor for postpartum hemorrhage.[12]

and it is due to iron deficiency, the deficiency has been present for a long period, and other system issues such as hypothyroidism may be present as well. In these cases, correction with iron supplementation may take longer. True iron-deficiency anemia typically presents with decreased RBC, hemoglobin, hematocrit, MCH, and MCHC in conjunction with a decreased iron saturation and ferritin. (See Iron Section.)

Thalassemia: Thalassemia is a genetic condition in which the bone marrow struggles to genetically express the components that make hemoglobin. There are two primary types: alpha-thalassemia and beta-thalassemia. Normal hemoglobin consists of two alpha chains and two beta chains. In thalassemia, there is a genetic decrease in the production of either the alpha or beta chains. This causes a lower production of hemoglobin and, in some cases, unstable hemoglobin that causes early cell death. Thalassemia is associated with higher rates of cellular hypoxia. Alpha-thalassemia is caused by reduced or absent synthesis of alpha-globin chains, and beta-thalassemia is caused by reduced or absent synthesis of beta-globin chains.

Copper and vitamin B6 (pyridoxine) deficiencies can mimic thalassemia or exacerbate symptoms. The key to distinguishing between thalassemia and copper deficiency is the Mentzer index (MCV/RBC count). True thalassemia generally has a Mentzer index <13. Thalassemia usually presents with high or normal RBC counts, low hemoglobin, low MCV, low MCH, high reticulocytes, and a low Mentzer index. (See Mean Corpuscular Hemoglobin Concentration (MCHC) Section.)

Sickle Cell Anemia: Sickle cell anemia is a genetic issue that causes hemoglobin to become curved and deformed. This is caused by abnormal genetic expression of hemoglobin B, which produces a hemoglobin S. A normal presentation in the CBC of sickle cell anemia is low hemoglobin with high MCH, MCV, and RBC counts, as well as higher WBC counts, especially lymphocytes and platelets.

Pyroluria: Also known as Mauve Factor, pyroluria is an increase in the urinary excretion of pyrroles, which are a component of hemoglobin. There are many theories as to what causes this genetic condition, which is associated with a breakdown in the production of hemoglobin. A byproduct called kryptopyrrole is produced. This byproduct has an affinity for zinc and vitamin B6 (pyridoxine), binding and excreting them through the urine. This, in turn, causes a functional deficiency in vitamin B6 and zinc, which can exacerbate anemia presentations and affect hemoglobin synthesis.

Copper Deficiency: One of the key enzymes in heme biosynthesis, ferroxidase, requires copper for its activity. Ferroxidase is involved in the conversion of ferrous iron (Fe^{2+}) to ferric iron (Fe^{3+}), a crucial step in heme synthesis. This conversion is necessary for incorporating iron into the heme molecule.

Vitamin B12 (Cobalamin) Deficiency: Certain medications have been shown to reduce hemoglobin levels; these include commonly used pregnancy medications such as metformin and antacids. These medications have been shown to reduce vitamin B12 levels. Certain dietary patterns, such as vegan diets, are also associated with higher rates of vitamin B12 deficiency. Vitamin B12 deficiency leads to the production of abnormally large and immature red blood cells. These cells, known as megaloblasts, do not mature properly. This condition is referred to as megaloblastic anemia. Megaloblastic red blood cells are fragile and have a shorter lifespan than normal red blood cells. Because of ineffective erythropoiesis and the shortened lifespan of red blood cells, the overall number of functional red blood cells is reduced, leading to low hemoglobin levels. Vitamin B9 (folate) and vitamin B12 are interrelated in hemoglobin synthesis. Folate helps regenerate vitamin B12.

Vitamin B6 (Pyridoxine) Deficiency: The synthesis of heme involves several enzymatic reactions, and vitamin B6 is specifically involved in the conversion of amino acids (glycine and succinyl-CoA) into δ-ALA.

Zinc Deficiency: Zinc is a cofactor for several enzymes involved in various stages of protein and nucleic acid metabolism. These enzymes play a role in the synthesis of heme, the iron-containing component of hemoglobin. One of the key enzymes in heme synthesis, δ-ALA dehydratase, requires zinc as a cofactor.

Environmental Toxin Exposure: Exposure to certain chemicals has been identified as a significant contributor to changes in hemoglobin synthesis, impacting red blood cell production and function. Lead, a well-documented toxic metal, interferes with heme synthesis and can substitute for iron in hemoglobin, leading to anemia. Benzene, an industrial solvent, induces bone-marrow suppression, resulting in disruptions to erythropoiesis and anemia. Mercury, cadmium, and arsenic, found in various environmental sources, have been associated with alterations in heme synthesis, affecting red blood cell function and contributing to anemia. Organophosphate pesticides, volatile organic compounds, and polycyclic aromatic hydrocarbons (PAHs) have also been linked to changes in hematological parameters, including hemoglobin levels. The duration and intensity of exposure, individual susceptibility, and specific mechanisms of each chemical influence their impact on hemoglobin synthesis.

Other Possible Causes: chronic intestinal inflammation or parasitic infections, internal bleeding, adrenal hypofunction, hemolysis, chronic infections, physical trauma or injury, hypothyroidism, progesterone deficiency, vitamin B1 (thiamine) deficiency, selenium deficiency

Treatment Strategies for Low Hemoglobin (HB)

See Red Blood Cell (RBC) Count Section.

Diet

Coffee and black tea consumption has been shown to increase the risk of anemia in pregnancy. In fact, women who consumed coffee daily were two and a half times more likely to develop anemia in pregnancy. Avoiding these drinks may help reverse low hemoglobin values by increasing nutrient absorption.[13] Consuming foods rich in heme iron (iron from animal sources) over nonheme iron (iron from plant sources) is crucial for increasing hemoglobin levels. Heme iron sources include red meat, poultry, and fish. Iron-deficiency anemia, and anemia in general, is more common in women consuming a more plant-based diet. Vegan diets, which exclude all animal products, can be associated with an increased risk of anemia during pregnancy. Plant-based sources of iron (nonheme iron) are less readily absorbed by the body than heme iron found in animal products. This lower absorption rate can make it challenging for pregnant women on vegan diets to meet their iron needs. (See Iron Section.)

Vitamin B12 (cobalamin) is primarily found in animal products and is vital for the formation of red blood cells. Vegan diets often lack this essential nutrient, which can contribute to anemia. For plant-based patients, the diet should include a variety of iron-rich plant foods such as legumes (beans, lentils), tofu, dark leafy greens (spinach, kale), fortified cereals, and dried fruits. Vitamin C-rich foods (citrus fruits, bell peppers) can enhance the absorption of nonheme iron. Combine iron-rich foods with vitamin C sources to improve iron absorption.

Lifestyle

Stress not only affects the risk of maternal anemia, but studies show that maternal stress also decreases the placental transfer of iron to the fetus.[14] This becomes a vicious cycle, as low iron can cause a decreased production of cortisol.[15] Minimizing exposure to chemicals associated with disruptions in hemoglobin synthesis involves awareness and proactive lifestyle choices. Lead, prevalent in old paint and certain water pipes, can be avoided by using lead-free paint and opting for filtered water. Benzene, found in tobacco smoke and industrial settings, can be reduced by avoiding smoking and ensuring proper ventilation in workspaces. Mercury in fish can be limited by choosing low-mercury seafood options.

Cadmium, present in tobacco smoke and some foods, underscores the importance of quitting smoking and adopting a balanced diet. Arsenic, found in contaminated water and certain foods, can be addressed by drinking clean water and diversifying dietary sources. Organophosphate pesticides on produce can be minimized by choosing organic options or washing fruits and vegetables thoroughly. Volatile organic compounds (VOCs) in household products and paints can be reduced by selecting low-VOC alternatives and maintaining good indoor ventilation. Polycyclic aromatic hydrocarbons (PAHs) in air pollution emphasize the need for avoiding heavily trafficked areas and using an in-home air filter if possible. Some environmental chemicals have short half-lives, and reduced exposure will reduce blood levels. Others have longer half-lives and may take years to fully leave the system. This is an example of controlling what we can and letting go of what we can't control.

Supplements

Identifying the underlying pattern is your key to proper management and treatment. Vegan individuals should take vitamin B12 (cobalamin) supplements, as this essential nutrient is not naturally found in plant foods. Iron supplements may also be needed. Iron supplementation is more effective in every-other-day doses. Every-other-day iron supplementation is as effective, if not more effective, as daily intake for treating iron-deficiency anemia, with lesser gastrointestinal side effects during pregnancy.[16] This has to do with hepcidin production after large-dose iron supplementation, which temporarily blocks iron absorption. Daily doses are more likely to keep hepcidin levels elevated, reduce overall absorption, and cause gastric upset. (See Iron Section.)

Additional Testing

comprehensive metabolic panel (CMP); comprehensive thyroid profile II; iron and TIBC; ferritin; vitamin B12 (cobalamin); progesterone; c-reactive protein (CRP); lactate dehydrogenase (LDH); copper, total; ceruloplasmin; comprehensive stool testing; heavy metal testing; oral zinc tolerance test

References

1. Mégier C, Peoc'h K, Puy V, Cordier AG. Iron Metabolism in Normal and Pathological Pregnancies and Fetal Consequences. Metabolites. 2022;12(2):129. Published 2022 Jan 29. doi:10.3390/metabo12020129
2. Young, M.F., Oaks, B.M., Rogers, H.P. et al. Maternal low and high hemoglobin concentrations and associations with adverse maternal and infant health outcomes: an updated global systematic review and meta-analysis. BMC Pregnancy Childbirth 23, 264 (2023). doi.org/10.1186/s12884–023-05489–6
3. Stephansson O, Dickman PW, Johansson A, Cnattingius S. Maternal hemoglobin concentration during pregnancy and risk of stillbirth. JAMA. 2000;284(20):2611–2617. doi:10.1001/jama.284.20.2611
4. Dana M, Fibach E. Fetal Hemoglobin in the Maternal Circulation-Contribution of Fetal Red Blood Cells. Hemoglobin. 2018;42(2):138–140. doi:10.1080/03630269.2018.1466712
5. Hansson SR, Nääv Å, Erlandsson L. Oxidative stress in preeclampsia and the role of free fetal hemoglobin. Front Physiol. 2015;5:516. Published 2015 Jan 13. doi:10.3389/fphys.2014.00516
6. Fang F, Hazegh K, Sinchar D, et al. Sex hormone intake in female blood donors: impact on haemolysis during cold storage and regulation of erythrocyte calcium influx by progesterone. Blood Transfus. 2019;17(4):263–273. doi:10.2450/2019.0053–19
7. Aguirre JD, Culotta VC. Battles with iron: manganese in oxidative stress protection. J Biol Chem. 2012;287(17):13541–13548. doi:10.1074/jbc.R111.312181
8. Marar T. Amelioration of glucose induced hemolysis of human erythrocytes by vitamin E. Chem Biol Interact. 2011;193(2):149–153. doi:10.1016/j.cbi.2011.06.004\
9. Rumbold A, Ota E, Hori H, Miyazaki C, Crowther CA. Vitamin E supplementation in pregnancy. Cochrane Database Syst Rev. 2015;2015(9):CD004069. Published 2015 Sep 7. doi:10.1002/14651858.CD004069.pub3
10. Boskovic R, Gargaun L, Oren D, Djulus J, Koren G. Pregnancy outcome following high doses of Vitamin E supplementation. Reprod Toxicol. 2005;20(1):85–88. doi:10.1016/j.reprotox.2005.01.003
11. Claster S, Wood JC, Noetzli L, et al. Nutritional deficiencies in iron-overloaded patients with hemoglobinopathies. Am J Hematol. 2009;84(6):344–348. doi:10.1002/ajh.21416
12. Haidar J (2010) Prevalence of anaemia, deficiencies of iron and folic acid and their determinants in Ethiopian women. J Heal, Population Nutri 28: 359.
13. American Academy of Pediatrics. "Mom's stress during pregnancy can affect baby's iron status." ScienceDaily. ScienceDaily, 29 April 2012. www.sciencedaily.com/releases/2012/04/120429085406.htm
14. Mario J.A. Saad, Samira L. Morais, Sara T.O. Saad; Reduced Cortisol Secretion in Patients with Iron Deficiency. Ann Nutr Metab 1 February 1991; 35 (2): 111–115. doi.org/10.1159/000177633
15. Chang CL, Yang JM, Wang KG. What kind of maternal factor might predict poor perinatal outcome in severe preeclampsia: a study based on doppler velocimetry? Zhonghua Yi Xue Za Zhi (Taipei) 1995;56(6):404–10
16. Karakoc G, Orgul G, Sahin D, Yucel A. Is every other day iron supplementation effective for the treatment of the iron-deficiency anemia in pregnancy? J Matern Fetal Neonatal Med. 2022 Mar;35(5):832–836. doi: 10.1080/14767058.2021.1910666. Epub 2021 Apr 18. PMID: 33866933

Hematocrit (HCT)

The hematocrit (HCT) test is a measure of the volume of packed red blood cells (RBCs) in a centrifuged sample.

Hematocrit = Individual Erythrocyte Volumes × Erythrocyte Count / 10

It is an essential component of a complete blood count (CBC) that is expressed as a percentage.

In much of conventional obstetrical and midwifery care, the classic H&H (hemoglobin and hematocrit) is all that is run in assessing for prenatal anemia. This is tragic, as many cases of low hemoglobin and hematocrit are not associated with iron deficiency, and the primary treatment for low H&H is iron supplementation.

Pregnancy

Percentages decrease by approximately 2% in the first half of pregnancy due to increasing plasma-to-RBC ratios. This decrease can be greater in multifetal gestations. More important than the percentage number is the drop that should occur from the first trimester through second trimester with hemodilution.

Postpartum

Changes may depend on birth experience. There may be an initial drop due to blood loss during delivery followed by a gradual return to pre-pregnancy levels. Generally, ranges recover and return to pre-pregnancy ranges by six weeks postpartum.

Hematocrit levels can be slightly higher in those living in altitudes above 5,000 feet.

STANDARD LAB RANGE: 34% – 46.6%

Trimester	Standard Pregnancy Ranges	**Functional Pregnancy Ranges**
Preconception	34–46.6%	**36–46.6%**
First Trimester	31–41%	**33–40%**
Second Trimester	30–39%	**32–39%**
Third Trimester	28–40%	**33–40%**
Postpartum	34–46.6%	**36–46.6%**

Causes of Elevated Hematocrit (HCT)

See Red Blood Cell (RBC) Count Section.

Elevated hematocrit of >44% increases the risk of adverse pregnancy outcomes.[1] Studies show that a hematocrit greater than 40% increases the risk of pregnancy complications, and a hematocrit that doesn't drop by approximately 2% from the first trimester to the late second trimester also increases the risk of pregnancy complications.

Dehydration: This is the most common cause of elevated hematocrit. Dehydration can cause a relative increase in the concentration of red blood cells, leading to higher hematocrit levels. This is often a temporary and reversible cause. If you find an elevated hematocrit, have the patient increase hydration and then retest.

Smoking/Vaping: Smoking is associated with an increase in carbon monoxide levels, which can stimulate the production of red blood cells. Chronic smoking may contribute to elevated hematocrit. This may also include secondhand smoke.

Hypothyroidism: Studies show that hypothyroidism can cause low RBC and hemoglobin but an increase in hematocrit. In hypothyroidism, mean corpuscular hemoglobin (MCH) and mean corpuscular hemoglobin concentration (MCHC) are also decreased.[2]

Other Possible Causes: congenital heart defects, asthma and respiratory diseases, hypoxia, sleep apnea, polycythemia, excess erythropoietin (EPO) production, iron overload/hemochromatosis

Treatment Strategies for Elevated Hematocrit (HCT)

See Red Blood Cell (RBC) Count Section.

Diet

Hydration is the key to lowering hematocrit in most cases. Encourage mamas to prioritize drinking water throughout the day, keeping a reusable water bottle handy. Herbal teas and coconut water are excellent choices for added variety. Emphasize the importance of hydrating fruits like watermelon, strawberries, and oranges as well as vegetables like cucumbers and bell peppers. Suggest snacking on yogurt, smoothies, or frozen treats made with hydrating ingredients. Encourage them to carry hydrating snacks and limit caffeinated and alcoholic beverages. Other dietary measures will depend on the underlying cause of the elevation in hematocrit. With the thickness of the blood, increasing foods that provide a slight blood-thinning property and reduce coagulation may also be of benefit. This can include vitamin E and vitamin C-rich foods, as well as fatty fish that provide omega-3 fatty acids. Antioxidants will also help to reduce the inflammation associated with higher hematocrit.

Lifestyle

Intense physical activity can lead to temporary increases in hematocrit due to changes in plasma volume. If patients are doing high-intensity workouts, have them decrease their routines or switch to less intense activities such as walking, yoga, and Pilates.

Supplements

Electrolyte supplements—which typically include minerals like sodium, potassium, chloride, calcium, and magnesium—may help with increasing plasma in the bloodstream.

Additional Testing

iron and TIBC; ferritin; comprehensive thyroid profile II; comprehensive metabolic panel (CMP); erythropoietin (EPO)

Causes of Low Hematocrit (HCT)

See Red Blood Cell (RBC) Count Section.

Microcytic Anemia: If RBC and hemoglobin are low with a low hematocrit, this generally indicates microcytic anemia, especially if the mean corpuscular volume (MCV) is also decreased.

Macrocytic Anemia: If RBC and hemoglobin are high or normal while the hematocrit is low, it could suggest macrocytic anemia. If MCV is high-normal or elevated, this may confirm macrocytic anemia.

Other Possible Causes: Another possible cause is vitamin B1 (thiamine) deficiency. Anything that can cause a decrease in the production of red blood cells can be a cause of lower hematocrit percentages.

Treatment Strategies for Low Hematocrit (HCT)

See Red Blood Cell (RBC) Count Section.

Low hematocrit treatment is primarily centered on increasing RBC production.

References

1. Nagao, T, Hirokawa, M. Diagnosis and treatment of macrocytic anemias in adults. J Gen Fam Med. 2017; 18: 200–204. doi.org/10.1002/jgf2.31

2. Dorgalaleh A, Mahmoodi M, Varmaghani B, et al. Effect of thyroid dysfunctions on blood cell count and red blood cell indice. Iran J Ped Hematol Oncol. 2013;3(2):73–77

Mean Corpuscular Volume (MCV)

MCV measures the volume occupied by a single red blood cell, or the average size of an individual red blood cell. It is an indice on the complete blood count (CBC) and is expressed in femtoliters (fL), which is equivalent to 10^{-15} liters.

MCV = Total Volume of Blood / Total Number of Red Blood Cells

The MCV is a tool to help distinguish between microcytic and macrocytic anemia types. This can help narrow down the differential etiology. It is essential to interpret MCV in conjunction with other parameters from the CBC to make accurate diagnoses and determine appropriate treatment plans.

MCV increases or decreases, along with increases and decreases in mean corpuscular hemoglobin (MCH), are significant findings for vitamin B12 (cobalamin), vitamin B9 (folate), vitamin B6 (pyridoxine), copper, and iron deficiencies.

MCV alone is an unreliable marker for iron deficiency due to increased erythrocytosis in pregnancy, which counterbalances the decrease in iron.

Pregnancy
MCV levels increase by approximately 4 fL throughout pregnancy, reaching a peak between 30 and 34 weeks. This is explained by an increase in production and release into circulation of immature red blood cells, which are larger in size. This does not indicate a vitamin B12 (cobalamin) or vitamin B9 (folate) deficiency issue unless the increase is greater than 4 fL or there are other symptoms with the associated change.

Postpartum
Changes may depend on birth experience, generally recovering by six weeks postpartum. If a woman experiences postpartum hemorrhage, characterized by significant blood loss during or after childbirth, there may be an impact on the red blood cell indices, including MCV. With blood loss and hypoxia, there is an increased production and release of immature red blood

cells that are larger in size, which increases the MCV value. Iron deficiency from blood loss can also cause a sharp decrease in MCV right after delivery.

STANDARD LAB RANGE: 79 – 97 fL

Trimester	Standard Pregnancy Ranges	**Functional Pregnancy Ranges**
Preconception	79 - 97	**80 - 95**
First Trimester	85 - 97.8	**85 - 95**
Second Trimester	85.8 - 99.4	**85 - 97**
Third Trimester	82.4 - 100.4	**85 - 99**
Postpartum	79 - 97	**80 - 99**

Causes of Elevated MCV

See Red Blood Cell (RBC) Count Section.

An elevated MCV is a marker for macrocytic anemia. In pregnancy, this is defined as an MCV >100 fL and a hemoglobin <11 g/dL. This form of anemia accounts for 40% of pregnancy anemia cases.[1]

Macrocytic anemia is divided into two distinct categories: megaloblastic and non-megaloblastic.

Megaloblastic means there are very large blood cells but not very many of them, and they are deformed. Megaloblastic anemia is caused by deficiency or impairment of utilization of vitamin B12 (cobalamin) or

Vitamin B9 (Folate) Deficiency: Folate deficiency usually only presents with an elevated MCV and MCH, but with a normal mean corpuscular hemoglobin concentration (MCHC).

Vitamin B12 (Cobalamin) Deficiency: A vitamin B12 (cobalamin) deficiency can present with elevated MCV and MCH, but with a normal MCHC, it can also include low hematocrit, elevated red blood cell distribution width (RDW), low white blood cell (WBC) counts, low neutrophils, low platelets, and low mean platelet volume (MPV). Vitamin B12 deficiency often mimics copper deficiency and vice versa. Vitamin B12 deficiency has also been shown to mimic HELLP syndrome. Heartburn medications are commonly used in pregnancy symptom management. These medications can cause vitamin B12 deficiency by decreasing the production of stomach acid and intrinsic factor needed for vitamin B12 absorption. A vegan diet that is low in vitamin B12 can also be associated with macrocytic anemia patterns. (See Red Blood Cell (RBC) Count Section.)

Gut Inflammation: H. (Helicobacter) pylori,[2] dysbiosis, celiac disease, Crohn's disease, and other inflammatory bowel disease (IBD) conditions increase the risk of B vitamin deficiencies and macrocytic anemia. Check the WBC differential for signs of gut pathology. (See Eosinophils Section.)

Hypothyroidism: Hypothyroidism has a strong correlation with anemia, having a cyclical relationship in anemia presentations. The most common form of anemia seen in hypothyroid patients is either normocytic or macrocytic. Thyroid hormones stimulate the production of erythropoietin (EPO) and regulate the RBC formation.[2] In cases of macrocytic anemia, you should run labs to assess thyroid function.

Adrenal Hyperfunction: Cushing's syndrome or excess cortisol production may lead to an increase in MCV, which represents the average size of red blood cells. This change can be related to changes in the maturation process of red blood cells.

Other Possible Causes: hereditary anemias, hypoxia, sleep apnea, vitamin C deficiency, liver inflammation, multiple sclerosis, hemolysis

vitamin B9 (folate). This is the primary cause of macrocytic anemia and should be tested in these cases. Often this is due to genetics.

—

Non-megaloblastic means the blood cells are very large, there are not many of them, and they are not deformed. Non-megaloblastic anemia may be the result of liver dysfunction, alcoholism, myelodysplastic syndrome (MDS), or hypothyroidism.

Treatment Strategies for Elevated MCV

See Red Blood Cell (RBC) Count Section.

Diet

Increasing the dietary intake of foods rich in vitamin B12 (cobalamin) and vitamin B9 (folate) is important. Red meat, organ meats, and legumes are necessary. Apple cider vinegar can help increase absorption. Bitter foods such as artichokes and arugula can help increase stomach acid production. Avoid iced beverages and smoothies, which can decrease stomach acid production. Avoid processed foods and meats, which can cause a decrease in nutrient absorption and lead to inflammation in the gut. Increase fermented and probiotic-rich foods. Fresh fruits and vegetables that are rich in vitamin C can help with folate metabolism.

Lifestyle

Stress management is important with macrocytic anemia. Stress decreases stomach acid production and can cause gastritis associated with overall poor nutrient absorption and increased heartburn.[3]

Supplements

Vitamin B12 (cobalamin) is available in several supplement forms, each with distinct characteristics. Cyanocobalamin, the most common form, is synthetic and requires conversion to active forms—methylcobalamin and adenosylcobalamin—in the body. Methylcobalamin and adenosylcobalamin are the active forms and do not require further conversion, making them preferred by individuals with potential conversion difficulties. Adenosylcobalamin is converted to methylcobalamin.

Methylcobalamin is now the most common form of supplementation. Hydroxocobalamin, with a longer half-life, is often used in cases when methylcobalamin is not effective in decreasing MCV levels.

Hydroxocobalamin is naturally produced by bacteria in the digestive tract. The choice between these forms may depend on individual preferences, tolerances, and health conditions. Genetic variants may change which form is best utilized. (See Additional Resources Section.) Generally, supplementation takes weeks or months to cause measurable effects. Often, oral vitamin B12 (cobalamin), such as lozenges or oral spray of 1,000 μg BID, is not effective in these cases. If B12 oral supplementation doesn't result in changes within 30 days, injectable B12 is a more favorable option with quicker results. Vitamin B9 (folate) supplementation may be needed if they are not already doing a quality prenatal vitamin. Caution should be used in folate supplementation; overdose is possible with changes to methylation function.

If the patient has had their gallbladder removed, is constipated, and has light-colored stools, an additional digestive enzyme complex with ox bile is appropriate.

Additional Testing

comprehensive thyroid profile II; comprehensive metabolic panel (CMP); vitamin B12 (cobalamin); methylmalonic acid; homocysteine; lactate dehydrogenase (LDH); comprehensive stool testing

> Sometimes the issue is genetic, in the processes of methylation. Supplementation in the acute stage may not be effective for these women.
>
> If nutrient therapy is being provided with no results, consider nutrient cofactors as well as gut health.

Causes of Low MCV

See Red Blood Cell (RBC) Count Section.

Copper Deficiency: Copper is responsible for several aspects of iron utilization in the body. A low MCV can be associated with long-term copper deficiency.[4] MCV is more often normal in acute copper-deficiency patterns, unless B vitamin components are also involved. Copper deficiency mimics B vitamin deficiencies. The most common cause of copper deficiency in pregnancy is zinc overload due to excess zinc supplementation. (See MCHC Section.)

Vitamin B6 (Pyridoxine) Deficiency: Vitamin B6 deficiency commonly causes microcytic anemia due to an inadequate synthesis of hemoglobin. A classic presentation of vitamin B6 deficiency in the CBC is low RBC, hematocrit, MCV, MCH, MCHC, and RDW, as well as low reticulocytes in the first trimester. (See Alanine Aminotransferase (ALT)(SGPT) Section.)

Heavy Metal Toxicity: Heavy metal toxicity decreases iron absorption, leading to iron-deficiency anemia, as well as causing increased cellular inflammation and anemia of inflammation patterns. An elevated eosinophil and basophil count may contribute to the diagnosis of heavy metal exposure. Different heavy metals may cause different patterns in lab work. If the serum iron and ferritin are normal but the MCV, hemoglobin, hematocrit, and MCH are all low, this may indicate chemical or heavy metal exposure.

Hypochlorhydria: In cases of microcytic anemia that are not corrected with nutrient supplementation, infections of H. pylori should be suspected. H. pylori can cause several nutritional deficiencies, by decreasing digestion and absorption. H. pylori affects stomach acid production. In cases of low stomach acid, vitamin C is converted to a less active form called dehydroascorbic acid, which prevents iron absorption. It is also associated with GI bleeds, which can cause a loss of blood.[5] Additionally, the stress hormone cortisol can decrease stomach acid production.

In pregnancy, heartburn is a common symptom, and many women will take antacid medications.[6] These medications can also decrease the levels of iron and vitamin B12 (cobalamin) in the body. This can

---

MCV is a marker for microcytic anemia. You'll see different resources saying anywhere from <80 fL to <85 fL is diagnostic for microcytic in pregnancy, due to the normal increase in MCV.

Microcytic anemia is defined as the presence of smaller-than-normal RBCs or less RBC production. Microcytic anemia is divided into three subtypes.

Hypochromic means the RBCs have less hemoglobin, causing them to be smaller than normal.

Normochromic means the RBCs have normal hemoglobin but lower RBC counts.

Hyperchromic means the RBCs have more hemoglobin than normal. This is a very rare condition known as sideroblastic anemia. This is primarily a genetic disorder related to iron utilization in the cells. It can be secondary to nutritional deficiency, antibiotics, heavy metals, and drug use. This pattern is characterized by a low MCV and MCH and elevated RDW.

be presented as either microcytic or macrocytic anemia. In some cases, as you correct iron-deficiency anemia, you find a sharp rise in the MCV, which indicates a hidden underlying vitamin B12 deficiency that was also present.

Excess Weight Gain: Erythropoiesis is sometimes increased in women with higher body mass in pregnancy, but without an increase in hemoglobin production. This causes microcytic anemia without iron deficiency, presenting with normal hemoglobin, low MCH, low MCHC, and low MCV but with normal or high RBC.

Other Possible Causes: intestinal parasites, vitamin C deficiency, iron deficiency, thalassemia and other genetic anemias, hyperthyroidism, chronic disease, certain medications (antibiotics)

Treatment Strategies for Low MCV

See Red Blood Cell (RBC) Count Section.

Diet

Increasing the dietary intake of iron and vitamin B6-rich foods is important. Apple cider vinegar can help increase absorption. Bitter foods such as artichokes and arugula can help increase stomach acid production. Avoid iced beverages and smoothies, which can decrease stomach acid production. Avoid processed foods and meats, which can cause a decrease in nutrient absorption and lead to inflammation in the gut. Increase fermented and probiotic-rich foods such as beet kvass. Beet kvass may improve gastric acid production and reduce heartburn symptoms. Patients should be instructed to consume between 1 and 2 tablespoons per day around meals. To minimize heavy metal exposure and potential contributors to low MCV, it is recommended that patients eat low-mercury fish, opt for organic produce, and wash fruits and vegetables thoroughly. They should also limit canned food consumption, especially canned fish and vegetables, instead opting for frozen.

Lifestyle

If heavy metal exposure is suspected, treatment will need to be postponed until after delivery for the safety of the baby. The patient should avoid smoking and exposure to secondhand smoke, and use cookware made from materials that do not leach heavy metals, such as cast iron and stainless steel. Have them test water quality, particularly if they are using well water, and consider a filtration system if necessary.

Supplements

If iron deficiency is identified, oral supplementation is warranted. In some cases, iron supplementation may not be successful in treatment. In these cases, iron infusions may be a better option. Digestive enzymes can be helpful for treating heartburn and increasing nutrient absorption. (See Iron Section.)

Additional Testing

comprehensive thyroid profile II; comprehensive metabolic panel (CMP); antinuclear antibodies (ANA); ferritin; iron and TIBC; c-reactive protein (CRP); copper, total; ceruloplasmin; comprehensive stool testing; heavy metal testing

> If a woman has a history of menorrhagia preconception, it is important to rule out the cause of excess bleeding, such as blood-clotting factors.
>
> Nutrient cofactors such as magnesium, molybdenum, essential fatty acids, vitamin C, and copper can decrease the utilization of other nutrients. Gut inflammation affects all aspects of nutrient absorption, and oral supplements may not be as effective in those with gut issues. Intravenous (IV) nutrient therapy may be an option in these cases.

References

1. Shi H, Chen L, Wang Y, et al. Severity of Anemia During Pregnancy and Adverse Maternal and Fetal Outcomes. JAMA Netw Open. 2022;5(2):e2147046. Published 2022 Feb 1. doi:10.1001/jamanetworkopen.2021.47046

2. Nasif WA, Ali ASE, Alamodi HS, et al. Impact of Helicobacter pylori on hematological parameters among Saudi population. Saudi Med J. 2021;42(6):643–648. doi:10.15537/smj.2021.42.6.20210103

3. Megha R, Farooq U, Lopez PP. Stress-Induced Gastritis. [Updated 2023 Apr 16]. In: StatPearls [Internet]. Treasure Island (FL): StatPearls Publishing; Jan 2023 www.ncbi.nlm.nih.gov/books/NBK499926

4. Wazir SM, Ghobrial I. Copper deficiency, a new triad: anemia, leucopenia, and myeloneuropathy. J Community Hosp Intern Med Perspect. 2017;7(4):265–268. Published 2017 Sep 19. doi:10.1080/20009666.2017.1351289

5. Maner BS, Moosavi L. Mean Corpuscular Volume. [Updated 2022 Jul 4]. In: StatPearls [Internet]. Treasure Island (FL): StatPearls Publishing; Jan 2023. www.ncbi.nlm.nih.gov/books/NBK545275

6. Jung SB, Nagaraja V, Kapur A, Eslick GD. Association between vitamin B12 deficiency and long-term use of acid-lowering agents: a systematic review and meta-analysis. Intern Med J. 2015;45(4):409–416. doi:10.1111/imj.12697

Mean Corpuscular Hemoglobin (MCH)

The mean corpuscular hemoglobin (MCH) test measures the average amount of hemoglobin present in a single red blood cell. It is an indice on the complete blood count (CBC).

The MCH value is calculated by dividing the total amount of hemoglobin in the blood by the total number of red blood cells.

MCH = Total Hemoglobin / Total RBC

An individual RBC can have 300 million hemoglobin molecules. MCH and mean corpuscular hemoglobin concentration (MCHC) increase and decrease along with mean corpuscular volume (MCV).[1] Changes in the MCH and MCHC are significant findings in the diagnosis of vitamin B12 (cobalamin), vitamin B9 (folate), iron, copper, and vitamin B6 (pyridoxine) deficiencies. MCV, MCH, and MCHC should be viewed together.

Pregnancy

MCH levels increase slightly throughout pregnancy, reaching a peak between 30 to 34 weeks. This is explained by an increase in production and release into circulation of immature red blood cells, which are larger in size and contain more hemoglobin than older RBCs. This change should coincide with slight differences in MCV and MCHC.

Postpartum

Changes may depend on birth experience, generally recovering by six weeks postpartum. After childbirth, there is a physiological adjustment known as postpartum diuresis, where the body eliminates excess fluid. This can result in a transient increase in hemoglobin concentration, including MCH levels, as the blood becomes more concentrated. Excessive bleeding during delivery may contribute to a drop in hemoglobin and MCH levels.

There is limited research into normal ranges for MCH, outside of overt disease.

STANDARD LAB RANGE: 26.6 – 33 pg

Trimester	Standard Pregnancy Ranges	**Functional Pregnancy Ranges**
Preconception	26.6 – 33	**27 – 32**
First Trimester	30 – 32	**30 – 32**
Second Trimester	30 – 33	**30 – 33**
Third Trimester	29 – 32	**29 – 32**
Postpartum	26.6 – 33	**27 – 32**

Causes of Elevated Mean Corpuscular Hemoglobin (MCH)

See the following sections: Red Blood Cell (RBC) Count, Mean Corpuscular Volume (MCV), and Mean Corpuscular Hemoglobin Concentration (MCHC).

Vitamin B9 (Folate) Deficiency: Folate deficiency usually only presents with an elevated MCV and MCH but with a normal MCHC. Additionally, testing serum folate and homocysteine can help identify folate deficiency as a cause.

Vitamin B12 (Cobalamin) Deficiency: Vitamin B12 (cobalamin) deficiency can present with elevated MCV and MCH but with a normal MCHC; it can also include low hematocrit, elevated RDW, low WBC counts, low neutrophils, low platelets, and low MPV. Vitamin B12 deficiency often mimics copper deficiency and vice versa; it can also mimic HELLP syndrome. Additionally, testing serum B12 and methylmalonic acid can help identify vitamin B12 deficiency as a cause.

Other Possible Causes: autoimmune disease, liver inflammation, nonalcohol fatty liver disease, alcohol use, hypothyroidism, polycythemia, excess erythropoietin (EPO) production, hypoxia, sleep apnea, dehydration

Treatment Strategies for Elevated Mean Corpuscular Hemoglobin (MCH)

See the following sections: Mean Corpuscular Volume (MCV), Red Blood Cell (RBC) Count, and Mean Corpuscular Hemoglobin Concentration (MCHC).

Diet

Ensure an adequate intake of vitamin B12 (cobalamin). While vitamin B12 is primarily found in animal products, fortified plant-based foods and supplements are available for those following vegetarian or vegan diets. Foods rich in vitamin B9 (folate) include leafy greens (spinach, kale, collard greens), asparagus, lentils, and fortified cereals. Blanching greens helps preserve folate content while reducing the risk of overcooking. It can also soften the greens, making them easier to digest, while also reducing oxalates and increasing mineral absorption.

Supplements

The recommended dosage of vitamin B12 (cobalamin) can vary based on the individual patient; this also includes which form is best. The typical oral dosage for vitamin B12 supplementation ranges from 250 to 1,000 µg per day. Injectable forms may also be prescribed in certain cases.

Additional Testing

comprehensive metabolic panel (CMP); iron and TIBC; ferritin; comprehensive thyroid profile II; homocysteine; vitamin B12 (cobalamin); methylmalonic acid; c-reactive protein (CRP); antinuclear antibodies (ANA)

Causes of Low Mean Corpuscular Hemoglobin (MCH)

See the following sections: Red Blood Cell (RBC) Count, Mean Corpuscular Volume (MCV), and Mean Corpuscular Hemoglobin Concentration (MCHC).

Iron Deficiency: Low MCH with low MCHC typically indicates low iron or low vitamin B6. Iron deficiency presents more commonly with decreased MCV, MCH, and MCHC with decreased RBC, hematocrit, serum iron, and ferritin.

Vitamin B6 (Pyridoxine) Deficiency: The presentation of iron deficiency and vitamin B6 deficiency can look similar; markers in the CMP as well as serum iron levels can help differentiate the patterns. In vitamin B6 anemia, MCV and MCH are decreased, but total iron and ferritin are normal. Aspartate aminotransferase (AST)(SGOT) will also generally be below 10 U/L. (See Aspartate Aminotransferase

(AST)(SGOT) Section.) A CRP level that does not decrease with antioxidant use may be associated with vitamin B6 deficiency.

Toxin Exposure: A decreased MCH, MCV, hemoglobin, hematocrit, and RBC as well as a decrease in lactate dehydrogenase (LDH), increased uric acid, increased bilirubin, and increased BUN is a classic presentation of toxin exposure. With certain heavy metals, calcium will be elevated and phosphorus low.

Other Possible Causes: internal bleeding (Crohn's flare), parasites, vitamin C deficiency, rheumatoid arthritis, hypothyroidism

Treatment Strategies for Low Mean Corpuscular Hemoglobin (MCH)

See the following sections: Mean Corpuscular Volume (MCV), Red Blood Cell (RBC) Count, and Mean Corpuscular Hemoglobin Concentration (MCHC).

Diet

Cruciferous vegetables may help reduce toxins in the body by increasing liver detox function. Incorporate foods that are rich in vitamin B6 (pyridoxine). This includes organ meats, fish, legumes, whole grains (amaranth, millet, quinoa), nuts, and seeds. If iron deficiency is the identified cause, supplementation may be required to raise levels based on gestational age. (See Iron Section.)

Lifestyle

If the pattern hints at a toxin exposure, it is best to try and find the source. This may be done by talking to the woman about food choices, lawn care (ask if they use glyphosates or Roundup for weeds), where they live, construction projects, or other possible sources of chemical exposure.

Supplements

If glyphosate exposure is identified, vitamin B12 1,000 µg in injection form may be useful in ameliorating toxic effects. N-acetyl cysteine (NAC) is a powerful chelating agent and can be used when endocrine-disruptive chemicals, heavy metals, or other toxins are suspected. The dosage would be 500 mg twice a day (BID).

Additional Testing

comprehensive metabolic panel (CMP); iron and TIBC; ferritin; c-reactive protein (CRP); lactate dehydrogenase (LDH); comprehensive thyroid profile II; toxin testing, comprehensive stool testing

Be cautious of any attempt to "detox" during pregnancy. The release of toxins into the bloodstream may have negative effects on the baby. Chelating agents that bind to toxins and neutralize are a better treatment approach.

Reference

1. Kauffmann T, Evans DS. Macrocytosis. [Updated 2022 Sep 26]. In: StatPearls [Internet]. Treasure Island (FL): StatPearls Publishing; Jan 2024. www.ncbi.nlm.nih.gov/books/NBK560908

Mean Corpuscular Hemoglobin Concentration (MCHC)

Mean corpuscular hemoglobin concentration (MCHC) measures the concentration of hemoglobin in a red blood cell relative to the size of the cell itself. It tells you what percentage of the blood cell is composed of hemoglobin. It is an indice on the complete blood count (CBC).

Some argue that this measure is more accurate in determining actual functional hemoglobin values, as it adjusts for the rate of red blood cell production and loose hemoglobin. This means it is less likely to account for free hemoglobin release from hemolysis of cells due to autoimmune or toxin exposure. Mean corpuscular hemoglobin (MCH) and MCHC should go up and down together; any variability in these values can indicate dysfunction.

Pregnancy

MCHC levels increase slightly throughout pregnancy, reaching a peak between 30 and 34 weeks. This is explained by an increase in overall production and release into circulation of immature red blood cells, which are larger in size and contain more hemoglobin than older RBCs. This change should coincide with slight mean corpuscular volume (MCV) and MCH increases.

Postpartum

Changes may depend on birth experience, generally recovering by six weeks postpartum.

STANDARD LAB RANGE: 31 – 36 g/dL

Trimester	Standard Pregnancy Ranges	**Functional Pregnancy Ranges**
Preconception	31-36	**31 – 36**
First Trimester	31-36	**31 – 36**
Second Trimester	31-36	**31 – 36**
Third Trimester	31-36	**31 – 36**
Postpartum	31-36	**31 – 36**

There is limited research into normal ranges for MCHC, outside of overt disease.

Causes of Elevated Mean Corpuscular Hemoglobin Concentration (MCHC)

See the following sections: Mean Corpuscular Volume (MCV), Red Blood Cell (RBC) Count, and Mean Corpuscular Hemoglobin (MCH).

Copper Deficiency: When there is a deficiency in copper and, consequently, impaired hemoglobin synthesis, the concentration of hemoglobin in red blood cells may be relatively higher compared to the decreased volume of the smaller cells. This can result in an elevated MCHC. If the MCH is low and the MCHC is high, this can indicate a copper deficiency, especially if neutropenia is also present. MCH and MCHC should rise and fall together. Copper deficiency can present as microcytic, macrocytic, or normocytic with the combination of neutropenia.[1] High MCHC with normal/low MCH is a differentiating pattern for copper issues. The most common cause of copper deficiency is zinc overload. The combination of decreased (zero) nucleated red blood cells (nRBC) and reticulocytes in early pregnancy is also a feature of first-trimester copper deficiency.

Other Possible Causes: Graves' disease, hemolytic anemia, autoimmune disease, dehydration, hypoxia, sleep apnea, polycythemia, excess erythropoietin (EPO) production, certain medications (diuretics), genetics, iron overload/hemochromatosis, vitamin B12 (cobalamin) deficiency, vitamin B9 (folate) deficiency

Treatment Strategies for Elevated Mean Corpuscular Hemoglobin Concentration (MCHC)

See the following sections: Mean Corpuscular Volume (MCV), Red Blood Cell (RBC) Count, and Mean Corpuscular Hemoglobin (MCH).

Diet

To address an elevated MCHC through dietary measures, it is essential to focus on increasing copper intake and promoting adequate hydration. Copper-rich foods include shellfish, organ meats, nuts, seeds, whole grains, legumes, and dark leafy greens. Incorporating these foods into a diet can help ensure sufficient copper levels. Also, staying well-hydrated is crucial to preventing dehydration, a common factor contributing to elevated MCHC. (See Copper Section.) Pregnant women should aim to consume adequate water throughout the day and be mindful of factors that may increase fluid loss, such as intense physical activity or hot weather. Maintaining a balanced and varied diet, along with staying hydrated, supports overall health and can positively influence MCHC.

Supplements

Copper supplements in the form of copper gluconate, copper sulfate, or copper chloride can reverse negative blood values within 4 to 12 weeks when copper deficiency is the culprit.[2] Check supplements for excess zinc intake.

Additional Testing

reticulocytes; vitamin B12 (cobalamin); methylmalonic acid; homocysteine; comprehensive metabolic panel (CMP); iron and TIBC; ferritin; copper, total; ceruloplasmin

Causes of Low Mean Corpuscular Hemoglobin Concentration (MCHC)

See the following sections: Mean Corpuscular Volume (MCV), Red Blood Cell (RBC) Count, and Mean Corpuscular Hemoglobin (MCH).

Iron Deficiency with or Without Anemia: Low MCH and MCHC are biomarkers for iron deficiency, often before serum hemoglobin levels decrease.

Vitamin B6 (Pyridoxine) Deficiency: Vitamin B6 is needed for hemoglobin synthesis, and a decrease in MCHC may be a marker of vitamin B6 deficiency. In the absence of vitamin B6, the production of hemoglobin and the maturation of red blood cells are impaired. This can result in smaller and paler red blood cells, a condition known as microcytic hypochromic anemia. Microcytic red blood cells contribute to lower MCHC values.

Other Possible Causes: lead exposure, heavy metal exposure, thalassemia, sideroblastic anemia, parasitic infection, autoimmune disease, heavy metal exposure, selenium deficiency

Treatment Strategies for Low Mean Corpuscular Hemoglobin Concentration (MCHC)

See the following sections: Mean Corpuscular Volume (MCV), Red Blood Cell (RBC) Count, and Mean Corpuscular Hemoglobin (MCH).

Diet

Pregnant women should focus on incorporating iron-rich foods such as lean meats, beans, lentils, and dark leafy greens, as iron is a fundamental component of hemoglobin. They should include vitamin B6-rich foods like poultry, fish, and bananas. And they should enhance iron absorption by including vitamin C-rich foods like citrus fruits and bell peppers in the diet.

Supplements

Vitamin B6 supplements are available in various forms, such as pyridoxine hydrochloride and pyridoxine-5'-phosphate, also known as P5P, or pyridoxal-5'-phosphate (PLP, the active form). PLP is considered more bioavailable. A typically high-dose vitamin B6 supplement of 10 to 25 mg three times per day has been safely used in pregnancy with no adverse effects.[3] That being said, a dosage of 25 mg per day is typically adequate to make changes.

Additional Testing

iron and TIBC; ferritin; comprehensive metabolic panel (CMP); antinuclear antibodies (ANA); heavy metal testing

References

1. Wazir SM, Ghobrial I. Copper deficiency, a new triad: anemia, leucopenia, and myeloneuropathy. J Community Hosp Intern Med Perspect. 2017;7(4):265-268. Published 2017 Sep 19. doi:10.1080/20009666.2017.1351289

2. Myint ZW, Oo TH, Thein KZ, Tun AM, Saeed H. Copper-deficiency anemia: review article. Ann Hematol. 2018;97(9):1527–1534. doi:10.1007/s00277–018-3407–5

3. Shrim A, Boskovic R, Maltepe C, Navios Y, Garcia-Bournissen F, Koren G. Pregnancy outcome following use of large doses of vitamin B6 in the first trimester. J Obstet Gynaecol. 2006;26(8):749–751. doi:10.1080/01443610600955826

Red Cell Size Distribution Width (RDW)

Red Cell Size Distribution Width (RDW) is a measure of the variability in red blood cell size. It is an analyte on the complete blood count (CBC).

An increase in value means a larger number of red blood cells are misshapen or vary in size. The lab analysis of the size is not based on the actual width of the cell, but the width of the curve of the red blood cell.

RDW-SD and RDW-CV are often analyzed as part of the red blood cell blood analysis.

RDW-CV = Coefficient of Variation
RDW-SD = Standard Deviation

RDW-CV is the one you will learn about in this section. It is found by the following formula:

RDW-CV = (Standard Deviation of MCV / MCV) × 100

This gives you a percentage value.

Pregnancy

There is a rise in RDW in the last four to six weeks of pregnancy, with no known etiology. Early increases in RDW are associated with pregnancy loss, so it is theorized that this may be a biological change close to parturition.[1]

Postpartum

There are no significant changes in the postpartum period after delivery. RDW levels drop within a few days of giving birth.

Some variability is *normal*, as it represents a healthy balance between young reticulocytes and older mature red blood cells in circulation. A release of nucleated red blood cells (nRBC) into circulation can cause larger variation in RDW, as will a decrease in red blood cell production.

STANDARD LAB RANGE: 11% – 15%

Trimester	Standard Pregnancy Ranges	**Functional Pregnancy Ranges**
Preconception	11–15%	**11–13%**
First Trimester	11.7–14.9%	**11–13%**
Second Trimester	12.3–14.7%	**11–14%**
Third Trimester	11.4–16.6%	**11–15%**
Postpartum	11–15%	**11–13%**

Causes of Elevated Red Cell Size Distribution Width (RDW)

See the following sections: Red Blood Cell (RBC) Count and Mean Corpuscular Volume (MCV).

Higher RDW levels (>14.5%) have been associated with higher risks of preeclampsia, gestational diabetes, and cholestasis.[2]

A sudden rise in RDW is a biomarker for intrahepatic cholestasis of pregnancy (ICP).[3]

A sudden rise in both RDW and mean platelet volume (MPV) is a biomarker for preterm labor risk.[4]

When the RDW is elevated, this

Vitamin B12 (Cobalamin) Deficiency: Vitamin B12 deficiency can present with an elevated MCV and MCH but with a normal MCHC; it can also include low hematocrit, elevated RDW, low WBC counts, low neutrophils, low platelets, and low MPV. Vitamin B12 deficiency often mimics copper deficiency and vice versa. B12 deficiency can also mimic HELLP syndrome. Vitamin B9 (folate) deficiency usually only presents with an elevated MCV and MCH but with a normal MCHC.

Iron Deficiency: In cases of iron deficiency, the synthesis of hemoglobin is compromised, leading to the formation of smaller red blood cells known as microcytic anemia. This deficiency prompts the bone marrow to release a mix of smaller and normal-sized red blood cells into circulation, creating a heterogeneous population with variations in size. The presence of immature red blood cells along with the smaller mature cells contributes to an elevated RDW. This usually occurs when iron deficiency has been present for some time.

Liver Inflammation: Alcoholism is known to increase RDW. You can also see this with intrahepatic cholestasis of pregnancy (ICP).

indicates that there is an increase in the variability of the red blood cell sizes: a larger percentage are not shaped the same. This may mean that there are more nucleated red blood cells (nRBC) entering circulation.

Autoimmune Disease: Lupus and psoriasis patients tend to have higher RDW values. This may be due to the destruction of RBCs and an increase in the production of smaller and younger cells.

T3 Syndrome, Subclinical Hypothyroidism: There is a connection between elevated RDW, thyroid-stimulating hormone (TSH), and free T3 (FT3) levels.

Other Possible Causes: myelodysplastic syndrome, sickle cell anemia, oxidative stress, hemolysis, genetics, thalassemia, hypoxia, sleep apnea

Treatment Strategies for Elevated Red Cell Size Distribution Width (RDW)

Diet

Address any underlying nutritional deficiencies by increasing dietary intake. Increase foods that help with liver function such as fresh herbs, cruciferous vegetables, and fatty fish. If the patient has cholestasis, apple cider vinegar, lemon, beet kvass, and bitter greens can also be good additions. Remove hydrogenated oils, processed foods, glyphosates, and high-fructose corn syrup. If a woman has markers of autoimmune disease, a gluten-free diet may be beneficial.

Supplements

Milk thistle is a helpful supplement for those with liver inflammation, such as in the case of ICP.[5] Antioxidant supplements may also be helpful in reducing older RBC apoptosis in inflammation and hemolysis conditions. (See Bile Acid, Serum Section.)

Additional Testing

comprehensive metabolic panel (CMP); bile acid, serum; glycated hemoglobin (hemoglobin A1c/HbA1c); homocysteine; vitamin B12 (cobalamin); nucleated red blood cells (nRBC); reticulocytes; copper, total; ceruloplasmin; lactate dehydrogenase (LDH); antinuclear antibodies (ANA)

Causes of Low Red Cell Size Distribution Width (RDW)

See the following sections: Red Blood Cell (RBC) Count and Mean Corpuscular Volume (MCV).

When the RDW is low, this indicates a decrease in the variability of the red blood cell sizes: a lower percentage are not shaped the same. There is a normal amount of variation in red blood cell size, as younger blood cells are slightly larger. But when the percentage is too low, this can indicate that there is not enough new RBC production.

Vitamin B6 (Pyridoxine) Deficiency: Vitamin B6 serves as a cofactor for enzymes involved in hemoglobin production, and its deficiency results in the formation of smaller-than-normal red blood cells. In the presence of vitamin B6 deficiency, bone marrow releases immature red blood cells into circulation earlier than usual, contributing to a more uniform size distribution of red blood cells, causing a lower RDW.

Other Possible Causes: aplastic anemia, thalassemia, inflammation and chronic disease, liver disease, polycythemia, excess erythropoietin (EPO) production

Treatment Strategies for Low Red Cell Size Distribution Width (RDW)

See the following sections: Red Blood Cell (RBC) Count, Mean Corpuscular Volume (MCV), and Mean Corpuscular Hemoglobin Concentration (MCHC).

Diet

Foods abundant in vitamin B6 include poultry such as chicken and turkey, fish like salmon and tuna, bananas, avocados, and nuts (especially walnuts).

For a complete list of nutrient food sources, visit my website and download my *Directory of Vitamin and Mineral Sources* e-book.

Supplements

Supplementation with vitamin B6 may help improve RDW levels.

Additional Testing

comprehensive metabolic panel (CMP); nucleated red blood cells (nRBC); reticulocytes; c-reactive protein (CRP)

References

1. Paliogiannis P, Zinellu A, Mangoni AA, et al. Red blood cell distribution width in pregnancy: a systematic review. Biochem Med (Zagreb). 2018;28(3):030502. doi:10.11613/BM.2018.030502

2. Kurban Y, Alan Y, Alan M, et al. A new marker in preterm labor: RDW and MPV. Obstet Gynecol Int J. 2020;11(6):366–372. DOI: 10.15406/ogij.2020.11.00538

3. Vural Yilmaz Z, Gencosmanoglu Turkmen G, Dağlar K, Yılmaz E, Kara O, Uygur D. Elevated red blood cell distribution width is associated with intrahepatic cholestasis of pregnancy. Ginekol Pol. 2017;88(2):75–80. doi:10.5603/GP.a2017.0015

4. Linda H. Goossen, 43—Hematology and hemostasis in the pediatric, geriatric, and pregnant populations, Editor(s): Elaine M. Keohane, Catherine N. Otto, Jeanine M. Walenga, Rodak's Hematology (Sixth Edition), Elsevier, 2020, Pages 813–831, ISBN 9780323530453, doi.org/10.1016/B978–0-323–53045-3.00052–0. (www.sciencedirect.com/science/article/pii/B9780323530453000520)

5. Alaca N, Özbeyli D, Uslu S, et al. Treatment with milk thistle extract (Silybum marianum), ursodeoxycholic acid, or their combination attenuates cholestatic liver injury in rats: Role of the hepatic stem cells. Turk J Gastroenterol. 2017;28(6):476–484. doi:10.5152/tjg.2017.16742

Reticulocytes

The reticulocyte blood test measures the number of reticulocytes in the bloodstream. This is sometimes found on the complete blood count (CBC) but not always.

Reticulocytes are nonnucleated young and immature red blood cells (RBCs). They are released from the bone marrow and mature in the bloodstream. During erythropoiesis, RBCs go through several steps and changes to become nonnucleated RBCs. They are generally larger than mature RBCs, and increased production and release into the bloodstream will affect other red blood cell indices. These cells do not have nuclei but do have a residual reticulum that disappears as the cell matures. This test is underutilized but can be a useful tool to understand how bone marrow is producing RBCs. Reticulocyte production is measured as a percentage of 1,000 RBCs.

Pregnancy

By 12 weeks gestation, there is a 90% increase in reticulocyte production. This decreases to 15% overall increased production by 34 weeks.

Postpartum

The increased production of reticulocytes is approximately 4% to 7% for the first three days postpartum, then declines abruptly between days four and seven. At eight weeks postpartum, the production of reticulocytes increases again, then declines again at 12 weeks. The production of reticulocytes remains lower than average for two years postpartum, only then returning to pre-pregnancy production levels.[1]

> Reticulocyte counts can be used to assess the treatment of anemia. Reticulocyte counts should increase within four to seven days of the start of anemia treatment if it is working.

STANDARD LAB RANGE: 0.5% – 2%

Trimester	Standard Pregnancy Ranges	**Functional Pregnancy Ranges**
Preconception	0.5–2%	**0.5–1.5%**
First Trimester	1–2%	**1–3%**
Second Trimester	1–2%	**1–2%**
Third Trimester	1–2%	**1–2%**
Postpartum	0.5–2%	**0.5–2%**
2YR Postpartum	0.5–2%	**0.5–1%**

Causes of Elevated Reticulocytes

See the following sections: Red Blood Cell (RBC) Count and Mean Corpuscular Volume (MCV)

Reticulocyte counts are higher in pregnancy or after the person moves to higher altitudes.

Hemolysis: An overproduction of reticulocytes may indicate hemolysis. As RBCs are destroyed, hypoxia stimulates an increase in RBC production and reticulocyte release. An additional increase of nucleated red blood cells (nRBC) may help identify this pattern.

Acute Iron Deficiency: In the early stages of iron deficiency, the body may respond by increasing the production of reticulocytes. This is an attempt to compensate for the reduced hemoglobin levels by releasing immature red blood cells into circulation more rapidly. As iron deficiency progresses and becomes more severe, the bone marrow's ability to produce reticulocytes may decrease. The reticulocyte count may normalize or even decrease as the bone marrow struggles to maintain red blood cell production in the face of limited iron availability. In this pattern, you may see very mild signs of iron-deficiency biomarkers in the CBC such as normal/increased RBC, decreased hemoglobin, decreased MCV, decreased MCH, and decreased MCHC.

Polycythemia: Polycythemia causes an increase in the overall production of blood cells.

Other Possible Causes: anemia, hypoxia, sleep apnea, thalassemia, excess erythropoietin (EPO) production, internal bleeding (IBD conditions)

Treatment Strategies for Elevated Reticulocytes

See Red Blood Cell (RBC) Count Section.

Diet

Although diet may not be profoundly effective for decreasing reticulocyte counts, it is still an essential part of patient care. Identifying the cause of increased production is key. Hypoxia may be caused by iron-deficiency anemia. If so, dietary treatment would be to increase iron-rich foods and possibly include supplementation.

Additional Testing

iron and TIBC; ferritin; nucleated red blood cells (nRBC); comprehensive metabolic panel (CMP); erythropoietin (EPO); c-reactive protein (CRP); lactate dehydrogenase (LDH)

Causes of Low Reticulocytes

See Red Blood Cell (RBC) Count Section.

Any nutritional deficiency or dysfunction that decreases the overall production of red blood cells can be a cause of decreased reticulocytes.

Chronic Iron Deficiency: Iron deficiency can lead to ineffective erythropoiesis, characterized by the production of small red blood cells with decreased hemoglobin. The bone marrow attempts to compensate for the lack of iron by producing more red blood cells, but these cells may be smaller and less mature, contributing to a decrease in reticulocyte counts.

Other Possible Causes: vitamin B12 (cobalamin) deficiency, vitamin B9 (folate) deficiency, copper deficiency, zinc deficiency, vitamin C deficiency, hypothyroidism, severe infections, environmental toxin exposure, heavy metal exposure, genetics

Treatment Strategies for Low Reticulocytes

See Red Blood Cell (RBC) Count Section.

Diet

When reticulocyte production is low, a diet rich in nutrients needed for proper red blood cell formation is crucial. Generally, for accuracy, identifying the exact nutritional deficiencies is important. Focus on these key nutrients: iron, vitamin B12 (cobalamin), vitamin B9 (folate), vitamin B6 (pyridoxine), copper, zinc, and vitamin C. Foods rich in iron such as meats, poultry, fish, organ meats like liver, and legumes provide the foundational component for hemoglobin synthesis.

Including eggs and fermented foods in the diet contributes vitamin B12, which is crucial for red blood cell maturation, and folate, found in green leafy vegetables like collard greens, supports DNA synthesis. Organ meats, particularly liver, stand out as potent sources of vitamin B6, zinc, and copper, further supporting optimal hematological health. Legumes, in addition to being iron-rich, provide an array of nutrients, including zinc and copper. To enhance iron absorption, incorporate vitamin C-rich foods like citrus fruits, strawberries, and bell peppers.

Supplements

Iron complex supplements may be useful in cases where multiple nutritional deficiencies are found to be contributing to decreased reticulocyte production. This may mean adding or changing prenatal supplements that provide a better array of nutrients in different forms.

Additional Testing

iron and TIBC; ferritin; vitamin B12 (cobalamin); methylmalonic acid; comprehensive metabolic panel (CMP); comprehensive thyroid profile II; copper, total; ceruloplasmin; heavy metal testing; oral zinc tolerance test

References

1. Kuo, Pao-Lin MD; Guo, How-Ran MD, ScD. Nucleated Red Blood Cells in Maternal Blood During Pregnancy. Obstetrics & Gynecology 94(3):464–468, Sept 1999

Nucleated Red Blood Cells (nRBC)

The nucleated red blood cells (nRBC) test measures the number of red blood cells with a nucleus present in a blood sample. It is sometimes found in the complete blood count (CBC) but not always.

Nucleated RBCs are immature red blood cells that still have a nucleus and DNA. As RBCs mature, they lose their nucleus and become concave in structure. Nucleated RBCs are generally only found in the bone marrow and are the precursors to reticulocytes. The other name for these cells is erythroblasts.

Many of the nucleated RBCs found in maternal circulation are from the fetus. There is a small amount of fetal blood and tissue cells in maternal circulation. These can include trophoblasts, lymphocytes, granulocytes, and nucleated red blood cells. Elevations in these cells past gestational norms can indicate placental dysfunction.

Pregnancy

Nucleated RBCs in the maternal circulation can be seen as early as six to eight weeks. This production steadily increases throughout pregnancy, with a sharper rise in the last few weeks before the onset of labor.[1] This rise in nucleated RBCs in the last few weeks of pregnancy may be the underlying connection to the increase in RDW. This is currently theoretical but could be a protective mechanism for blood loss during childbirth.

Postpartum

Nucleated RBCs in maternal circulation drop rapidly postpartum, returning to preconception levels within the first three days. There may be a slight number of residual nRBCs in circulation, but this level should continue to decline until it reaches 0% by six weeks postpartum.

> Nucleated red blood cells are typically found ONLY in the bone marrow, fetus, and maternal circulation during pregnancy.

STANDARD LAB RANGE: 0.0/100 WBC (0%)

Trimester	Standard Pregnancy Ranges	**Functional Pregnancy Ranges**
Preconception	0	**0**
First Trimester	Not Established	**<4**
Second Trimester	Not Established	**Not Established Research**
Third Trimester	Not Established	**<13**
Postpartum	0	**0 – 1**

Causes of Elevated Nucleated Red Blood Cells (nRBC)

See Red Blood Cell (RBC) Count Section.

—

WBC >4/100 (4%) in the first trimester can be a predictive biomarker for high-risk pregnancy complications associated with placental dysfunction.[2]

—

WBC >13/100 (13%) may be associated with pregnancy complications. Studies have shown that an elevation of nRBC counts may be a predictive marker for idiopathic IUGR and other pregnancy complications.[3]

Hypoxia: Hypoxia, a condition characterized by low levels of oxygen in tissues, can stimulate the bone marrow to produce an increased number of nRBCs. Hypoxia triggers the release of erythropoietin (EPO), which acts on the erythroid progenitor cells to stimulate the production of red blood cells. As a result, the bone marrow becomes more active, generating a higher number of red blood cell precursors, including nucleated red blood cells. Nucleated red blood cells have a higher oxygen-carrying capacity than mature red blood cells, as they contain more hemoglobin. The increase in nRBCs is part of a compensatory mechanism to counteract the effects of hypoxia. Hypoxia can also trigger a stress response in the fetus, prompting the release of immature red blood cells, including nRBCs, into maternal circulation.

Recent Move to Higher Altitudes: Moving to higher altitudes, where the atmospheric pressure is lower and oxygen levels are reduced, can lead to a condition known as hypobaric hypoxia. This type of hypoxia results from the decreased partial pressure of oxygen at higher altitudes. EPO production is strongly associated with altitude changes.[4] During a shift from low altitude to high altitude, EPO levels continue to rise for up to three days before eventually returning to normal after three weeks. EPO triggers increased RBC turnover and a doubling of nucleated red blood cells in circulation within seven days of altitude shift.[5]

Placental Dysfunction: The presence of nRBCs in maternal blood may be indicative of issues with fetal and placental health. Placental dysfunction can be associated with conditions such as placental insufficiency or intrauterine growth restriction, which may result in fetal distress. In response to stress, fetal bone marrow accelerates the production of red blood cells, including nRBCs, as a compensatory mechanism to improve oxygen delivery. Placental dysfunction may be associated with inflammation and oxidative stress. Inflammatory processes can affect the fetal hematopoietic system and contribute to the release of immature red blood cells. Various conditions can impair placental function, including preeclampsia, gestational diabetes, and certain infections. These conditions may disrupt the normal exchange of gases and nutrients across the placenta, influencing fetal hematopoiesis.

Other Possible Causes: polycythemia, excess erythropoietin (EPO) production, thalassemia, sleep apnea, asthma or lung disease, hemolytic anemia, sickle cell anemia, severe infection, ketoacidosis, heavy metal exposure, intestinal bleeding, cancer

Treatment Strategies for Elevated Nucleated Red Blood Cells (nRBC)

See Red Blood Cell (RBC) Count Section.

Diet

Nutritional deficiencies associated with poor RBC formation and function should be assessed and addressed, with nutritional protocols already outlined under the red blood cell (RBC) indice sections.

Lifestyle

Moderate exercise signals the production of RBCs to increase oxygen delivery to muscles. Excess exercise can signal muscle hypoxia and increase the production and release of nRBCs into circulation to improve muscle oxygenation. Reducing strenuous exercise and choosing more moderate exercise such as yoga, walking, and Pilates may help improve nRBC levels.

Additional Testing

erythropoietin (EPO); comprehensive metabolic panel (CMP); heavy metal testing

Causes of Low Nucleated Red Blood Cells (nRBC)

See Red Blood Cell (RBC) Count Section.

Causes of decreased production of nRBCs in pregnancy are not typically addressed as a specific medical issue. Any condition in which there is an overall reduction in RBC production can cause a decrease in nRBC release into circulation.

Treatment Strategies for Low Nucleated Red Blood Cells (nRBC)

See Red Blood Cell (RBC) Count Section.

References

1. Kuo PL, Guo HR. Nucleated red blood cells in maternal blood during pregnancy. Obstet Gynecol. 1999;94(3):464-468. doi:10.1016/s0029-7844(99)00281-1

2. Song GA, Lee SG, Baek DH, Je GH, Han JY. Obstetrical Outcomes of Increased Nucleated RBC in Maternal Blood during Early Pregnancy. Korean Journal of Obstetrics & Gynecology 2001;44(10):1817–1822, Oct 2001

3. Davari-Tanha F, Kaveh M, Nemati S, Javadian P, Salmanian B. Nucleated red blood cells count in pregnancies with idiopathic intra-uterine growth restriction. J Family Reprod Health. 2014;8(2):77–81

4. Ri-Li G, Witkowski S, Zhang Y.et al Determinants of erythropoietin release in response to short-term, hypobaric hypoxia. J Appl Physiol 2002922361–2367

5. Windsor JS, Rodway GW. Heights and haematology: the story of haemoglobin at altitude. Postgrad Med J. 2007;83(977):148–151. doi:10.1136/pgmj.2006.049734

Erythropoietin (EPO)

An erythropoietin (EPO) blood test measures the amount of erythropoietin in a blood sample. It is an individual analyte.

Erythropoietin is a glycoprotein hormone that is primarily produced by the kidneys. It is responsible for stimulating the maturation of red blood cells. The production of EPO is regulated by the amount of oxygen present in cells. When oxygen levels are low, hypoxia and EPO production increase, which leads to an increase in RBC production.

The fibroblasts of the renal cortex are the primary site of EPO production. It is regulated by the transcription of hypoxia-inducible factor (HIF). HIF is degraded when oxygen levels are normal but will accumulate and bind to EPO gene promoter regions, increasing EPO secretion, when oxygen levels are low.

Pregnancy

During the first trimester, erythropoietin production is slightly increased but slightly blunted in response to maternal hypoxia.[1] EPO levels are relatively low in pregnancy when compared to the degree of maternal anemia. Erythropoietin levels steadily rise throughout the remainder of pregnancy. This is triggered by a combination of hemodilution, mild anemia, increased glomerular filtration rate, and overall decreased oxygen in the kidneys. During pregnancy, the placenta also contributes to erythropoietin production in response to lower oxygen levels in the placental cells, and more significantly in fetal hypoxia.

Postpartum

During delivery, EPO levels decrease slightly but increase in response to blood loss in pregnancy. In normal birth experiences, they should remain stable through the third trimester into postpartum.

STANDARD LAB RANGE: 2.6 – 18.5 mIU/mL

Trimester	Standard Pregnancy Ranges	**Functional Pregnancy Ranges**
Preconception	2.6 - 18.5	**2.6 - 18.5**
First Trimester	12 - 25	**12 - 25**
Second Trimester	8 - 67	**13 - 44**
Third Trimester	14 - 222	**13 - 62**
Postpartum	14 - 222	**3 - 70**

Causes of Elevated Erythropoietin (EPO)

Erythropoietin levels have been known to increase two to four times normal ranges during maternal anemia,[2] in some cases reaching levels as high as 10,000 mUI/mL in acute hypoxic stress.[3] Abnormally elevated EPO levels are seen in gestational diabetes mellitus.[4]

Elevated EPO levels are seen in preeclampsia, due to increased placental production in response to placental hypoxia.[5]

Iron-Deficiency Anemia: In this scenario, there is low hemoglobin, low ferritin, low hepcidin, and increased erythropoietin.

Hyperthyroidism: In those with hyperthyroidism, elevated EPO levels as well as an increase in RBC production and RBC indices have been seen. Thyroid hormones have been found to increase the production of EPO through the augmentation of HIF.[6] Secondarily, increased metabolic rates due to hyperthyroid function increases oxygen consumption in the tissues. This increase in oxygen demand signals an increase in EPO production.

Hypoxia: Although anemia is the most common cause of hypoxia in pregnancy, other conditions such as chronic asthma, cardiovascular disease, living at higher altitudes, sleep apnea, infections, and metabolic disorders can decrease the oxygen found in tissues, thus increasing EPO production.

Secondary Polycythemia Vera (PV): Secondary PV refers to an increase in RBC production in response to systemic conditions rather than primary bone-marrow disorder. This is generally a compensation for conditions that cause hypoxia in the tissues. Unlike primary PV, secondary PV production of RBC is driven by and increased in EPO.

Other Possible Causes: anemia of chronic inflammation, hemolytic anemia, abnormal blood clotting/ischemia, thalassemia, vitamin B6 (pyridoxine) deficiency, copper deficiency, zinc overload, intestinal bleeding (IBD conditions), kidney disease, genetics, multiple gestation, cancer

Treatment Strategies for Elevated Erythropoietin (EPO)

See Iron Section.

Diet

Testing for iron status is important, but generally focus on nutrient guidelines that help to increase RBC function and tissue oxygenation. If iron deficiency is identified, this may mean increasing iron-rich foods. Fresh pomegranate juice has been shown to decrease fasting serum erythropoietin levels in those with diabetes.[7] Additionally, flavonoid and antioxidant consumption helps reduce oxidative stress, and certain flavonoids have been shown to boost cellular oxygen by preserving mitochondrial oxidative phosphorylation.[8] As of the writing of this book, specific flavonoids found in tea, grapes, berries, and several fruits and vegetables are being studied for their clinical use in mitochondrial medicine.

Hypoxia is a complicated condition with various underlying causes that are not related to micronutrient deficiencies. Dietary fat intake has been associated with lipid bilayer structural changes that may have a substantial impact on the transfer of oxygen across cell membranes, thus causing cellular hypoxia, even when adequate RBC and oxygen are present in circulation. Avoiding trans fat and eating high polyunsaturated fat diets may be of benefit. Dietary cholesterol is important for maintaining cell structure as well as hormone synthesis.

Additional Testing
complete blood count (CBC); comprehensive metabolic panel (CMP); comprehensive thyroid profile II; reverse T3 (rT3); thyroid peroxidase antibodies (TPOAb); thyroglobulin antibody (TgAb); thyroid receptor antibodies (TRAb); iron and TIBC; ferritin; nucleated red blood cells (nRBC); reticulocytes

Causes of Low Erythropoietin (EPO)

Heavy Metal Exposure: Lead and other heavy metals have been associated with depressed kidney function, causing a decrease in erythropoietin production and thus anemia.

Primary Polycythemia Vera (PV): When RBC counts and indices are elevated and erythropoietin is low, this is a diagnostic marker of primary polycythemia vera. Approximately 95% of primary PV cases are associated with a genetic mutation in the JAK2 gene.[9]

Hypothyroidism: Thyroid hormones are needed for the genetic expression of EPO, and hypothyroidism has been associated with decreased production. Secondary to this, hypothyroidism has been shown to cause resistance to EPO in erythropoiesis. In these cases, patients who are given EPO medications show decreased responses.[10]

Progesterone Deficiency: There is an interesting cyclical relationship between EPO and progesterone. Studies show that progesterone upregulates EPO production, and EPO decreases progesterone levels.[11][12]

Vitamin D Deficiency: Erythropoietin cells express receptors for calcitriol. There is an associated between vitamin D deficiency and decreased EPO production. There are other mechanisms that may be attributable to this.[13]

Vitamin A Deficiency: Studies have found that vitamin A supplementation increases EPO production.[14]

Other Possible Causes: anemia of chronic inflammation, autoimmune disease, iron overload/hemochromatosis, genetics

Treatment Strategies for Low Erythropoietin (EPO)

Diet

High-protein diets are associated with a decrease in EPO excretion through the urine. Decreasing protein intake does seem to help increase EPO levels.[15] This may be due more to the high iron content of most high-protein diets.

Other Possible Causes

complete blood count (CBC); comprehensive metabolic panel (CMP); iron and TIBC; ferritin; comprehensive thyroid profile II; c-reactive protein (CRP); antinuclear antibodies (ANA); progesterone; vitamin D, 25-hydroxy (25-hydroxycalciferol, 25OH-D)

References

1. Beguin Y, Lipscei G, Thoumsin H, Fillet G. Blunted erythropoietin production and decreased erythropoiesis in early pregnancy. Blood. 1991;78(1):89–93.

2. Vazenmiller D, Ponamaryova O, Muravlyova L, et al. The Levels of Hepcidin and Erythropoietin in Pregnant Women with Anemia of Various Geneses. Open Access Maced J Med Sci. 2018;6(11):2111–2114. Published 2018 Nov 23. doi:10.3889/oamjms.2018.471

3. Obeagu E I, Obeagu G U. A Review on Erythropietin in Pregnancy. J Gynecol Women's Health 2018; 8(3): 555740. DOI: 10.19080/JGWH.2018.08.555740

4. Mohd Idris MR, Nordin F, Mahdy ZA, Abd Wahid SF. Gestational Diabetes Mellitus in Pregnancy Increased Erythropoietin Level Affecting Differentiation Potency of Haematopoietic Stem Cell of Umbilical Cord Blood. Front Med (Lausanne). 2021;8:727179. Published 2021 Aug 19. doi:10.3389/fmed.2021.727179

5. Goldstein JD, Garry DJ, Maulik D. Obstetric conditions and erythropoietin levels. Am J Obstet Gynecol. 2000;182(5):1055–1057. doi:10.1067/mob.2000.105389

6. Ma Y, Freitag P, Zhou J, Brüne B, Frede S, Fandrey J. Thyroid hormone induces erythropoietin gene expression through augmented accumulation of hypoxia-inducible factor-1. Am J Physiol Regul Integr Comp Physiol. 2004;287(3):R600-R607. doi:10.1152/ajpregu.00115.2004

7. Banihani SA, Shuaibu SM, Al-Husein BA, Makahleh SS. Fresh Pomegranate Juice Decreases Fasting Serum Erythropoietin in Patients with Type 2 Diabetes. Int J Food Sci. 2019;2019:1269341. Published 2019 Apr 18. doi:10.1155/2019/1269341

8. Zhang Q, Wang J, Zhang H, Zeng T. Dihydromyricetin inhibits oxidative stress and apoptosis in oxygen and glucose deprivation/reoxygenation-induced HT22 cells by activating the Nrf2/HO-1 pathway. Mol Med Rep. 2021;23(6):397. doi:10.3892/mmr.2021.12036

9. Pillai AA, Fazal S, Mukkamalla SKR, et al. Polycythemia. [Updated 2023 May 20]. In: StatPearls [Internet]. Treasure Island (FL): StatPearls Publishing; Jan 2024. www.ncbi.nlm.nih.gov/books/NBK526081

10. Dilek M, Akpolat T, Cengiz K. Hypothyroidism as a cause of resistance to erythropoietin. Nephron. 2002;92(1):248. doi:10.1159/000064459

11. Ogawa A, Terada S, Sakuragawa N, Masuda S, Nagao M, Miki M. Progesterone, but not 17beta-estradiol, upregulates erythropoietin (EPO) production in human amniotic epithelial cells. J Biosci Bioeng. 2003;96(5):448–453. doi:10.1016/S1389–1723(03)70130–3

12. Tsompos C, Panoulis C, Toutouzas K, Zografos G, Papalois A. The Effect of Erythropoietin on Progesterone Levels during Ischemia Reperfusion Injury in Rats. J South Asian Feder Obs Gynae 2014; 6 (2):65–70

13. Santoro D, Caccamo D, Lucisano S, et al. Interplay of vitamin D, erythropoiesis, and the renin-angiotensin system. Biomed Res Int. 2015;2015:145828. doi:10.1155/2015/145828

14. Zimmermann MB, Biebinger R, Rohner F, et al. Vitamin A supplementation in children with poor vitamin A and iron status increases erythropoietin and hemoglobin concentrations without changing total body iron. Am J Clin Nutr. 2006;84(3):580–586. doi:10.1093/ajcn/84.3.580

15. Rosenberg ME, Howe RB, Zanjani ED, Hostetter TH. The response of erythropoietin to dietary protein in human renal disease. J Lab Clin Med. 1989;113(6):735–742

Iron

Serum iron measures the amount of iron in the bloodstream. This can be found in an iron and TIBC panel or as a single analyte.

The amount of iron in the bloodstream depends on various factors, including whether the patient has been fasting before the test, if they recently ate, and if they have taken certain medications. Approximately 75% of the iron in the body is found in hemoglobin, 10% is found in myoglobin, and the rest is found distributed in the bloodstream, bound to transferrin and stored in hemosiderin and ferritin.[1] The liver has the largest capacity to store iron, so it is very sensitive to overload.[2]

Iron absorption is complex and reliant on several enzymes, hormones, and nutrients. There are two types of absorbable dietary iron: heme and nonheme iron. Heme iron is derived from hemoglobin and myoglobin in animal food sources. Generally, 25% to 35% of heme iron is absorbed from the diet. Nonheme iron is generally less absorbed with an average of between 1% and 10%, depending on food source and cooking methods.[3] Nonheme iron (Fe^{3+}) must be broken down into Fe^{2+} and requires additional steps to be absorbed. Vitamin C and acidic pH cause Fe^{3+} to convert to Fe^{2+}. Heme iron is Fe^{2+} bound to heme.

Iron needs to be in the iron ferrous form, Fe^{2+}, or bound to heme to be absorbed through the gut. This is regulated by several nutrients and hormones. Gastric acid in the proximal duodenum helps the ferric reductase enzyme convert Fe^{3+} iron ferric to Fe^{2+} iron ferrous, increasing absorption. Once absorbed, the iron is either exported into the bloodstream or stored as ferritin.

Ferroportin is a cellular transport protein that helps release iron from the epithelial cells into the bloodstream; it is highly regulated by copper.

Hepcidin is a hormone that regulates iron absorption into the bloodstream. To prevent iron overload, hepcidin levels rise when serum iron levels increase. Estrogen and testosterone levels regulate hepcidin production. When iron stores are high, hepcidin binds to ferroportin and causes the protein to be degraded, blocking iron export to the bloodstream. When iron stores are low, hepcidin is low, increasing the expression of iron transport proteins and increasing iron absorption through the gut and into the cells for storage and release into the bloodstream.

Once in circulation, iron is bound to transferrin and then transported to the bone marrow to become red blood cells, to the liver for iron storage as ferritin and hemosiderin, to the thyroid to be a structural component of the thyroid peroxidase enzyme (TPO), and to other tissues in the body such as the placenta.

Ceruloplasmin is a protein that carries copper throughout the body. In iron metabolism, it works as a ferroxidase that helps to oxidize Fe^{2+} to make Fe^{3+} for binding to transferrin. Transferrin delivers the iron to the cells. Vitamin C helps convert Fe^{3+} to Fe^{2+} in the body as well as in the gut, increasing absorption of serum iron into the cells for use.

Pregnancy

In pregnancy, iron absorption changes by trimester and both maternal and fetal needs. Over the course of pregnancy, a woman needs to consume approximately 450 mg of iron for the increase in maternal RBC formation and maternal function; 250 mg in ferritin storage, which will be lost during a normal delivery; and 350 mg in the last trimester that will be stored as ferritin in the baby for the first three months of life when they do not readily absorb iron from breast milk or formula.[4] In the first trimester, iron absorption drops drastically due to an increase in hepcidin production, with a woman only requiring 1 mg of iron per day. The loss of menses and the preconception diet should have set a mother up for this drop with adequate ferritin storage. Iron absorption increases again between 20 and 24 weeks, after a normal anemic phase signals the release of stored iron, decreasing ferritin in the cells, decreasing hepcidin, and increasing absorption. There is a significant reduction in hepcidin production from 24 weeks to 40 weeks to signal a significant increase in iron absorption in the system.

During pregnancy, there is also a change in the absorption of heme versus nonheme iron. Nonheme iron absorption drops to about 2% in the first trimester, increasing to approximately 7% at 12 weeks gestation. At 24 weeks, nonheme iron absorption is between 28% and 47%. At 36 weeks, nonheme iron absorption is between 57% and 76%.[5] This is primarily driven by changes in hepcidin. In the first trimester, hepcidin levels average between 19 and 20 ng/mL, and by the third trimester hepcidin levels average between 1 and 2 ng/mL.[6]

Heme iron absorption seems to maintain about the same rate throughout pregnancy, except for during the first trimester. Heme is also more likely to be absorbed intact and transported directly to the placenta for fetal use.

Postpartum

The average amount of blood lost during a vaginal birth is 500 mL; the average amount of blood lost during a surgical delivery is 1,000 mL. It is estimated that 250 mg of iron are lost during a *normal* vaginal birth, and double that for a surgical birth. Hepcidin levels increase significantly within 24 hours after birth. Lactation requires a daily dietary allowance of 10 mg of iron. Iron levels should return to normal ranges by eight weeks postpartum.

Serum iron values can vary between 10% and 40% within a single day or day to day based on supplementation, iron absorption status, dietary intake, and other factors. Serum iron should always be assessed with other indices.

STANDARD LAB RANGE: 27 – 159 μg/dL

Trimester	Standard Pregnancy Ranges	**Functional Pregnancy Ranges**
Preconception	27–159	**50 – 170**
First Trimester	72–143	**50 – 170**
Second Trimester	44–178	**50 – 170**
Third Trimester	30–193	**50 – 170**
Postpartum	27–159	**50 – 170**

There is little research and information on serum iron as a biomarker of disease in pregnancy. Most research revolves around iron-deficiency anemia or serum ferritin and less around iron-deficiency as an independent factor. (See Ferritin Section.)

Causes of Elevated Iron

See Red Blood Cell (RBC) Count Section.

Iron Overload/Hemochromatosis: Hemochromatosis is a condition in which too much iron is absorbed into the body. Primary hemochromatosis is genetic. A variant in the HFE (high Fe^{2+}) gene is the most common genetic cause of hemochromatosis. Hepcidin deficiency is a hallmark of hemochromatosis.[7] Hemochromatosis is rarely diagnosed in women, as the menstrual cycle works as "bloodletting" and helps to reduce iron loads in the body. Most women are diagnosed postpartum or postmenopausal. Hemochromatosis can cause multiorgan maternal complications such as cardiovascular problems, hypertension, preeclampsia, and gestational diabetes.[8]

If the serum iron is normal or increased with a decreased RBC, hemoglobin, or hematocrit, there is an issue in utilizing iron. It is important to rule out vitamin B12 (cobalamin), vitamin B9 (folate), vitamin B6 (pyridoxine), and/or copper factors. Patterns associated with these deficiencies are discussed in the Red Blood Cell (RBC), Mean Corpuscular Volume (MCV), Mean Corpuscular Hemoglobin (MCH), and other RBC indices sections.

Secondary hemochromatosis often occurs after blood transfusions in those with thalassemia or sickle cell conditions. This can also occur in those who consume too much iron in the form of cast-iron-skillet use, or high liver or other heme iron intake. Secondary hemochromatosis is also known as iron overload. The classic presentation for hemochromatosis is high serum iron (usually >200 µg/dL), low total iron-binding capacity (TIBC), low unsaturated iron-binding capacity (UIBC), and in women transferrin saturation >45% with ferritin >200 ng/mL. If the liver is involved, liver enzymes and bilirubin will be elevated.

Preexisting Polycystic Ovarian Syndrome (PCOS): Women with PCOS often have higher serum iron and ferritin levels, especially when insulin resistance is present. They also often have elevated dehydroepiandrosterone (DHEA). DHEA has been implicated in the regulation of hepcidin. Some studies have observed elevated serum ferritin levels in women with PCOS.[9] If a mother has a preexisting elevated DHEA from conditions such as PCOS, the addition of fetal DHEA may cause higher androgen levels in pregnancy and affect iron absorption.

Sideroblastic Anemia: This is primarily a genetic disorder in iron utilization in the cells. It can be secondary to nutritional deficiency, antibiotics, heavy metals, and drug use. This pattern is characterized by a low RBC, MCV, MCH, and RDW and elevated serum iron and transferrin saturation with normal ferritin and TIBC. There are different types of sideroblastic anemia, but all of them are characterized by the presence of nonheme iron accumulating in the mitochondria of erythroid precursor cells. These deposits create a "ring" around the nucleus.

Hemolytic Anemia: A classic presentation of hemolytic anemia is high serum iron, transferrin saturation, and ferritin and normal TIBC/UIBC with low RBC, low or normal hemoglobin, high reticulocytes, high nucleated red blood cells (nRBC), low platelets, low MPV, and low neutrophils.

Vitamin B6 (Pyridoxine) Deficiency: Vitamin B6 forms pyridoxine phosphate, which is the coenzyme for the first, rate-limiting step of heme production. A deficiency in vitamin B6 can cause sideroblastic anemia. Higher serum iron levels are often found in this presentation.[10] Low aspartate aminotransferase (AST)(SGOT) and alanine aminotransferase (ALT)(SGPT) in the comprehensive metabolic panel

(CMP) as well as low lactate dehydrogenase (LDH) may also indicate vitamin B6 deficiency.

Vitamin D Overdose: There is an interesting connection between vitamin D and hepcidin. Studies show that high-dose vitamin D supplementation can decrease hepcidin production.[11] This pattern would be possible if serum vitamin D, 25-hydroxy (25-hydroxycalciferol, 25OH-D) levels were high in conjunction with elevated serum iron.

Other Possible Causes: vitamin B9 (folate) or vitamin B12 (cobalamin) deficiencies, selenium overdose, molybdenum deficiency, high iron mineral exposure (pots and pans, well water)

Treatment Strategies for Elevated Iron

See Red Blood Cell (RBC) Count Section.

Diet

In cases of iron overload, or high serum iron, the patient may need to reduce iron intake, specifically heme iron. Significant increases of serum iron or ferritin have not been shown with the consumption of nonheme iron. Therefore, in cases of high serum iron, a more plant-based diet may be beneficial. Dietary antioxidants can be helpful in chelating iron in the digestive system and decreasing absorption. These include pomegranates, blueberries, radishes, eggplants, and other fruits and vegetables that contain anthocyanin, as well as cranberries.

Anthocyanins' water-soluble pigments are responsible for the red, purple, and blue colors in many fruits and vegetables. These compounds are flavonoids, which are a type of polyphenolic compound with antioxidant properties. Rutin is a naturally occurring flavonoid in many foods, especially buckwheat, apricots, cherries, grapes, grapefruit, plums, and oranges. Rutin is a safe and effective iron chelator in pregnancy. Other herbs containing flavonoids that work as potent iron chelators may not be safe in supplemental doses in pregnancy, making dietary therapy important. Fortified foods, such as certain cereals and processed products, may contain added iron. Have patients read labels and choose products that are not fortified with iron. Check prenatal vitamins for added iron as well. For those with iron overload and an excess production of red blood cells, hydration is important for keeping the blood thinner.

Lifestyle

Avoid cooking acidic foods in cast-iron skillets. Limit cooking time to less than 15 minutes in a cast-iron skillet or switch cookware to stainless steel or ceramic-coated. For those who use a well for drinking water, test the water for iron content. The most effective treatment for those with hereditary hemochromatosis is blood donation. This should be done with lifestyle changes that also limit the exposure to excess iron.

Supplements

Reduce vitamin C supplementation to <500 mg, or remove completely. Pectin has been shown to chelate iron in the intestines and reduce absorption. In a small study, iron absorption decreased by half with an average loading dose of 15 grams.[12] Milk thistle, 140 mg silymarin, consumed with meals can help reduce the amount of iron absorbed by 40%, as well as help to protect the liver from higher iron levels.[13] Green tea polyphenols have been shown to help reduce oxidative stress and iron overload associated with thalassemia conditions.[14]

Inositol is a supplement commonly given to women with PCOS and insulin resistance. Inositol is an iron chelator and can bind to iron in the digestive system. Myo-inositol may also be associated with a reduction of hypertensive disorders of pregnancy. Avoid N-acetyl cysteine (NAC) supplements. In some animal model studies, NAC supplementation was shown to cause harm in those with iron overload. Other studies have found NAC protective when combined with iron chelators such as deferiprone.[15]

Additional Testing

complete blood count (CBC); comprehensive metabolic panel (CMP); lactate dehydrogenase (LDH); ferritin; peripheral blood smear; reticulocytes; nucleated red blood cells (nRBC); vitamin D, 25-hydroxy (25-hydroxycalciferol, 25OH-D)

Causes of Low Iron

See Red Blood Cell (RBC) Count Section.

Vitamin A Deficiency: Vitamin A maintains iron homeostasis by modulating liver hepcidin expression.[18] Vitamin A levels are inversely related to hepcidin levels and c-reactive protein (CRP).[19] So in cases of vitamin A deficiency, hepcidin levels are elevated and block iron absorption. This may be a consideration if patients are not having ferritin or serum iron recovery with proper iron supplementation, especially in the third trimester when there is a sixfold increase in vitamin A receptors in the uterine tissues and a subsequent increase in dietary need.

Vitamin C Deficiency: Vitamin C facilitates the conversion of Fe^{3+} to Fe^{2+} within the intestinal lumen, as well as in the bloodstream. Iron must be in the Fe^{2+} form to enter cells.

Studies on the prevalence of iron-deficiency anemia in the US are limited. Studies on predominately minority-based populations found iron deficiency in approximately 27% of women tested. Other studies have found the rate of iron deficiency to be between 10% and 21%. In a study done on women carrying multiples, 45% of them were anemic, but only 18% had iron deficiency. Another study on adolescent pregnant women found that 35% had anemia, but only 6.1% had iron deficiency.[16] It is estimated that approximately 20% of all anemia cases in the US are associated with true iron-deficiency anemia, while 50% of anemia cases in developing countries are associated with iron-deficiency anemia. This means that in all cases of anemia, serum iron and ferritin levels should be assessed to determine whether iron deficiency is the cause of anemia patterns. (See Red Blood Cell (RBC) Count Section.)

Low serum iron in pregnancy has been associated with cognitive issues in babies, regardless of anemia status. Low maternal iron intake at conception is associated with an increased risk of poor memory and focus in children.[17]

Hemoglobin is traditionally used as the marker of iron deficiency in conventional medical practices, because iron is a component of hemoglobin, and in iron-deficiency cases, hemoglobin is generally decreased

Zinc Deficiency: It has been thought that zinc and iron competed for absorption through the DMT-1 transporter in the intestines. However, studies have shown that inhibiting the DMT-1 transporter did not affect zinc absorption, just iron absorption. Instead, zinc stabilizes the DMT-1 transporter and supports iron absorption.[20] DMT-1 primarily transports Fe^{2+} across cell membranes and into cells. This cellular transport protein is responsible for the absorption of iron into the epithelial cells of the gut, as well as into systemic cells in the body.

Zinc in dietary form does not affect iron absorption. But large doses of zinc, in supplementation form >25 mg, does have an impact on iron absorption, specifically nonheme iron (not heme iron). Therefore, a deficiency in zinc, as well as high doses of supplemental zinc, can impair iron absorption. Zinc deficiency diets have been associated with iron accumulation in the tissues of both mothers and fetuses during pregnancy. In zinc deficiency patterns, there can be higher ferritin with lower serum iron. (See Ferritin Section.)

Selenium Deficiency: Higher serum selenium is associated with an increased serum iron level, MCHC, and hemoglobin level and a decreased risk of anemia.[21]

Copper Deficiency: Copper plays several roles in iron absorption and utilization in the body. Copper stimulates ferroportin expression and activates hepcidin, a hormone that regulates iron absorption and release. It also serves as a structural component of ceruloplasmin and forms ferric iron from Fe^{2+} so it can bind to transferrin through the multicopper ferroxidase enzymes. Copper also controls the uptake of iron into the mitochondria. Many steps in iron absorption and utilization are affected by copper levels.

In pregnancy, copper levels increase significantly, and there is a natural decrease in zinc levels to balance this rise. This is why many of the normal lab patterns in pregnancy mimic zinc deficiency patterns. Copper levels double by term with three distinct peaks in levels: at 22 weeks, 27 weeks, and 35 weeks.[22] In this pattern, you may see lower serum iron with normal stored iron parameters. Iron levels will not be corrected with iron supplementation. (See Copper Section.)

Inflammatory Bowel Disease (IBD): Patients with IBD are commonly found to have iron-deficiency anemia secondary to chronic

but not always. This is not a reliable marker of iron deficiency. Iron use in hemoglobin production is prioritized in biology, and often the hemoglobin levels are only decreased in cases of severe or prolonged iron deficiency. Serum iron levels decrease early in iron-deficiency settings and are one of the earliest markers of iron deficiency in pregnancy. Used with transferrin saturation (iron saturation) and ferritin, it is a very accurate measure of iron deficiency before anemia is present.

If the serum iron is decreased with a decrease in RBC, hemoglobin, hematocrit, MCH, and MCHC in conjunction with a decreased transferrin saturation and ferritin, iron-deficiency anemia is the diagnosis. Identifying the underlying cause is important.

blood loss, and impaired iron absorption due to tissue inflammation.[23] Iron deficiency is often an overlooked complication of conditions such as Crohn's disease, celiac disease, ulcerative colitis, parasitic infections, and other IBD conditions. Patients with preexisting gut pathology should be closely monitored for iron deficiency.

Decreased Testosterone Production: There are many reasons a woman may have lower testosterone levels during pregnancy, when testosterone increases by 70%. Its production is dependent on fetal dehydroepiandrosterone (DHEA) production and the expression of the aromatase enzyme by the placenta.[24] It has been well established that testosterone influences iron absorption and metabolism, by regulating hepcidin production. Lower DHEA and testosterone production can be seen in older moms.

High Phytates: Phytates, also known as phytic acid or inositol hexaphosphate, are naturally occurring compounds found in certain plant-based foods, particularly grains, legumes, nuts, and seeds. While they serve as antioxidants and may have some health-promoting properties, they can also bind to minerals like iron, zinc, calcium, and magnesium, forming phytate-mineral complexes. Phytates have a strong affinity for minerals, particularly iron. When phytates bind to iron, they form insoluble complexes, making the iron less available for absorption in the intestines. Nonheme iron, which is the predominant form of iron in plant-based foods, is more susceptible to the inhibitory effects of phytates compared to the heme iron found in animal products. Heme iron is generally better absorbed in the presence of phytates.

Inflammation: Low serum levels of iron have been negatively correlated with some traditional inflammatory markers such as high-sensitivity c-reactive protein (hs-CRP), tumor necrosis factor (TNF), and adiponectin, and inflammatory cytokines can decrease serum iron concentrations with no evidence of iron deficiency.[25]

Other Possible Causes: certain medications (antacids), hypothyroidism, adrenal hypofunction, cancer

Treatment Strategies for Low Iron

See Red Blood Cell (RBC) Count Section.

Diet

Remove antinutrients. Phytates are found in whole grains, seeds, nuts, and legumes. Phytic acid is the stored form of phosphorus. Humans lack the enzymes needed to break down phytic acid. Soaking grains and legumes before cooking is the most effective way to reduce phytic acid in these foods. The soaking process releases enzymes, which break down phytic acid and release the stored phosphorus.[26] Twenty-four hours of soaking reduces phytic acid levels by between 16% and 21%. Fermenting grains can reduce phytates by 88.3%; this includes techniques like making sourdough bread. Consuming vitamin C-rich foods alongside meals can counteract the inhibitory effects of phytates. Vitamin C forms a soluble complex with iron, making it more easily absorbed. Have iron-rich foods for breakfast when iron absorption is at its peak. Vitamin A-rich foods such as liver, pasture-raised chicken eggs, salmon, dairy, orange fruits, and veggies are usually adequate in increasing and maintaining levels.

Dietary practices that encourage better digestion may also be beneficial. This includes cooking foods, avoiding cold foods and drinks, and adding in fermented vegetables. Beet kvass and beet juice can have a positive impact on serum iron levels as well as RBC indices.

Lifestyle

Use cast-iron cookware. When cooking, add some vinegar, cooking wine, or citrus to the foods to increase iron content. Focus on gut health. In cases of iron deficiency, identify gut dysfunction that may inhibit absorption.

Supplements

Traditionally, iron deficiency in pregnancy has been treated with daily high-dose iron supplements. Even the CDC (Centers for Disease Control and Prevention) recommends that all pregnant women take 30 mg of iron every day during their pregnancies. There is mixed consensus about whether this daily dosage is accurate based on physiology, and more research suggests that every-other-day dosing may be more beneficial.[27] With large-dose supplementation, there is an acute surge in hepcidin. This rise can take between 24 and 48 hours to return to normal. High-dose iron supplements taken consecutively can keep hepcidin levels elevated, reducing overall absorption, increasing gastric upset, and requiring more frequent large doses of iron.

Iron supplementation has been shown to decrease beneficial bacteria in the gut, which are important for the inoculation of the infant immune system at birth and the suppression of group B streptococcus (GBS) bacteria. Those taking additional iron during pregnancy may need to increase both dietary and supplemental probiotics to help reduce the risk of dysbiosis.[28] Generalized iron supplementation without accurate diagnosis raises the risk of iron overload complications. For increased iron absorption from supplements, it is best to take them in the morning with 1,000 mg of vitamin C.

Additional Testing

complete blood count (CBC); comprehensive metabolic panel (CMP); lactate dehydrogenase (LDH); ferritin; c-reactive protein (CRP); copper, total; ceruloplasmin; oral zinc tolerance test

References

1. Anderson GJ, Frazer DM. Hepatic iron metabolism. Semin Liver Dis. 2005;25(4):420–432. doi:10.1055/s-2005–923314

2. Skolmowska D, Głąbska D. Analysis of Heme and Non-Heme Iron Intake and Iron Dietary Sources in Adolescent Menstruating Females in a National Polish Sample. Nutrients. 2019;11(5):1049. Published 2019 May 10. doi:10.3390/nu11051049

3. Institute of Medicine (US) Committee on Nutritional Status During Pregnancy and Lactation. Nutrition During Pregnancy: Part I Weight Gain: Part II Nutrient Supplements. Washington (DC): National Academies Press (US); 1990. 14, Iron Nutrition During Pregnancy. www.ncbi.nlm.nih.gov/books/NBK235217

4. Barrett JF, Whittaker PG, Williams JG, Lind T. Absorption of non-haem iron from food during normal pregnancy. BMJ. 1994;309(6947):79–82. doi:10.1136/bmj.309.6947.79

5. Lammi-Keefe C, Couch S, Kirwan J. Handbook of Nutrition and Pregnancy. 2nd Edition. Humana Press; 2018

6. Sun P, Zhou Y, Xu S, et al. Elevated first-trimester hepcidin level is associated with reduced risk of iron-deficiency anemia in late pregnancy: a prospective cohort study. Front Nutr. 2023;10:1147114. Published 2023 Aug 15. doi:10.3389/fnut.2023.1147114

7. Ambrin Gull Shamas, "Primary Hereditary Haemochromatosis and Pregnancy", GastroHep, vol. 2023, Article ID 2674203, 12 pages, 2023. doi.org/10.1155/2023/2674203

8. Shamas, Ambrin. (2023). Primary Hereditary Haemochromatosis and Pregnancy. GastroHep. 2023. 1-12. 10.1155/2023/2674203.

9. Mathew M, Sivaprakasam S, Phy JL, Bhutia YD, Ganapathy V. Polycystic ovary syndrome and iron overload: biochemical link and underlying mechanisms with potential novel therapeutic avenues. Biosci Rep. 2023;43(1):BSR20212234. doi:10.1042/BSR20212234

10. Ashorobi D, Chhabra A. Sideroblastic Anemia. [Updated 2023 Jul 17]. In: StatPearls [Internet]. Treasure Island (FL): StatPearls Publishing; Jan 2023. www.ncbi.nlm.nih.gov/books/NBK538287

11. Moran-Lev, H., Weisman, Y., Cohen, S. et al. The interrelationship between hepcidin, vitamin D, and anemia in children with acute infectious disease. Pediatr Res 84, 62–65 (2018). doi.org/10.1038/s41390-018-0005–0

12. Monnier L, Colette C, Aguirre L, Mirouze J. Evidence and mechanism for pectin-reduced intestinal inorganic iron absorption in idiopathic hemochromatosis. Am J Clin Nutr. 1980;33(6):1225–1232. doi:10.1093/ajcn/33.6.1225

13. Hutchinson C, Bomford A, Geissler CA. The iron-chelating potential of silybin in patients with hereditary haemochromatosis. Eur J Clin Nutr. 2010;64(10):1239–1241. doi:10.1038/ejcn.2010.136

14. Settakorn K, Kongkarnka S, Chompupoung A, et al. Effects of green tea extract treatment on erythropoiesis and iron parameters in iron-overloaded β-thalassemic mice. Front Physiol. 2022;13:1053060. Published 2022 Dec 23. doi:10.3389/fphys.2022.1053060

15. Sripetchwandee J, Pipatpiboon N, Chattipakorn N, Chattipakorn S. Combined therapy of iron chelator and antioxidant completely restores brain dysfunction induced by iron toxicity. PLoS One. 2014;9(1):e85115. Published 2014 Jan 6. doi:10.1371/journal.pone.0085115

16. Clara Camaschella; Treating iron overload with hepcidin. Blood 2006; 107 (7): 2595. doi: doi.org/10.1182/blood-2006–01-0189

17. Georgieff MK. Iron deficiency in pregnancy. Am J Obstet Gynecol. 2020;223(4):516–524. doi:10.1016/j.ajog.2020.03.006

18. Arruda SF, Siqueira EM, de Valência FF. Vitamin A deficiency increases hepcidin expression and oxidative stress in rat. Nutrition. 2009;25(4):472–478. doi:10.1016/j.nut.2008.11.030

19. Silva AP, Pereira ADS, Simões BFT, et al. Association of vitamin A with anemia and serum hepcidin levels in children aged 6 to 59 mo. Nutrition. 2021;91–92:111463. doi:10.1016/j.nut.2021.111463

20. Kondaiah P, Yaduvanshi PS, Sharp PA, Pullakhandam R. Iron and Zinc Homeostasis and Interactions: Does Enteric Zinc Excretion Cross-Talk with Intestinal Iron Absorption?. Nutrients. 2019;11(8):1885. Published 2019 Aug 13. doi:10.3390/nu11081885

21. Zhou, Q., Zhang, B., Chen, X., Chen, Q., & Hao, L. (2021). Association of serum selenium with anemia-related indicators and risk of anemia. Food science & nutrition, 9(6), 3039–3047. doi.org/10.1002/fsn3.2261

22. Vukelić J, Kapamadzija A, Petrović D, et al. Variations of serum copper values in pregnancy. Srp Arh Celok Lek. 2012;140(1–2):42–46

23. Kaitha S, Bashir M, Ali T. Iron-deficiency anemia in inflammatory bowel disease. World J Gastrointest Pathophysiol. 2015;6(3):62–72. doi:10.4291/wjgp.v6.i3.62

24. Kallak TK, Hellgren C, Skalkidou A, et al. Maternal and female fetal testosterone levels are associated with maternal age and gestational weight gain. Eur J Endocrinol. 2017;177(4):379–388. doi:10.1530/EJE-17–0207

25. Peng, Y. F., & Wei, Y. S. (2017). Associations between serum bilirubin levels and essential trace elements status in an adult population. Oncotarget, 8(46), 81315–81320. doi.org/10.18632/oncotarget.18351

26. Gupta RK, Gangoliya SS, Singh NK. Reduction of phytic acid and enhancement of bioavailable micronutrients in food grains. J Food Sci Technol. 2015;52(2):676–684. doi:10.1007/s13197–013-0978-y

27. Nicole U. Stoffel, Christophe Zeder, Gary M. Brittenham, Diego Moretti, Michael B. Zimmermann. Iron absorption from supplements is greater with alternate day than with consecutive day dosing in iron-deficient anemic women. Haematologica 2020;105(5):1232–1239; doi.org/10.3324/haematol.2019.220830

28. Yilmaz B, Li H. Gut Microbiota and Iron: The Crucial Actors in Health and Disease. Pharmaceuticals (Basel). 2018;11(4):98. Published 2018 Oct 5. doi:10.3390/ph11040098

29. Yang Y, Wang R, Jiang H, Hu M, Tang A, Xiang Z. Changes of iron metabolism during pregnancy and the establishment of reference intervals for pregnant Chinese women. Annals of Clinical Biochemistry. 2019;56(5):556–563. doi:10.1177/0004563219835853

Total Iron-Binding Capacity (TIBC)

Total iron-binding capacity (TIBC) measures the amount of total binding proteins and their capacity to bind to serum iron in the bloodstream. It is often used in conjunction with other iron tests to assess the body's iron status in an iron and TIBC panel.

The body makes transport proteins in response to a person's need for iron. When iron storage is low, transport protein production increases. When iron storage is high, there is a reduction in the production of transport proteins. Transferrin is a transport protein that is responsible for between 50% and 70% of all iron-binding, and generally the TIBC is described as a measure of transferrin-binding capacity because it is the primary transport protein.

Pregnancy

Transferrin production steadily increases throughout pregnancy, almost doubling by the peak in the third trimester. This causes an elevation in the TIBC. More transferrin in the bloodstream means there is more of a capacity for iron-binding.

Postpartum

TIBC remains elevated through at least six weeks postpartum. There is limited data on when these values return to normal and may be more associated with birth outcomes and blood loss in childbirth.

STANDARD LAB RANGE: 250 – 450 µg/dL

Trimester	Standard Pregnancy Ranges	**Functional Pregnancy Ranges**
Preconception	250 - 450	**250 - 450**
First Trimester	135 - 408	**135 - 408**
Second Trimester	302 - 519	**302 - 519**
Third Trimester	380 - 597	**380 - 597**
Postpartum	Not Established	**250 - 450**

Causes of Elevated Total Iron-Binding Capacity (TIBC)

See Iron Section.

TIBC is elevated when there is iron deficiency, as it represents a large portion of unbound transport proteins and lower serum iron levels. It can also represent an elevated production of transferrin and transport proteins.

If the serum iron is decreased with a decrease in RBC, hemoglobin, hematocrit, MCH, and MCHC in conjunction with a decrease in transferrin saturation (iron saturation) and ferritin and an increase in TIBC/UIBC, then iron-deficiency anemia is the diagnosis. Identifying the underlying cause is important.

Insulin Resistance: Elevated TIBC and higher transferrin levels are a biomarker for insulin resistance. Transferrin and ferritin are inversely related. If both are elevated, this is a predictive biomarker for insulin resistance and diabetes onset.[1] Iron status affects the insulin sensitivity by modulating the transcription and membrane expression/affinity of insulin receptor expression. It has been well documented that higher ferritin levels and iron excess can be a stimulator of insulin resistance and type 2 diabetes. In these cases, transferrin affects insulin's ability to bind to receptors, causing insulin resistance. Higher serum insulin levels affect hepcidin production. In cases of insulin resistance, you may see low hemoglobin and serum iron levels with elevated TIBC and ferritin.

Magnesium Deficiency: Magnesium is required to "glue" iron to transferrin.[2, 3] Higher/normal serum iron with a higher TIBC may show that there is a magnesium deficiency. There is enough iron and lots of open-transport protein, but they are not bonding.

Other Possible Causes: iron deficiency, internal bleeding (Crohn's disease flare), preconception oral contraception use, hemolytic anemia, hypothyroidism, heavy metal exposure

Treatment Strategies for Elevated Total Iron-Binding Capacity (TIBC)

See Iron Section.

Diet

If iron deficiency is the cause, address guidelines in the Iron Section. In cases of insulin resistance, it is important to regulate blood sugar levels. Breakfast consumption is key, and consuming most of the calories in the first half of the day is beneficial. Slow and mindful eating practices (like intuitive eating) can help limit overeating. Overeating is just as detrimental to insulin resistance as consuming high-sugar foods. This is based on the idea of glycemic loading. (See Glucose Section.)

Supplements

Magnesium supplementation of 375 mg was used in studies to benefit insulin resistance patterns. In pregnancy, magnesium needs increase, though few studies have highlighted the actual increase in maternal needs. Supplementation should be done based on patient presentation. There are several forms of supplemental magnesium on the market. Not all of them are highly absorbed, and some work better than others for specific patterns. Magnesium oxide is the elemental form of magnesium. It contains a large amount of magnesium per dose, but this form is poorly absorbed, with an absorption rate of about 4%.[4]

Magnesium oxide requires hydrochloric acid (HCl) for absorption. Magnesium citrate, which is often used as a laxative, is another popular form. It has a better absorption rate than oxide, at about 8%, but can cause severe diarrhea. Chelated forms of magnesium are often better absorbed. The rate of absorption of chelated magnesium sources is roughly between 23% and 25%. These include magnesium glycinate and magnesium malate, as well as other forms. Dosages should be adjusted based on the symptoms of the patient. If diarrhea and digestive upset occur, reduce the dosage or discontinue.

Additional Testing

complete blood count (CBC); comprehensive metabolic panel (CMP); lactate dehydrogenase (LDH); iron and TIBC; ferritin; comprehensive thyroid profile II; heavy metal testing; comprehensive stool testing

Causes of Low Total Iron-Binding Capacity (TIBC)

See Iron Section.

A low TIBC occurs when there is more than adequate iron in the bloodstream and the transport proteins have a reduced availability to bind additional iron. This can be due to iron excess or a reduced production of transferrin.

Low Estrogen: Estrogen levels increase throughout pregnancy, reaching a peak in the third trimester. These levels can be sixfold higher at peak.[5] The hepatic expression of transferrin is increased by estrogen and corticosteroids. Estrogen has been shown to upregulate transferrin production and downregulate hepcidin production.[6] During pregnancy, estrogen production is the placenta's responsibility. Aromatase enzyme production in the placenta converts fetal DHEA to estrogens for maternal and fetal use. Aromatase, also known as CYP19A1 or estrogen synthase, is the enzyme responsible for the conversion of androgens into estrogen. Aromatase is found in granulosa cells, the brain, adipose tissue, the placenta, blood vessels, skin, and bone. During pregnancy, the production of aromatase by the placenta increases by up to thirteenfold.

Iron Overload/Hemochromatosis: Excess iron in the bloodstream will cause a lower TIBC. In conditions of iron overload, transferrin becomes saturated with excess iron. (See Iron Section.)

Other Possible Causes: low-protein diet, liver disease, inflammation, hemolysis, thalassemia

Treatment Strategies for Low Total Iron-Binding Capacity (TIBC)

See Iron Section.

Diet

Isoflavonoids—like genistein, which is found in soy and other legumes—have been shown to increase the production of aromatase.[7] Vitamin D has been shown to modulate the aromatase enzyme, and deficiencies may affect estrogen production during pregnancy. Transferrin is a protein produced by the liver, and protein intake is crucial to transferrin production. According to the American College of Obstetricians and Gynecologists (ACOG), the recommended dietary allowance (RDA) for protein during pregnancy is between 70 and 100 grams per day for an average-weight woman. If a woman is low in protein, she may need more than 100 grams to correct deficiencies.

To achieve a daily protein intake of 100 grams, incorporating a diverse range of protein-rich foods is essential. Meats such as chicken, turkey, and lean beef along with fish and seafood like salmon and tuna offer substantial protein content. Dairy products such as full-fat Greek yogurt and cottage cheese as well as eggs and various plant-based proteins like lentils, chickpeas, tofu, and quinoa contribute to nutrient-dense protein intake. Additionally, nuts and seeds, such as almonds and chia seeds, offer healthy plant-based protein sources. Integrating a mix of these foods into meals and snacks throughout the day ensures a balanced approach to meeting protein goals.

If needed, protein supplements like whey or plant-based protein powders can be considered. If iron overload is discovered, incorporating high-protein foods that are lower in iron may be required. Opting for lean protein sources such as poultry, fish, and eggs provides a substantial protein boost without the higher iron content found in red meats. Plant-based proteins like tofu, legumes, and certain grains, while rich in protein, tend to have lower iron levels compared to their meat counterparts. Nuts and seeds, particularly almonds and chia seeds, contribute protein without being high in iron.

If you are looking for a resource to help patients reach these protein goals, please visit my website and download my e-book, *Protein Packed Pregnancy.*

Supplements

If vitamin D is deficient, supplementation should be done to help bring levels up. (See Vitamin D, 25-Hydroxy (25-Hydroxycalciferol, 25OH-D) Section.)

Additional Testing

complete blood count (CBC); iron and TIBC; ferritin; comprehensive metabolic panel (CMP); lactate dehydrogenase (LDH); progesterone

References

1. Kim JD, Lim DM, Park KY, Park SE, Rhee EJ, Park CY, Lee WY, Oh KW. Serum Transferrin Predicts New-Onset Type 2 Diabetes in Koreans: A 4-Year Retrospective Longitudinal Study. Endocrinol Metab. 2020;35(3):610–617

2. Parent ME, Zemel MB. Magnesium potentiation of iron-transferrin binding. Life Sci. 1989;44(15):1007–1012. doi:10.1016/0024–3205(89)90551–1

3. Milinković N, Zeković M, Dodevska M, et al. Magnesium supplementation and iron status among female students: The intervention study. J Med Biochem. 2022;41(3):316–326. doi:10.5937/jomb0–33898

4. Firoz M, Graber M. Bioavailability of US commercial magnesium preparations. Magnes Res. 2001;14(4):257–262

5. Soldin OP, Guo T, Weiderpass E, Tractenberg RE, Hilakivi-Clarke L, Soldin SJ. Steroid hormone levels in pregnancy and 1 year postpartum using isotope dilution tandem mass spectrometry. Fertil Steril. 2005;84(3):701–710. doi:10.1016/j.fertnstert.2005.02.045

6. Badenhorst CE, Forsyth AK and Govus AD (2022) A contemporary understanding of iron metabolism in active premenopausal females. Front. Sports Act. Living 4:903937. doi: 10.3389/fspor.2022.903937

7. Ye L, Chan MY, Leung LK. The soy isoflavone genistein induces estrogen synthesis in an extragonadal pathway. Mol Cell Endocrinol. 2009;302(1):73–80. doi:10.1016/j.mce.2009.01.003

Unsaturated Iron-Binding Capacity (UIBC)

UIBC is the measure of transport proteins that are unsaturated. This measure is used in conjunction with total serum iron to calculate the total iron-binding capacity (TIBC). It is found as a part of an iron and TIBC panel.

> TIBC (μg/dL) = UIBC (μg/dL) + Iron (μg/dL)

The body makes transport proteins in response to iron levels. About 30% of transport proteins are used at any given time, and the UIBC measures the unbound transport protein content.

Pregnancy
UIBC changes in conjunction with TIBC.

Postpartum
Same as TIBC.

STANDARD LAB RANGE: 131 – 425 μg/dL

Trimester	Standard Pregnancy Ranges	**Functional Pregnancy Ranges**
Preconception	131 – 425	**131 – 425**
First Trimester	131 – 425	**131 – 425**
Second Trimester	131 – 425	**131 – 425**
Third Trimester	131 – 425	**131 – 425**
Postpartum	131 – 425	**131 – 425**

Causes of Elevated Unsaturated Iron-Binding Capacity (UIBC)

See Total Iron-Binding Capacity (TIBC) Section.

Treatment Strategies for Elevated Unsaturated Iron-Binding Capacity (UIBC)

See Total Iron-Binding Capacity (TIBC) Section.

Causes of Low Unsaturated Iron-Binding Capacity (UIBC)

See Total Iron-Binding Capacity (TIBC) Section.

Treatment Strategies for Low Unsaturated Iron-Binding Capacity (UIBC)

See Total Iron-Binding Capacity (TIBC) Section.

Transferrin Saturation (Iron Saturation)

Transferrin saturation (iron saturation) is a laboratory test that measures the percentage of transferrin that is saturated or filled with iron. This test is part of an iron and TIBC panel and is useful in assessing how effectively the body is utilizing the available iron.

The transferrin saturation is calculated by multiplying serum iron by 100 and dividing the results by the TIBC.

(Serum Iron x 100) / TIBC

If the results are >50%, the transport proteins are saturated with iron, indicating iron overload. If the results are <15%, there is more space on the transferrin than there is iron, so there is low saturation. This indicates a need for more iron.

Pregnancy

Transferrin saturation tends to decrease slightly during pregnancy. Pregnancy leads to an expansion of blood volume to supply the growing placenta and fetus. While the total amount of iron in the body increases, the concentration of iron in the blood (serum iron) may not rise proportionally, leading to a lower transferrin saturation. While the total iron-binding capacity (TIBC) may increase due to the rise in transferrin, the increase in demand for iron may result in a lower transferrin saturation.

Postpartum

In the immediate postpartum period, there is often a transient rise in transferrin saturation as blood volume decreases and concentrates following childbirth. Blood loss during childbirth, individual ferritin levels before giving birth, and the occurrence of postpartum anemia all contribute to the overall iron status. Additionally, dietary choices and nutritional support play a pivotal role in shaping iron levels and transferrin saturation during the postpartum recovery period. For breastfeeding mothers, the demands of lactation further impact iron mobilization and may change the values slightly. However, values should never be outside of reference ranges.

STANDARD LAB RANGE: 15% - 50%

Trimester	Standard Pregnancy Ranges	**Functional Pregnancy Ranges**
Preconception	15-50%	**15 - 45%**
First Trimester	15-50%	**20 - 45%**
Second Trimester	15-50%	**20 - 45%**
Third Trimester	15-50%	**20 - 45%**
Postpartum	15-50%	**15 - 45%**

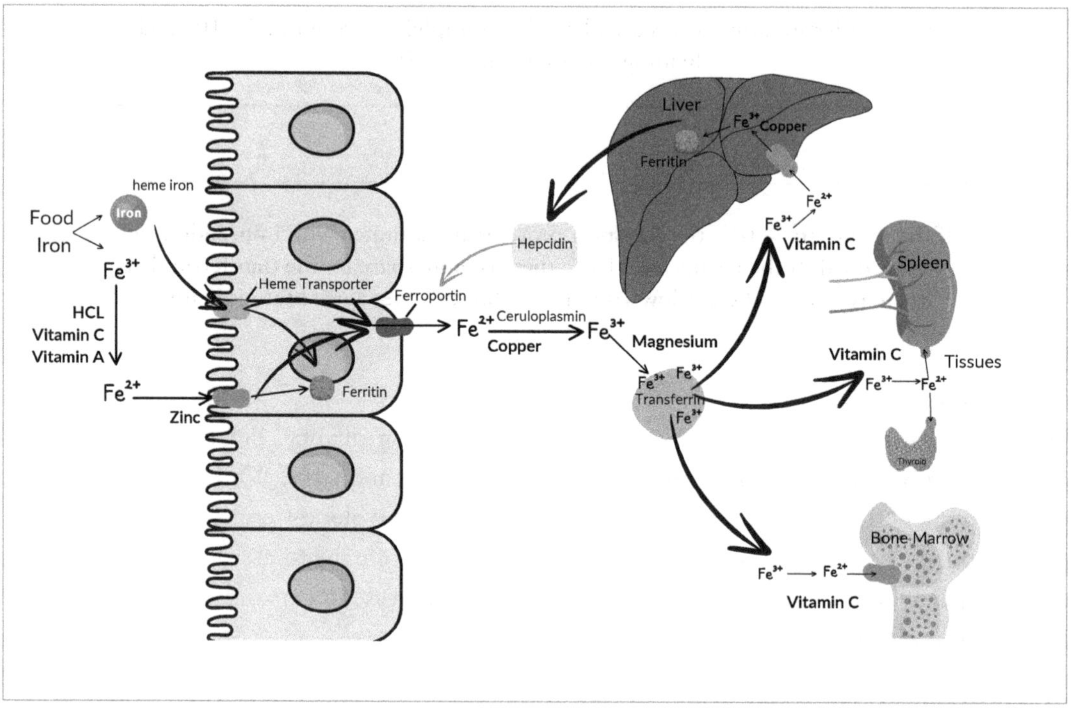

Figure 7: Iron Absorption and Utilization

Causes of Elevated Iron Transferrin Saturation (Iron Saturation)

See Iron Section.

Iron Overload/Hemochromatosis: Elevated transferrin saturation is indicative of an increased percentage of transferrin that is saturated or filled with iron. This condition is often associated with iron overload. Iron overload/hemochromatosis should be suspected if transferrin saturation is >45% in women.[1] There are two main types of hemochromatosis: hereditary and secondary.

Hereditary hemochromatosis is a genetic disorder typically caused by mutations in the HFE gene. Secondary hemochromatosis, on the other hand, is acquired and usually occurs as a result of other medical conditions that necessitate frequent blood transfusions, such as certain types of anemias or thalassemia. Both types of hemochromatosis share the common feature of elevated transferrin saturation. Classic presentation for hemochromatosis is high serum iron (usually >200 µg/dL), low total iron-binding capacity (TIBC), low unsaturated iron-binding capacity (UIBC), and in women transferrin saturation >45% with ferritin > 200 ng/mL. If the liver is involved, liver enzymes and bilirubin will be elevated.

Other Possible Causes: low-protein diet, liver disease, inflammation, hemolysis, thalassemia, genetics

Treatment Strategies for Elevated Iron Transferrin Saturation (Iron Saturation)

See Iron Section.

Additional Testing

complete blood count (CBC); comprehensive metabolic panel (CMP); c-reactive protein (CRP); lactate dehydrogenase (LDH)

Causes of Low Iron Transferrin Saturation (Iron Saturation)

See Iron Section.

A decreased transferrin saturation, particularly when the TIBC is normal or increased, correlates with other indicators of iron deficiency in pregnancy. It can also indicate iron deficiency in patients with a normal ferritin

An average transferrin saturation with values between 19% and 27% has been found in normal pregnancies through the first and second trimesters.[3 4] Organizations such as the University of California San Francisco and Mount Sinai use a transferrin saturation of 20% for the lower range of transferrin saturation in pregnancy.

Iron Deficiency: The most common cause of low transferrin saturation is iron deficiency. When the body lacks sufficient iron, there is a decrease in the amount of iron carried by transferrin, leading to lower saturation levels.

concentration in whom iron deficiency is suspected on a clinical or statistical basis.[2]

Other Possible Causes: chronic inflammation, inflammatory bowel disease (Crohn's disease, celiac disease), hypothyroidism, vitamin C deficiency, copper deficiency, zinc deficiency, vitamin A deficiency, low testosterone, high phytate diet

Treatment Strategies for Low Iron Transferrin Saturation (Iron Saturation)

See Iron Section.

Additional Testing

complete blood count (CBC); comprehensive metabolic panel (CMP); lactate dehydrogenase (LDH); ferritin; c-reactive protein (CRP); oral zinc tolerance test

References

1. Alisa Sokoloff, Scott Brook, Marvin Cooper; Iron Studies in Hemochromatosis During Pregnancy. Blood 2009; 114 (22): 5099. doi.org/10.1182/blood.V114.22.5099.5099

2. Means RT. Iron Deficiency and Iron Deficiency Anemia: Implications and Impact in Pregnancy, Fetal Development, and Early Childhood Parameters. Nutrients. 2020;12(2):447. Published 2020 Feb 11. doi:10.3390/nu12020447

3. Yang Y, Wang R, Jiang H, Hu M, Tang A, Xiang Z. Changes of iron metabolism during pregnancy and the establishment of reference intervals for pregnant Chinese women. Ann Clin Biochem. 2019;56(5):556–563. doi:10.1177/0004563219835853

4. Singhal U, Mohsin S, Saini K, Singhal KC. Serum level of iron and transferrin in normal and anaemic pregnant women. Indian J Physiol Pharmacol. 1993;37(1):71 74

Ferritin

The ferritin blood test measures the level of ferritin in the blood. It can be found in certain iron panels or as a separate analyte.

Ferritin is one of the stored forms of iron. It is produced and used by almost all living organisms, including algae. In our bodies, it helps to keep iron in a safe and nontoxic form until it is needed. Small amounts of ferritin are released into circulation to help carry iron safely through the bloodstream. It is a protector of iron deficiency and iron excess. Serum ferritin is a secondary measure of ferritin stores within the tissues. It is generally accepted that serum ferritin correlates with tissue ferritin stores. In certain cases, this may not be accurate, such as with cell damage, acute illness, or chronic inflammatory disease.

Ferritin is a complex protein. Twenty-four ferritin subunits come together to form an apoferritin, a ferritin without iron attached. Each apoferritin can bind up to 4,500 iron atoms. Fe^{2+} is oxidized to Fe^{3+} before binding and storage, and ferritin also works to reduce Fe^{3+} to Fe^{2+} before release.

The synthesis of ferritin is controlled by the levels of iron in the bloodstream, as well as oxidative stress and inflammatory chemicals. Ferritin synthesis and iron storage begin in the enterocytes of the gut during iron absorption and are stimulated by either inflammation or hypoxia.

Pregnancy

During the first trimester, with the cessation of the menstrual cycle and the decrease in iron absorption, ferritin levels may increase slightly, remain the same, or decrease slightly. From 12 weeks, ferritin levels begin to consistently decrease, reaching the lowest point between 35 and 38 weeks. They then increase in the last month of pregnancy before delivery. This is primarily due to the changes in iron absorption and utilization throughout pregnancy. (See Iron Section.)

Postpartum

A drop in ferritin is normal after delivery, as the iron stores are used to rebuild red blood cells after blood loss. Ferritin levels should begin to increase by six weeks postpartum.

> This is a value for which you will see a lot of variation on what constitutes "normal" among sources and research studies.

STANDARD LAB RANGE: 15 – 150 ng/mL

Trimester	Standard Pregnancy Ranges	**Functional Pregnancy Ranges**
Preconception	15–150	**30 – 150**
First Trimester	6–130	**30 – 80**
Second Trimester	2–130	**30 – 80**
Third Trimester	0–166	**15 – 80**
Postpartum	Not Established	**15 – 80**

Causes of Elevated Ferritin

See Iron Section.

Chronic alcohol consumption, metabolic syndrome, obesity, diabetes, malignancy, infection, and inflammatory conditions explain 90% of the causes of elevated serum ferritin levels inside and outside of pregnancy. Ferritin level testing in early pregnancy can set a baseline of ferritin levels throughout pregnancy. In other cases, iron overload/hemochromatosis may be a cause.

Elevated serum ferritin concentrations in early gestation are associated with an increased risk of gestational diabetes.[1] There is an observed 1.5-fold increased risk of gestational diabetes in women who have serum ferritin

Iron Overload/Hemochromatosis: Hemochromatosis and iron overload are often silent, with no symptomology. Excess iron and ferritin can cause tissue damage, bacterial overgrowth, arthritis, and other complications. If hemochromatosis is identified with severely elevated ferritin, a referral to a hematologist may be warranted. (See Iron Section.)

Infection: During infections, a release of ferritin is thought to be a defense mechanism that deprives bacterial growth of iron and protects immune cell function.[4] When the body detects the presence of pathogens such as bacteria or viruses, immune cells release inflammatory cytokines that stimulate the liver to produce more ferritin. This elevated ferritin serves a dual purpose: it helps sequester iron, limiting its availability to pathogens, and it acts as an acute-phase reactant, contributing to the overall inflammatory response. While this elevation is a natural and protective response to infection, persistently high ferritin levels may be indicative of chronic inflammation or underlying health conditions, requiring further investigation.

Inflammation/Cellular Damage: Elevated ferritin is also a biomarker of tissue damage and chronic inflammation. Ferritin can be elevated as destroyed cells release their ferritin stores into circulation.[5] Additionally, in conditions characterized by persistent inflammation—such as autoimmune disorders, chronic infections, or certain inflammatory diseases—inflammatory cytokines prompt the liver to release increased amounts of ferritin. The purpose of elevated ferritin

levels >45 ng/mL in the first trimester.[2] Ferritin levels >80 ng/mL increase the risk of gestational diabetes 2.4-fold.

Several studies have linked elevated first-trimester ferritin with higher risks of hypertension and preeclampsia in pregnancy, with varying cutoff between 80 and 130 ng/mL. Other studies have also shown a connection to higher ferritin levels at 30 weeks as a predictive marker of preterm birth and low fetal birth weight.[3]

Currently, there is no consensus on what the upper end of the range for the first trimester should be. Studies do seem to indicate that lower serum ferritin levels in pregnancy are more protective than elevated levels.

in chronic inflammation is to sequester iron, thereby limiting its availability in the bloodstream. Ferritin levels can serve as an important biomarker in assessing the severity and persistence of chronic inflammatory conditions. In cases of chronic inflammation, serum iron levels and saturation may be decreased with elevated ferritin.

Thalassemia/Sickle Cell Anemia: In these conditions, there is a lower production of RBCs but an elevation of stored iron because of issues in utilization. This causes a "backing up" of iron and increased storage as ferritin. In these anemia cases, as well, we can see a shortened red blood cell lifespan and increased hemolysis, causing a release of stored ferritin into the bloodstream.

Vitamin A Deficiency: Vitamin A deficiency anemia is associated with a reduction in serum iron, low TIBC, low transferrin saturation, and increased serum ferritin. This is due to a lower mobilization of iron stores, with increased deposition of iron in the liver and spleen.[6]

Excess Physical Activity: Intense physical activities, especially when performed excessively, may contribute to oxidative stress and inflammation in the body, potentially impacting iron metabolism. Generally, this will cause decreased serum iron levels with increased ferritin.

Other Possible Causes: rheumatoid arthritis (particularly those with a preexisting diagnosis of juvenile RA), Graves' disease, autoimmune diseases, copper deficiency, vitamin B6 (pyridoxine) deficiency, sleep apnea, insulin resistance, certain cancers

Treatment Strategies for Elevated Ferritin

See Iron Section.

Diet

In all cases of elevated ferritin, focus on increasing foods that are higher in antioxidants. If iron levels are also elevated, reduce consumption of iron-rich foods, especially heme iron, which is found in red meat. Limiting intake of iron-fortified foods can also be beneficial. If iron levels are low, focus on reducing inflammation. Incorporating high-flavonoid foods into the diet may offer a promising approach for individuals dealing with elevated ferritin levels. Flavonoids, a diverse group of plant compounds with antioxidant and anti-inflammatory properties, have been studied for their potential to modulate iron metabolism and mitigate oxidative stress.

Foods rich in flavonoids include berries (such as blueberries, strawberries, and raspberries), citrus fruits, apples, onions, tea, dark chocolate, and leafy greens. These flavonoid-rich foods may reduce inflammation and oxidative stress, which are often associated with elevated ferritin levels. Including a variety of colorful fruits and vegetables in the daily diet not only ensures a diverse flavonoid intake but also provides essential vitamins and minerals that support overall health.

Lifestyle

Excessive physical exercise has been shown to decrease serum iron levels and increase serum ferritin levels. Reducing high-intensity workouts—such as CrossFit, running, and high-intensity interval training—and opting for more moderate exercises—such as brisk walking, hiking, or yoga—provides an opportunity for physical activity that is gentler on the body while still promoting overall well-being. These activities not only help maintain cardiovascular health and muscle flexibility but may also contribute to stress reduction, an essential factor in mitigating inflammation. Additionally, by incorporating a variety of exercises, individuals can achieve a balanced and sustainable fitness routine, potentially avoiding the negative impact of excessive high-intensity workouts on iron levels.

Supplements

If serum iron levels are also elevated, reduce/remove vitamin C supplements. Avoid NAC supplements. In some animal model studies, NAC supplementation was shown to cause harm in those with iron overload. Studies specifically on iron overload associated with beta-thalassemia found that 600 mg/day of alpha-lipoic acid decreased serum ferritin levels.[7] Green tea extract is also beneficial in those with iron overload and utilization issues associated with beta-thalassemia. Green tea extract, which is rich in epigallocatechin-3-gallate (EGCG), is known to possess radical scavenging and iron-chelating activities.[8] Dosages of EGCG in studies vary but average to approximately 50 mg/kg. In cases of iron overload, copper demand is increased. Increasing copper intake via supplementation has been shown to reduce the negative effects of elevated iron levels. Before and during supplementation, copper levels should be tested and monitored.[9]

Additional Testing

complete blood count (CBC); comprehensive metabolic panel (CMP); iron and TIBC; c-reactive protein (CRP); glycated hemoglobin (hemoglobin A1c/HbA1c); antinuclear antibodies (ANA); comprehensive thyroid profile II; thyroid peroxidase antibodies (TPOAb); thyroglobulin antibody (TgAb); thyrotropin-receptor antibody; lactate dehydrogenase (LDH); gamma-glutamyl transpeptidase (GGT)

Causes of Low Ferritin

See Iron Section.

A 2014 study from *The New England Journal of Medicine* stated that ferritin levels <30 ng/mL were indicative of iron deficiency, and levels <10 ng/mL indicated iron-deficiency anemia.[10] After pregnancy and childbirth, it may take a full 12 weeks to recover ferritin stores.

Ferritin levels <27.23 ng/mL are a predictive biomarker of pregnancy anemia, regardless of CBC indices in the first trimester.[11]

At the lowest point in pregnancy (between 35 and 38 weeks gestation), ferritin levels can be as low as between 15 and 20 ng/mL and be a normal presentation.[12]

Ferritin <15 ng/mL in the early third trimester is associated with small-for-gestational-age growth.[13]

Ferritin <8 ng/mL 48 hours after delivery increases the risk of postpartum depression.[14]

Hypothyroidism: Thyroid hormones are required for the utilization of iron in the liver. Hypothyroidism can cause low ferritin, and hyperthyroidism can cause increased ferritin. In pregnancy, there is a direct correlation between elevated first-trimester TSH and low first-trimester ferritin.[15] Several studies have pointed to hypothyroidism as a primary cause of iron-deficiency anemia in pregnancy that is not corrected with iron supplementation. Thyroid hormones play a direct role in the genetic expression of ferritin. Secondary to low ferritin levels, hypothyroidism causes hypochlorhydria and decreases dietary iron absorption, which leads to iron deficiency. (See Thyroid-Stimulating Hormone (TSH) Section.)

Low Progesterone: Ferritin heavy chain (FHC) is a ferroxidase enzyme produced in the liver and placenta that synthesizes a unit of ferritin. Ferritin is composed of 24 heavy and light subunits. Increases of FHC production in the maternal body rise in conjunction with rising surges of progesterone.[16] (See Progesterone Section.)

Vitamin D Deficiency: Vitamin D suppresses hepcidin production. When vitamin D is low, there is more hepcidin and, thus, a higher degradation of ferroportin, causing a decrease in iron absorption and a decrease in ferritin storage.[17]

Other Possible Causes: iron deficiency, protein-deficient diets, lead exposure, polycythemia, inflammatory bowel disease (celiac disease, Crohn's), zinc deficiency

Treatment Strategies for Low Ferritin

See Iron Section.

Diet

Increase foods that provide a complex of nutrients needed for ferritin production, such as organ meats, legumes (soaked properly), eggs, cooked green leafy veggies, seafood, nuts, and seeds. Studies show that increasing millet, teff, and lentils in the diet can improve ferritin levels over the course of six weeks. Millet porridge or lentil dal may be good options for vegan patients with low ferritin.[18]

Supplements

Vitamin D supplementation may be beneficial if vitamin D deficiency is identified. (See Vitamin D, 25-Hydroxy (25-Hydroxycalciferol, 25OH-D) Section.) If progesterone deficiency is present, progesterone supplementation may also be helpful. (See Progesterone Section.) If hypothyroidism is present, supporting thyroid function may also be beneficial. (See Thyroid-Stimulating Hormone (TSH) Section.) If iron deficiency is present, iron supplementation may be beneficial. However, if iron supplementation at a moderate dosage every other day does not increase both serum iron levels and ferritin, additional supplementation is *not* recommended. Unabsorbed iron can cause enterocyte cytotoxicity and destroy the gut microbiome.[19] This can, in turn, allow for the overgrowth of pathogenic bacteria, increasing the risk of infection.

In cases where moderate iron supplementation does not increase serum iron or ferritin levels, gut support is recommended. This can include pre- and probiotic supplements. L-glutamine is an amino acid supplement commonly used for gut pathologies. It can help balance the microbiome and increase the integrity of the gut lining. Studies have not shown an increase in iron absorption when taken with L-glutamine. It is a common supplement among those with IBD conditions. Currently, glutamine has been assigned to pregnancy category C by the Food and Drug Administration (FDA). More recent studies have found some protective properties to the use of L-glutamine in pregnancy. Currently, there is not enough evidence to say for sure that L-glutamine supplementation is safe, and it should only be recommended when the benefits outweigh any potential risks.

Additional Testing

complete blood count (CBC); iron and TIBC; comprehensive metabolic panel (CMP); progesterone; comprehensive thyroid profile II; thyroid peroxidase antibodies (TPOAb); thyroglobulin antibody (TgAb); vitamin D, 25-hydroxy (25-hydroxycalciferol, 25OH-D); comprehensive stool testing; oral zinc tolerance test

References

1. Durrani L, Ejaz S, Tavares LB, et al. Correlation Between High Serum Ferritin Level and Gestational Diabetes: A Systematic Review. Cureus. 2021;13(10):e18990. Published 2021 Oct 23. doi:10.7759/cureus.18990

2. Soheilykhah S, Mojibian M, Jannati Moghadam M. Serum ferritin concentration in early pregnancy and risk of subsequent development of gestational diabetes: A prospective study. Int J Reprod Biomed. 2017;15(3):155–160.

3. Lanyao Yang, Lanlan Wu, Yao Liu, Hengying Chen, Yuanhuan Wei, Ruifang Sun, Siwen Shen, Bowen Zhan, Jianjun Yang, Guifang Deng. (2022). Diabetes, Metabolic Syndrome and Obesity: Targets and Therapy 15, pages 2867–2876.

4. Kernan KF, Carcillo JA. Hyperferritinemia and inflammation. Int Immunol. 2017;29(9):401–409. doi:10.1093/intimm/dxx031

5. Douglas B Kell, Etheresia Pretorius, Serum ferritin is an important inflammatory disease marker, as it is mainly a leakage product from damaged cells, Metallomics, Volume 6, Issue 4, April 2014, Pages 748–773, doi.org/10.1039/c3mt00347g

6. Michelazzo FB, Oliveira JM, Stefanello J, Luzia LA, Rondó PH. The influence of vitamin A supplementation on iron status. Nutrients. 2013 Nov 7;5(11):4399–413. doi: 10.3390/nu5114399. PMID: 24212089; PMCID: PMC3847738

7. Sharifi-Zahabi E, Abdollahzad H, Mostafa Nachvak S, et al. Effects of alpha-lipoic acid on iron overload, lipid profile and oxidative stress indices in β-thalassemia major patients: A cross-over randomised controlled clinical trial. Int J Clin Pract. 2021;75(6):e14062. doi:10.1111/ijcp.14062

8. Settakorn K, Kongkarnka S, Chompupoung A, et al. Effects of green tea extract treatment on erythropoiesis and iron parameters in iron-overloaded β-thalassemic mice. Front Physiol. 2022;13:1053060. Published 2022 Dec 23. doi:10.3389/fphys.2022.1053060

9. Wang T, Xiang P, Ha JH, et al. Copper supplementation reverses dietary iron overload-induced pathologies in mice. J Nutr Biochem. 2018;59:56–63. doi:10.1016/j.jnutbio.2018.05.006

10. Camaschella C, Longo D. Iron-Deficiency Anemia. New England Journal of Medicine. 2015;372(19):1832–1843. doi:10.1056/NEJMra1401038.

11. Raden Tina, Dewi Judistiani, Tita Husnitawati Madjid, Budi Handono, Hadyana Sukandar, Setyorini Irianti, Lani Gumilang, Sefita Aryuti Nirmala, Budi Setiabudiawan, "First-Trimester Ferritin Is Superior over Soluble Transferrin Receptor and Hepcidin in Predicting Anemia in the Third Trimester: Result from a Cohort Study in Indonesia", Anemia, vol. 2020, Article ID 8880045, 6 pages, 2020. doi.org/10.1155/2020/8880045

12. Mégier C, Peoc'h K, Puy V, Cordier AG. Iron Metabolism in Normal and Pathological Pregnancies and Fetal Consequences. Metabolites. 2022;12(2):129. Published 2022 Jan 29. doi:10.3390/metabo12020129

13. Col Madendag I, Eraslan Sahin M, Madendag Y, et al. The Effect of Iron-Deficiency Anemia Early in the Third Trimester on Small for Gestational Age and Birth Weight: A Retrospective Cohort Study on Iron-Deficiency Anemia and Fetal Weight. Biomed Res Int. 2019;2019:7613868. Published 2019 Nov 22. doi:10.1155/2019/7613868

14. Wassef A, Nguyen QD, St-André M. Anaemia and depletion of iron stores as risk factors for postpartum depression: a literature review. J Psychosom Obstet Gynaecol. 2019;40(1):19–28. doi:10.1080/0167482X.2018.1427725

15. R V, Dhiman P, Kollipaka R, P S, V H. Association of Hypothyroidism With Low Serum Ferritin Levels and Iron-Deficiency Anemia During the First Trimester of Pregnancy. Cureus. 2022;14(8):e28307. Published 2022 Aug 23. doi:10.7759/cureus.28307

16. L J Zhu and others, Ferritin heavy chain is a progesterone-inducible marker in the uterus during pregnancy, Endocrinology, Volume 136, Issue 9, 1 September 1995, Pages 4106–4115, doi.org/10.1210/endo.136.9.7649119

17. Mogire RM, Muriuki JM, Morovat A, Mentzer AJ, Webb EL, Kimita W, Ndungu FM, Macharia AW, Cutland CL, Sirima SB, Diarra A, Tiono AB, Lule SA, Madhi SA, Prentice AM, Bejon P, Pettifor JM, Elliott AM, Adeyemo A, Williams TN, Atkinson SH. Vitamin D Deficiency and Its Association with Iron Deficiency in African Children. Nutrients. 2022 Mar 25;14(7):1372. doi: 10.3390/nu14071372. PMID: 35405984; PMCID: PMC9002534

18. Anitha S, Kane-Potaka J, Botha R, et al. Millets Can Have a Major Impact on Improving Iron Status, Hemoglobin Level, and in Reducing Iron-Deficiency Anemia: A Systematic Review and Meta-Analysis. Front Nutr. 2021;8:725529. Published 2021 Oct 14. doi:10.3389/fnut.2021.725529

19. Rusu IG, Suharoschi R, Vodnar DC, et al. Iron Supplementation Influence on the Gut Microbiota and Probiotic Intake Effect in Iron Deficiency: A Literature-Based Review. Nutrients. 2020;12(7):1993. Published 2020 Jul 4. doi:10.3390/nu12071993

Copper, Total

The copper, total test measures the total amount of copper present in a blood sample from all sources, free and bound. It is a single indice.

Free copper levels are calculated like this:

Total Serum Copper (µg/dL) - [3.15 × Ceruloplasmin (mg/dL)]

Copper is a dietary mineral and element on the periodic table that is essential as a cofactor for cuproenzymes that catalyze oxidation reactions. Approximately 95% of total serum copper is found as ceruloplasmin. Only small amounts of copper are stored in the body, with the average person having a storage of between 50 and 120 mg, mostly in the skeleton and muscles.

Copper (II), cupric, is the stable form of copper. This form must be converted to copper (I), cuprous, before it can be absorbed through the gut. Much of the reduction and absorption of copper is regulated by amino acids.[1] Dietary copper is absorbed at approximately 50% to 75%. The body will absorb between 1 and 2 mg/day of copper. CTR1 and DMT1 uptake copper into the enterocytes. About 80% of copper transport is via CRT1. Cu (I) is converted to Cu (II) to enter the bloodstream.

In the cells, the antioxidant I copper chaperone (ATOX1) helps maintain copper homeostasis by binding and transporting copper to ATPase proteins. ATPases are plasma membrane transporters that transport Cu (II) into the bloodstream. Once in the bloodstream, copper is bound to albumin and/or transcuprein to be transported to the liver for processing or to the kidneys for excretion. Only 2% of dietary copper is excreted through the kidneys; the majority is excreted through bile. Once in the liver, it is converted into enzymes such as superoxide dismutase and ceruloplasmin. The uptake, homeostasis, and export of copper in other cells is regulated by CRT1, ATOX1, and ATPases, including placental cells.

Copper-dependent enzyme cytochrome c oxidase (CCO) plays a role in energy production. Cuproenzyme lysyl oxidase (LOX) is needed for the cross-linking of collagen and elastin fiber that helps form connective tissue, including the cross-linking needed to help maintain cervical structure during pregnancy. Multiple copper oxidases aid in iron homeostasis. Other copper enzymes are needed for neurotransmitter synthesis and the health of myelin. Melanin biosynthesis also requires copper. Depigmentation is a noted side effect of severe copper deficiency. Superoxide dismutase functions as an antioxidant that helps to reduce reactive oxygen species. Copper/zinc superoxide dismutase (SOD1) is the most expressed SOD form in the body. Copper regulates post-translational gene expression. Copper also regulates white blood cell formation by affecting colony-stimulating factors.

Currently, there is no specific biomarker for copper deficiency. Blood levels of copper in conjunction with ceruloplasmin levels are reduced only in severe copper-deficiency scenarios.[2] Both of these indices are affected by pregnancy and may be less useful in detecting deficiencies.

Pregnancy

Serum copper levels double preconception levels by full term, with significant increases seen at approximately 22, 27, and 35 weeks of gestation. Levels decrease during the first stage of labor.

Postpartum

Serum copper levels drop significantly in the first week postpartum, averaging 25% of peak pregnancy levels. The decrease in copper levels continues to reach pre-pregnancy levels by six weeks postpartum.

STANDARD LAB RANGE: 63 – 121 μg/dL

Trimester	Standard Pregnancy Ranges	**Functional Pregnancy Ranges**
Preconception	63 – 121	**90 – 140**
First Trimester	112 – 199	**150 – 305**
Second Trimester	165 – 221	**190 – 330**
Third Trimester	130 – 240	**222 – 380**
Postpartum	63 – 121	**90 – 140**

Causes of Elevated Copper, Total

Excess copper reacts with hydrogen peroxide to create reactive oxygen species, which damages tissues.

Infection and/or Inflammation: In cases of acute infection or inflammation, both serum copper and ceruloplasmin activity increases. These changes in copper metabolism are the result of an increase in interleukin-1 (IL-1). Copper upregulation is needed to help increase white blood cell production to fight infections and reduce inflammation.[3]

Hemolysis: The destruction of cells can cause a release of copper from hemoglobin into the bloodstream.

Long-Term Oral Contraceptive Use: Oral contraceptives have been well documented to cause an increase in serum copper levels. Use prior to pregnancy may be a cause of abnormally elevated copper levels in early pregnancy. These elevated copper levels can also cause zinc deficiencies.

Other Possible Causes: excess copper supplementation, water contamination, genetics (Wilson disease), cancer

Treatment Strategies for Elevated Copper, Total

Diet

Limiting copper-rich foods may not be necessary in these cases, as the issue is less one of overabsorption and more one of utilization/excretion or excess supplementation.

Increasing vitamin C-rich foods may be beneficial. The copper content of food varies greatly based on the copper content of the soil, agricultural practices, and food processing. Generally, a low copper diet means restricting organ meats, shellfish, legumes, grains, and chocolate. Checking the water supply for copper levels is also important, especially if they are using well water.

Supplements

High-dose supplementation of vitamin C (>10 mg/kg) and copper (>1 mg/kg) have been shown to increase oxidative stress reactions in the body, in addition to causing kidney inflammation and damage. Vitamin C works as a copper-chelating agent and increases urinary excretion of copper by affecting the proximal tubules. Combined supplementations should be avoided.[4] Zinc supplementation of 50 mg/day may help reduce copper absorption in cases of Wilson disease. For those who are following a low copper diet due to Wilson disease or excess copper, it is important that they supplement with vitamin B6 (pyridoxine).

Additional Testing
complete blood count (CBC); comprehensive metabolic panel (CMP); ceruloplasmin; water testing

Causes of Low Copper, Total

In pregnancies that present with recurrent miscarriage, preterm labor, spontaneous pregnancy loss, and premature rupture of membranes, copper levels are measurably lower than those of normal pregnancies.[5] Serum copper levels <108 in the first trimester, <130 in the second trimester, and <171 in the third trimester are associated with negative pregnancy outcomes.[6]

Adrenal Hyperfunction: There is evidence that elevated cortisol causes a decrease in serum copper levels. Serum copper levels are reduced in response to adrenocorticotropic hormone (ACTH) and glucocorticoids. Both serum copper and ceruloplasmin are decreased.

Iron Overload/Hemochromatosis: Lower serum copper levels are found in those with hemochromatosis and in cases of iron overload. The DMT1 transporter is responsible for the absorption of iron as well as copper. High intake of iron, as in high-dose supplementation, may impair copper absorption. Additionally, the internal regulation of high iron levels requires higher copper and ceruloplasmin levels. Some studies have shown an increase in urinary excretion of copper in cases of iron overload.[7]

Zinc Overload: Zinc and copper should have a 1:1 ratio in the body, except during pregnancy, when copper levels increase and zinc levels decrease. It is common to see lower copper levels in those taking oral zinc supplements, particularly high-dose supplements. This may be the most commonly seen cause of low copper levels during pregnancy. Zinc blocks copper absorption and may also increase copper excretion through the urine. In this case, you may also see neutropenia and sideroblastic anemia presentations.[8] This has become more common with patients taking high-dose zinc supplements for the prevention or treatment of viral infections.[9]

Hypothyroidism: Some studies have shown an association between low copper levels and hypothyroidism. Hypothyroidism is characterized by low serum copper and ceruloplasmin.[10] Thyroid hormones help with the genetic expression of ATP7A and ATP7B.

Other Possible Causes: protein-deficient diets, low copper diets, excess vitamin C supplementation, inflammatory bowel diseases (celiac disease, Crohn's), gastric surgery, genetics

Treatment Strategies for Low Copper, Total

Diet

Incorporate foods that are high in copper such as organ meats, shellfish, nuts and seeds, whole grains, legumes, darky leafy greens, cocoa, and certain fruits like avocados. The current RDA for copper in pregnancy is around 1,000 μg/day and 1,300 μg/day while breastfeeding. The upper limit is currently 10,000 μg/day. Factors such as maternal age, genetics, and medications may affect the amount needed to maintain healthy levels. Increasing vitamin C-rich foods may be beneficial. The copper content of food varies greatly based on the copper content of the soil, agricultural practices, and food processing. Generally a low copper diet means restricting organ meats, shellfish, legumes, grains, and chocolate. Checking the water supply for copper levels is also important, especially if they are using well water.

Supplements

Usually, adequate levels can be maintained with a diet alone. Copper is readily available in food sources. Supplementation may be the best option in some cases. Cupric oxide, copper gluconate, copper sulfate, and copper amino acid chelates are commonly found in supplements. Cupric oxide has a low absorption rate and high excretion rate and is not considered a good supplement form. It is low-cost and often found in cheaper supplements.[11] High-dose supplementation of 10 mg/day of cupric gluconate for 12 weeks was not shown to cause toxicity.[12] As of 2022, the research on absorption of copper supplements is limited, and bioavailability and toxicity studies have not been completed.[13]

Additional Testing

complete blood count (CBC); comprehensive metabolic panel (CMP); ceruloplasmin; ferritin; iron and TIBC; comprehensive thyroid profile II

References

1. Kar S, Sen S, Maji S, et al. Copper(II) import and reduction are dependent on His-Met clusters in the extracellular amino terminus of human copper transporter-1. J Biol Chem. 2022;298(3):101631. doi:10.1016/j.jbc.2022.101631

2. Collins JF. Copper. In: Ross AC, Caballero B, Cousins RJ, Tucker KL, Ziegler TR, eds. Modern Nutrition in Health and Disease. 11th ed. Philadelphia: Wolter Kluwer; Lippincott Williams & Wilkins; 2014:206–216

3. Liu Y, Zhu J, Xu L, Wang B, Lin W, Luo Y. Copper regulation of immune response and potential implications for treating orthopedic disorders. Front Mol Biosci. 2022;9:1065265. Published 2022 Dec 5. doi:10.3389/fmolb.2022.1065265

4. Jiang R, Sui Y, Hong J, et al. The Combined Administration of Vitamin C and Copper Induces a Systemic Oxidative Stress and Kidney Injury. Biomolecules. 2023;13(1):143. Published 2023 Jan 10. doi:10.3390/biom13010143

5. Grzeszczak K, Kwiatkowski S, Kosik-Bogacka D. The Role of Fe, Zn, and Cu in Pregnancy. Biomolecules. 2020;10(8):1176. Published 2020 Aug 12. doi:10.3390/biom10081176

6. Vukelić J, Kapamadzija A, Petrović D, et al. Variations of serum copper values in pregnancy. Srp Arh Celok Lek. 2012;140(1–2):42–46

7. Klevay LM. Iron overload can induce mild copper deficiency. J Trace Elem Med Biol. 2001;14(4):237–240. doi:10.1016/S0946–672X(01)80009–2

8. Wahab A, Mushtaq K, Borak SG, Bellam N. Zinc-induced copper deficiency, sideroblastic anemia, and neutropenia: A perplexing facet of zinc excess. Clin Case Rep. 2020;8(9):1666–1671. Published 2020 May 28. doi:10.1002/ccr3.2987

9. Francis Z, Book G, Litvin C, Kalivas B. The COVID-19 Pandemic and Zinc-Induced Copper Deficiency: An Important Link. Am J Med. 2022;135(8):e290-e291. doi:10.1016/j.amjmed.2022.03.008

10. Valenzise M, Sferlassas C, Porcaro F, Messina MF, Wasniewska M, Cinguegrani M, De Luca M. Hypoceruloplasminemia as a Marker of Severe Hypothyroidism. 54th Annual Meeting of the European Society for Paediatric Endocrinology (ESPE). Barcelona, Spain. Abstracts. Horm Res Paediatr. September 2015; 84 (Suppl. 1): 302. doi.org/10.1159/000437032

11. National Center for Biotechnology Information. PubChem Compound Summary for CID 164827, Cupric Oxide. pubchem.ncbi.nlm.nih.gov/compound/Cupric-Oxide. Accessed Mar 25, 2024

12. Pratt WB, Omdahl JL, Sorenson JR. Lack of effects of copper gluconate supplementation. Am J Clin Nutr. 1985;42(4):681–682

13. Burkhead JL, Collins JF. Nutrition Information Brief-Copper. Adv Nutr. 2022;13(2):681–683. doi:10.1093/advances/nmab157

Ceruloplasmin

The ceruloplasmin test measures the total amount of ceruloplasmin in the bloodstream. It is a separate indice.

Ceruloplasmin is a ferroxidase that is responsible for 95% of copper transport in the bloodstream. It is synthesized in the liver, monocytes, and placental cells. The ceruloplasmin gene (CP) is responsible for the instructions for synthesizing ceruloplasmin. The initial unbound form is called apoceruloplasmin. Apoceruloplasmin undergoes post-translational modification and folding to be able to bind to and store copper. Once mature, ceruloplasmin can bind to six copper molecules. Ceruloplasmin has a half-life of about five or six days.

Ceruloplasmin also has ferroxidase actions, which facilitate the conversion of ferrous iron (Fe^{2+}) to ferric iron (Fe^{3+}). Ferric iron can then be bound to transferrin for transport. Ceruloplasmin also has antioxidant properties, helping to protect the cells from oxidative stress.

Another isoform of ceruloplasmin, zyklopen, has been discovered in placental cells. Its actions are unclear but do not seem to be essential for the placental transfer of iron.[1]

Pregnancy

During pregnancy, there is an increase in ceruloplasmin levels that mimics the increase and changes seen in conjunction with serum copper levels. Levels begin to rise as early as four weeks of gestation.[2]

Postpartum

Ceruloplasmin levels mimic serum copper levels in the postpartum period, decreasing significantly from pregnancy ranges until six weeks postpartum.

> There is limited research or data on the reference ranges for ceruloplasmin in pregnancy. Until there is further research, the ranges used are those recommended by the American College of Obstetricians and Gynecologists (ACOG).

STANDARD LAB RANGE: 19 – 39 mg/dL

Trimester	Standard Pregnancy Ranges	**Functional Pregnancy Ranges**
Preconception	19 – 39	**19 – 39**
First Trimester	30 – 49	**30 – 49**
Second Trimester	40 – 53	**40 – 53**
Third Trimester	43 – 78	**43 – 78**
Postpartum	19 – 39	**19 – 39**

Causes of Elevated Ceruloplasmin

See Copper, Total Section.

Elevated ceruloplasmin levels are seen in cases of preeclampsia and other inflammatory conditions in pregnancy. This may be due to the placental expression of ceruloplasmin, as well as inflammation and cell damage.[3 4]

Inflammation and/or Infection: Ceruloplasmin is an acute-phase reactant due to its elevated expression during times of inflammation, infection, or trauma. In cases of inflammation, both serum copper and ceruloplasmin are elevated.

Iron-Deficiency Anemia: In cases of iron-deficiency anemia, ceruloplasmin levels may increase. Ceruloplasmin has also been shown to affect iron absorption in the gut. The increase in ceruloplasmin may be a mechanism in which the body attempts to increase iron absorption.[5]

Other Possible Causes: autoimmune disease, rheumatoid arthritis, liver disease, genetics, cancer

Treatment Strategies for Elevated Ceruloplasmin

See Copper, Total Section.

Causes of Low Ceruloplasmin

See Copper, Total Section.

Wilson Disease: Wilson disease is a genetic condition associated with low serum ceruloplasmin and an accumulation of copper in the tissues. In Wilson disease, there is a genetic decrease in the production of ATP7B. Copper cannot be processed into ceruloplasmin or excreted through the bile. This buildup of copper in the cells causes an increase in oxidative stress. This then causes free copper to spill back into the bloodstream, causing higher serum copper levels with lower serum ceruloplasmin. The brain is sensitive to the accumulation of copper, and neurological symptoms usually present with copper overload.

Another place where copper deposits are often seen in cases of excess is the Descemet's membrane of the cornea. This causes Kayser-Fleischer rings, dark circles around the cornea. Wilson disease will present with high serum copper, high urine copper, low serum ceruloplasmin, and elevated liver enzymes. Other conditions that can be seen are an enlarged liver and spleen, damage to the proximal tubules of the kidneys and associated biomarkers, and hemolytic anemia.

Copper Deficiency: Serum copper and ceruloplasmin levels will be decreased in cases of moderate to severe copper deficiency only. This may not allow you to detect mild copper deficiencies. In mild deficiency patterns, there can be a decrease in cuproenzyme production and function, while maintaining normal serum copper and ceruloplasmin levels.[6] Cuproenzymes include superoxide dismutase, dopamine β-hydroxylase, tyrosinase, lysyl oxidase, and nitrite reductase. It is estimated that there are around 30 different coenzymes in the body.

Other Possible Causes: adrenal hyperfunction, hypothyroidism, iron overload/hemochromatosis, zinc overload, excess copper intake, water contamination, inflammatory bowel disease (celiac, Crohn's), liver damage, gastric surgery, excess vitamin C intake, vitamin B6 (pyridoxine) deficiency, genetics

Treatment Strategies for Low Ceruloplasmin

See Copper, Total Section.

A medical specialist should treat Wilson disease.

Additional Testing

comprehensive thyroid profile II; iron and TIBC; ferritin; complete blood count (CBC); copper, total; comprehensive metabolic panel (CMP); comprehensive stool testing

References

1. O'Brien KO. Maternal, fetal and placental regulation of placental iron trafficking. Placenta. 2022;125:47–53. doi:10.1016/j.placenta.2021.12.018

2. Rao PB, Modi P, Modi A. Serum Ceruloplasmin Levels in Pregnant Women. Int. J. Pharm. Sci. Res. 2015;3(2):57–60. ISSN:23480262

3. Sak S, Barut M, Çelik H, et al. Copper and ceruloplasmin levels are closely related to the severity of preeclampsia. J Matern Fetal Neonatal Med. 2020;33(1):96–102. doi:10.1080/14767058.2018.1487934

4. Bellos I, Papantoniou N, Pergialiotis V. Serum ceruloplasmin levels in preeclampsia: a meta-analysis. J Matern Fetal Neonatal Med. 2018;31(17):2342–2348. doi:10.1080/14767058.2017.1340449

5. Cherukuri S, Potla R, Sarkar J, Nurko S, Harris ZL, Fox PL. Unexpected role of ceruloplasmin in intestinal iron absorption. Cell Metab. 2005;2(5):309–319. doi:10.1016/j.cmet.2005.10.003

6. Olivares M, Méndez MA, Astudillo PA, Pizarro F. Present situation of biomarkers for copper status. Am J Clin Nutr. 2008;88(3):859S-62S. doi:10.1093/ajcn/88.3.859S

Fasting Glucose

Serum glucose measures the amount of glucose in the bloodstream. It is an analyte found on both the basic metabolic panel and the comprehensive metabolic panel (CMP). This test should always be done while fasting for accuracy.

Levels are influenced by the amount of carbohydrates and sugar in the diet, stress, inflammation, and hormones. The amount of glucose in the bloodstream is regulated by insulin.

Sugars are the simplest forms of carbohydrates. The term *sugar* is typically used to refer to table sugar but encompasses two groups of carbohydrates: monosaccharides and disaccharides. These saccharides are naturally found in fruits, vegetables, and grains and are especially high in starchy fruits and vegetables.

Monosaccharides are single-molecule sugars. These are simple sugars that are extremely easy to digest and absorb. They include glucose, fructose, and galactose.

Glucose is also known as dextrose and is found in many different plants. It is the building block of other sugars and starches.

Fructose is converted to glucose by the liver. It is found mostly in fruits but also in some vegetables, as well as honey.

Galactose is a component of lactose and is found in dairy products.

Disaccharides are multiple-molecule sugars. These sugars are more complex and require digestion to break them down into monosaccharides before absorption. These include sucrose, lactose, and maltose.

Sucrose is composed of glucose and fructose molecules and is naturally found in fruits and vegetables. It is also the structural form of table sugar.

Lactose is composed of glucose and galactose and is a milk sugar.

Maltose is composed of multiple glucose molecules and is naturally found in grains.

To be used in cellular metabolism, carbohydrates are broken down into their base molecule: glucose.

The breakdown of carbohydrates into simple sugars starts in the mouth with enzymes in the saliva. These simple sugars are absorbed through the small intestines and into the blood with the help of cellular transporters called GLUTs (glucose transporters). There are multiple types of GLUTs found in the membranes of every cell. They are the doors that open to allow sugar molecules in and out.

Once digested, GLUT 1 moves glucose through the intestinal cells and into the blood. This does not require insulin but does require a sodium ion.

Red blood cells can have an inverse association with glucose. If their cells are deficient in glucose fuels, they produce more GLUT 1 in their membranes to allow more glucose to enter without needing insulin. If there is enough stored glucose in the cells, they reduce the amount of GLUT 1 in the cell membranes. These cells are the first to take up glucose when needed. They self-regulate their glucose intake because they do not need insulin to unlock the GLUT molecules. GLUT 1 becomes the primary glucose transporter in the placenta at peak insulin need during the third trimester.

When glucose levels in the small intestines hit a certain threshold, GLUT 2 is produced by the small intestines, pancreas, and liver. GLUT 2 takes the excess glucose straight to the liver to be processed into the storage form of glucose, called glycogen. This process is also not reliant on insulin. Glucose is brought to the pancreas, which stimulates insulin production. The more GLUT 2 produced in the small intestines, the more insulin is stimulated to open the necessary transports for glucogenesis, glucose metabolism.

GLUT 3 is found in the brain, nerves, and placenta. These means of transport, also not dependent on insulin, are always open. They respond to even the slightest amount of glucose in the body.

Found in muscle and fat, GLUT 4 is the only one that needs an insulin key to open. GLUT 4 is also expressed in endometrial tissues, ovaries, and placental tissues in pregnancy.

Our brains need glucose to work properly, and our cells need glucose for energy production. Insulin attaches to cells, like a key, to signal the GLUT 4 to let glucose into the cells. Any unused glucose is transported into the fat cells by insulin for storage as glycogen.

Fructose intake has been overlooked in previous years because it does not directly affect blood sugar levels. Many with diabetes and blood sugar issues have switched to using fructose-based sugars as substitutes, because their blood sugar is less likely to spike.

Like glucose, fructose is absorbed through the small intestines with the aid of GLUTs. Unlike glucose, it does not need to be bound with a sodium molecule to pass through the intestines and into the blood, and fructose does not need insulin to be let into muscle and fat cells. Most of the fructose consumed goes straight to the liver to be processed. Fructose metabolism is almost identical to alcohol metabolism in the liver.

Once digested and in the small intestines, rising levels of fructose signal the production of GLUT 2. They can carry not only glucose and fructose but also extremely large amounts of these sugars. GLUT 2 transports glucose and fructose to the pancreas and liver. The liver is stimulated to produce more GLUT 2 in response to the large amounts of fructose. All GLUT 2 fructose ends up in the liver for processing. Although GLUT 2 does not need insulin to work, insulin stimulates the production of more GLUT 2 in the liver. When the pancreas senses high levels of fructose or glucose in the blood, it produces insulin to signal the liver to uptake fructose for processing.

GLUT 5 is another transport molecule. It is produced in the small-intestine cells once fructose levels reach a certain threshold. Unlike GLUT 2, which can move both fructose and glucose, GLUT 5 only works with fructose. When fructose levels are high, GLUT 5 opens, allowing fructose to cross into the bloodstream. Fructose can then travel to other cells that have open GLUT 5: the brain, muscles, and fat cells. GLUT 5 production is affected by diabetes, insulin resistance, and intestinal inflammation.

Only a small amount of fructose is ever free-flowing in the blood and taken up by GLUT 5, but this fructose is the immediate fuel source for certain cells such as the brain. The majority is processed in the liver, where fructose is broken down into glucose, glycogen, and lactate.

Glycogen is the storage form of glucose. The production of glycogen is stimulated by insulin. Glycogen is primarily stored in the liver and muscles, but a small portion is also stored in other organs, the brain, and red blood cells. Glycerol is a sugar alcohol that makes up the backbone of triglycerides in the body. This is the body's way of regulating times of high and low sugar consumption. The body's blood sugar levels need to remain within narrow parameters. The body naturally does this with the use of all these different mechanisms. It is normal to use energy immediately and store the remainder for later.

The types of foods and amounts we eat contribute to stress on the sugar processing cycles. Our body is quite capable of handling the sugars that are found naturally and in small doses. However, the average American consumes 82 grams of sugar daily. Some studies show even higher amounts of consumption in children and adolescents. Most of this comes from sweetened beverages like sodas, sweet teas, Gatorade, and Vitaminwater.

Normal amounts of sugar are necessary, especially in pregnancy. Refined sugars, or large amounts of food in one sitting, can throw our bodies into a pro-inflammatory spin.

Insulin is produced by specialized cells in the pancreas known as β cells, which are found in the islets of Langerhans. Insulin is primarily involved in the regulation of glucose metabolism. Cortisol is a steroid hormone produced by the adrenal glands that plays a significant role in the body's response to stress. It can have both direct and indirect effects on insulin production and regulation of blood sugar levels. When there are issues with serum glucose, it may be important to address stress responses, whether physical or emotional.

Pregnancy

Glucose levels undergo several changes during pregnancy, primarily due to the various hormonal and metabolic adaptations that occur to support the growing fetus and the changing needs of the mother's body.

During the first trimester, cells are quickly dividing to create the fetus and placenta. This requires quick and instant energy in the form of glucose. During early pregnancy, human chorionic gonadotrophin (hCG) promotes insulin sensitivity. This means that maternal cells become more responsive to insulin, and the body utilizes glucose more effectively. Sugar grows babies. This increased sensitivity to insulin is thought to help facilitate nutrient transfer from the mother to the developing fetus. This is one of the primary drivers of hypoglycemia and nausea in the first trimester.

Pregnancy is a state of insulin resistance. As pregnancy advances, the placenta begins to produce placental lactogen. Lactogen affects insulin sensitivity in the maternal tissues, creating a state of insulin resistance. The presence of zinc heavily influences lactogen function.[1] Insulin resistance leads to a maternal prioritization of fats over carbohydrates for energy and spares carbohydrates for the fetus. Thus, the development of insulin resistance serves as a physiological adaptation of the mother to ensure adequate carbohydrate supply for the rapidly growing fetus.[2] This state of insulin resistance can be seen in the second trimester, and as pregnancy progresses, the sensitivity of insulin receptors decreases by 50%. In addition, throughout the course of pregnancy, to compensate for the increased demand for sugar in fetal growth and maturity, insulin production can be up to fifteenfold what it was preconception,[3] with an average of 3- to 3.5-fold increase in fasting insulin levels.[4]

Insulinase is an enzyme that plays a role in glucose metabolism during pregnancy. It is produced in the placenta and has the ability to degrade insulin. Insulinase production begins to increase as the placenta matures and grows during the second trimester. This increase is necessary to accommodate the rising energy demands of the developing fetus. By the third trimester, insulinase production is at its peak. The placenta is fully developed and supporting the growing fetus. Insulin degradation is highest during this period, contributing to significant insulin resistance in pregnant women. This insulin resistance helps to ensure that glucose is readily available to the fetus, even as maternal insulin levels rise.

Compared to preconception levels, fasting glucose levels decrease by a median of 3 mg/dL in the first trimester. This returns to normal preconception levels in the second trimester. During the third trimester, there is another slight decrease in serum glucose levels due to an increase in insulin production.[5]

Postpartum

After birth, fasting glucose levels typically decrease gradually over the first few days and weeks of postpartum. This decline is partly due to the cessation of placental lactogen and insulinase. As these hormones diminish, insulin sensitivity improves, leading to lower fasting glucose levels. However, in women with gestational diabetes or impaired glucose tolerance, there may be a more significant and prolonged decrease in glucose levels postpartum as their bodies adjust to no longer being pregnant. Breastfeeding can also affect fasting glucose levels. Initially, breastfeeding may lead to a slight decrease in fasting glucose levels due to increased energy expenditure associated with lactation. Additionally, the hormone prolactin, which stimulates milk production, can enhance insulin sensitivity, further contributing to lower glucose levels. Significant blood loss can trigger a release of stress hormones like cortisol and catecholamines, which can elevate blood glucose levels through gluconeogenesis.

STANDARD LAB RANGE: 70 – 99 mg/dL*

Trimester	Standard Pregnancy Ranges	**Functional Pregnancy Ranges**
Preconception	70 – 99	**80 – 95**
First Trimester	Not Established	**70 – 85**
Second Trimester	70 – 95	**75 – 90**
Third Trimester	70 – 95	**75 – 90**
Postpartum	70 – 99	**80 – 95**

*Some labs and countries use mmol (millimole)/L measurements for glucose ranges.

GLUCOSE CONVERSION TABLE

mg/dL	mmol/L	mg/dL	mmol/L
50	2.8	125	6.9
60	3.3	130	7.2
70	3.9	135	7.5
75	4.2	140	7.8
80	4.4	145	8
85	4.7	150	8.3
90	5	160	8.9
95	5.3	170	9
100	5.5	180	10
105	5.8	190	10.5
110	6.1	200	11.1
115	6.4	225	12.5
120	6.7	250	13.9

Causes of Elevated Fasting Glucose

First-trimester fasting blood glucose levels may be a predictive marker of gestational diabetes and poor pregnancy outcomes. A fasting blood glucose level >4.6 mmol/L (approximately 82 mg/dL) was associated with an increased risk of gestational diabetes mellitus (GDM) later in pregnancy.[6] Other studies have found a cutoff around 84 and 85 mg/dL in the first trimester as a predictive marker

Insulin Resistance: Pregnancy is a state of insulin resistance, especially in the third trimester. This natural maternal insulin resistance can worsen preexisting insulin resistance and diabetes, causing increased blood glucose levels. Women with preexisting polycystic ovarian syndrome (PCOS) and/or insulin resistance are at a higher risk of gestational diabetes.[10] Lower CO_2 may be present due to systemic acidity. (See Carbon Dioxide (CO_2) Section.)

Diabetes: Preexisting diabetes, whether type 1 or type 2, significantly increases the risk of developing GDM during pregnancy. Women with preexisting diabetes already have underlying insulin resistance or insufficient insulin production, which can be exacerbated by the metabolic changes that occur during pregnancy.

Adrenal Hyperfunction: The release of cortisol is under the control of the hypothalamic-pituitary-adrenal (HPA) axis. The hypothalamus releases corticotropin-releasing hormone (CRH). It then acts on the

of GDM later in pregnancy.[7, 8]

The Hyperglycemia and Adverse Pregnancy Outcome (HAPO) study found strong associations between higher levels of maternal glucose between 24 and 32 weeks, within what is currently considered normoglycemia, and adverse pregnancy outcomes. Lower ranges of fasting blood sugar, <90 mg/dL, is considered protective for both maternal and fetal health in pregnancy but also with childhood metabolic health, as those with higher fasting glucose levels showed long-term effects on childhood metabolic function.[9]

First-trimester screening of fasting glucose via the comprehensive metabolic panel offers the opportunity to detect and treat undiagnosed pregestational diabetes. This becomes a major problem, as the prevalence of diabetes increases rapidly. Otherwise, these high-risk women would not receive any special treatment until the beginning of the third trimester. If blood sugar dysregulation issues are addressed early, overt GDM may be prevented

anterior pituitary to release adrenocorticotropic hormone (ACTH), which subsequently acts on the adrenal cortex. In a negative feedback loop, sufficient cortisol inhibits the release of both ACTH and CRH. The HPA axis follows a circadian rhythm. Thus, cortisol levels will be high in the morning and low at night.[11] One of the primary jobs of cortisol is to regulate blood sugar levels. High cortisol levels increase gluconeogenesis and decrease glycogen synthesis. Elevated cortisol also increases insulin resistance.

Fasting increases cortisol levels. In those with insulin resistance, fasting for more than 12 hours can make fasting glucose levels worse. You may also see this in acute stress reactions. Patients with a fear of needles who have fasted more than 12 hours for a blood draw, or who have had a bad experience with a blood draw, can have inaccurate fasting glucose readings. It is normal for the rise in cortisol first thing in the morning to signal the liver to release stored glucose to keep fasting levels regulated and balanced. This triggers the β cells of the pancreas to increase insulin production to grab this glucose and get it to the cells. If there is too much cortisol being produced or nighttime hypoglycemia, this may be a larger release of glycogen.[12] This causes a presentation called "dawning phenomenon," in which morning fasting glucose levels are elevated, but other glucose levels throughout the day are normal.

Thyroid Dysfunction: Thyroid hormones affect glucose homeostasis by impacting pancreatic β-cell development and glucose metabolism through several organs including the liver, gastrointestinal tract, pancreas, adipose tissue, skeletal muscles, and the central nervous system.[13] Several studies have shown links between thyroid hormones and pancreatic β-cell development and function. Specifically, triiodothyronine (T3) stimulates β-cell proliferation. T3 has also been shown to increase glucose-stimulated insulin secretions. Other studies have shown that administration of T3 helps to improve glucose intolerance.[14]

On the other hand, excess thyroid hormones increase glucose absorption by the gut and gluconeogenesis and glycogenolysis by the liver, as well as stimulating insulin secretion and inducing hyperinsulinemia, while simultaneously accelerating insulin degradation and decreasing the half-life of insulin.[15] All of these actions cause an increase in blood glucose levels. So in cases of hyperglycemia, assessing overall thyroid function may be important.

via dietary, lifestyle, and supplemental management.

Vitamin D Deficiency: Studies show that people with lower vitamin D levels have more insulin dysregulation issues.[16] The active form of vitamin D, through its receptors directly or through the regulation of intracellular calcium, helps to secrete insulin.[17] Vitamin D increases the sensitivity of the insulin receptor to insulin. Vitamin D also upregulates the expression of GLUT 4 proteins.

Vitamin B1 (Thiamine) Deficiency: Thiamine is essential for insulin synthesis and secretion.[18] An enzyme called thiaminase I (EC2.5.1.2)—present in raw fish, shellfish, tea, and coffee—decreases thiamine absorption.[19] Higher intake of thiamine during pregnancy is associated with a lower incidence of GDM.[20] Women who are struggling with hyperemesis gravidarum (HG) are more likely to develop thiamine deficiency. In cases of HG with memory issues, thiamine deficiency should be assessed and treated immediately. A blood thiamine level <180 nmol/L can be used to diagnose thiamine deficiency. Pregnant women have the highest rates of thiamine deficiency. One study found that 34% of pregnant women assessed in the United Kingdom had low thiamine levels.[21]

Magnesium Deficiency: Magnesium is required for both proper glucose utilization and insulin signaling. Insulin aids in magnesium uptake into insulin-sensitive tissues.[22] Magnesium works to support GLUT 4 function.

Vitamin A Deficiency: Vitamin A enhances β-cell formation and glucose metabolism. A deficiency in vitamin A is associated with decreased β-cell formation and decreased lifespan. This decreases the production of insulin, causing elevated glucose levels.[23]

Iron Overload/Hemochromatosis: Iron influences insulin function, and iron overload can cause insulin resistance. Iron interferes with the ability of insulin to function, and specifically with glucose production in the liver. In fact, the most common symptom of iron overload is insulin resistance.[24] (See Iron Section.)

Zinc Deficiency: Zinc is highly concentrated in the islet cells of the pancreas, where insulin is produced. Zinc is a trace element that serves as a cofactor for various enzymes in the human body, including those involved in glycolysis.[25] Hexokinase is the enzyme responsible for the initial step of glycolysis, which involves phosphorylating glucose to form glucose-6-phosphate. Zinc does not directly bind to hexokinase but is required for the enzyme's activity. Phosphoglucoisomerase catalyzes the isomerization of glucose-6-phosphate into fructose-6-phosphate, an essential step in the glycolytic pathway. Zinc also acts as a cofactor for phosphoglucoisomerase, facilitating its function.

Zinc is known to influence insulin sensitivity. It appears to enhance the action of insulin. In insulin-sensitive areas of the body such as skeletal muscle and adipose tissue, insulin stimulates the translocation of GLUT 4 to the cell membrane, allowing for glucose uptake. Zinc may indirectly affect GLUT 4 by improving insulin sensitivity, thus promoting the efficient translocation of GLUT 4 to the cell membrane in response to insulin. Zinc can impact the activity of kinases and phosphatases, which are involved in the regulation of GLUT 4 translocation. By affecting these signaling pathways, zinc indirectly modulates the movement of GLUT 4 to the cell membrane. Low zinc = low glycolysis, and low GLUT 4 = high blood sugar.

Other Possible Causes: acute trauma, infections, inflammation, progesterone deficiency, certain medications (corticosteroids, beta-blockers, antidepressants), excess growth hormone, sleep apnea, severe liver disease, pancreatitis, renal disease, vitamin C overdose

Treatment Strategies for Elevated Fasting Glucose

Diet

As a resource for dietary management of elevated glucose levels, I highly recommend the book *Real Food for Gestational Diabetes* by Lily Nichols. Dietary management looks different for each person. Everyone should minimize or eliminate refined carbohydrates (bread, baked goods, cookies, added sugars), fast-acting sugars (fruit juice, soda), and refined hydrogenated fats, which can increase blood glucose and triglyceride levels. Choose complex and nutrient-dense carbohydrates (such as whole grains or sweet potatoes) for steady blood sugar rises. Increase dietary fats to balance carbohydrate intake, focusing on monounsaturated fats such as olive oil, avocado oil, and coconut oil as well as foods that offer a fatty acid complex such as fish, bone-in and skin-on meat cuts, full-fat dairy, nuts, and seeds. Eat smaller meals; a large meal can increase blood glucose levels, even if the meal is healthy and balanced due to glycemic loading. Snacks between meals can help prevent fasting rises in glucose. Include small healthy snacks before bed to limit the dawning phenomenon.

Lifestyle

Management of physical and emotional stress is especially important in cases of elevated fasting glucose. Identify whether the stress originates from emotional or inflammation triggers. Emotional stress can increase physical stress and vice versa. Proper exercise, effective breathing, and other activities known to reduce stress may be important tools in the management of adrenal causes of elevated glucose.

For more resources on emotional stress management, visit my website to download my *Stress Reduction Strategies* e-book.

Supplements

Studies have shown that a dose of up to 4 grams of inositol per day has been well tolerated by pregnant women without any adverse effects.[26] A 2022 review found that myo-inositol was a safe and effective treatment strategy for increasing insulin sensitivity and reducing GDM-related complications.[27] There has been mixed research on the success of using vitamin D for elevated fasting glucose. The key is to test and confirm deficiency before administering supplementation. It is possible that the correlation between vitamin D deficiency and GDM originates in early gestation, and that treatment in the acute phase is not effective due to the damage already being done.

Supplementation with high-dose vitamin B1 (thiamine) may prevent deterioration in fasting glucose and insulin, and improve glucose tolerance in patients with hyperglycemia.[28] Dosages in studies vary between 100 and 900 mg per day of thiamine.[29] Generally, a dosage of 100 mg per day is used in the treatment of low thiamine.[30] Magnesium supplementation has been shown to reduce fasting glucose levels over the course of 4 to 16 weeks. The form of magnesium matters as well as the dosage. The most effective form of magnesium in managing blood glucose levels is magnesium chloride in a dosage of approximately 250 mg per day.[31] The administration of ALA 100 to 300 mg per day may help reduce fasting glucose levels.[32]

Additional Testing

fasting insulin; serum thiamine; vitamin D, 25-hydroxy (25-hydroxycalciferol, 25OH-D); complete blood count (CBC); ferritin; iron and TIBC; c-reactive protein (CRP); comprehensive thyroid profile II; reverse T3 (rT3); progesterone; oral zinc tolerance test; oral glucose tolerance test (OGTT)

Causes of Low Fasting Glucose

If the fasting glucose is <75 mg/dL and there are symptoms of hypoglycemia such as nausea and vomiting in pregnancy, fasting hypoglycemia should always be suspected. If fasting glucose is <70 mg/dL, fasting hypoglycemia is certain. Generally, in cases of hypoglycemia, lactate dehydrogenase (LDH) will also be decreased. LDH activity reflects the exchange of chloride with glucose and glucose with zinc and sodium, aka glycolysis. This is more common in the first and second trimesters.

Adrenal Hypofunction: Adrenal insufficiency is characterized by a decreased production of cortisol and aldosterone by the adrenal glands. The lack of cortisol can cause a decrease in glucose production by the liver, a decrease in glucose intake by cells, and decreased glucose uptake by peripheral tissues, leading to hypoglycemia.[33 34]

Vitamin C Deficiency: Vitamin C deficiency induces hypoglycemia, and high-dose vitamin C, especially in IV form, can cause a rise in blood sugars.[35]

Vitamin B6 (Pyridoxine) Deficiency: Vitamin B6 is a cofactor for several enzymes involved in glycogenolysis, including glycogen phosphorylase. This enzyme is responsible for breaking the glycosidic bonds in glycogen, releasing glucose-1-phosphate. Vitamin B6 helps activate these enzymes, allowing them to perform their functions efficiently. Vitamin B6 is also involved in the regulation of gluconeogenesis, which is the synthesis of glucose from noncarbohydrate sources. By influencing the activity of enzymes involved in gluconeogenesis, vitamin B6 indirectly affects the balance between glycogenolysis and gluconeogenesis, helping to maintain blood glucose levels within a normal range. Low B6 = low glycogenolysis, and low gluconeogenesis = low blood sugar.

Vitamin B7 (Biotin) Deficiency: Biotin plays an important role in various metabolic pathways, including gluconeogenesis. Biotin serves as a cofactor for several carboxylase enzymes involved in gluconeogenesis, such as pyruvate carboxylase and propionyl-CoA carboxylase. These enzymes are responsible for adding a carboxyl group to specific molecules, which is an essential step in gluconeogenesis. For example, pyruvate carboxylase catalyzes the conversion of pyruvate to oxaloacetate, an intermediate in gluconeogenesis. Biotin is required for the carboxylation reactions to occur, facilitating the conversion of these precursors into glucose. Biotin also plays a role in the metabolism of fatty acids. Fatty acids can be broken down into acetyl-CoA, which can then enter the gluconeogenesis pathway as a precursor for glucose synthesis. Low biotin = low gluconeogenesis = low blood sugar.

Zinc Overload: Some studies show lower blood sugar levels in those taking high-dose zinc supplements >30 mg per day.[36]

Other Possible Causes: carrying multiples, low carbohydrate diet (specifically in the first trimester), genetics, secondary hypothyroidism caused by hypopituitarism, overexercising, history of bariatric surgery, alcohol use, malnutrition, certain medications (beta-blockers, antibiotics, metformin), overmanaged diabetes, infections, autoimmune disease, cancer

Treatment Strategies for Low Fasting Glucose

Diet

In cases of hypoglycemia in pregnancy, frequent meals that contain complex carbohydrates and proteins will help keep blood sugars up. Generally, this is more common in the first trimester. Heavy proteins like meat are often hard to process in hypoglycemia cases. Dairy and starchy foods such as potatoes can be good food sources for those struggling with hypoglycemia. Trail mix is a good snack option. The biggest key is to keep eating.

In acute hypoglycemic stages, having 15 grams of sugar and waiting 15 minutes is a trick recommended by the American Diabetes Association. This means consuming 15 grams of sugar—about one tablespoon of honey, a three-quarter cup of orange juice, half a banana, a peach, or another piece of fruit—waiting 15 minutes, and either testing blood sugar levels or assessing symptoms. If blood sugar levels are still low, repeat until symptoms improve. Often in hypoglycemia, the goal is consuming more calories more frequently.

Lifestyle

Continuous glucose monitors are becoming more readily available and may help to identify patterns of dietary intake and fasting surrounding changes in blood sugar levels. When a patient is using one, make sure to have them also write in a journal information such as food intake, timing, drinks (including teas and coffees), water intake, exercise, stress, and other symptoms. This may more easily help to identify symptoms and measurement patterns, as well as finding the most effective dietary protocols.

Additional Testing

fasting insulin; complete blood count (CBC); antinuclear antibodies (ANA)

References

1. Voorhees JL, Rao GV, Gordon TJ, Brooks CL. Zinc binding to human lactogenic hormones and the human prolactin receptor. FEBS Lett. 2011;585(12):1783–1788. doi:10.1016/j.febslet.2011.04.019

2. Sonagra AD, Biradar SM, K D, Murthy D S J. Normal pregnancy: a state of insulin resistance. J Clin Diagn Res. 2014 Nov;8(11):CC01–3. doi: 10.7860/JCDR/2014/10068.5081. Epub 2014 Nov 20. PMID: 25584208; PMCID: PMC4290225

3. Lammi-Keefe C, Couch S, Kirwan J. Handbook of Nutrition and Pregnancy. 2nd Edition. Humana Press; 2018

4. Parrettini S, Caroli A and Torlone E (2020) Nutrition and Metabolic Adaptations in Physiological and Complicated Pregnancy

5. Riskin-Mashiah S, Damti A, Younes G, Auslander R. Normal fasting plasma glucose levels during pregnancy: a hospital-based study. J Perinat Med. 2011 Mar;39(2):209–11. doi: 10.1515/jpm.2010.142. Epub 2011 Jan 18. PMID: 21241203

6. Parrettini S, Caroli A, Torlone E. Nutrition and Metabolic Adaptations in Physiological and Complicated Pregnancy: Focus on Obesity and Gestational Diabetes. Front Endocrinol (Lausanne). 2020;11:611929. Published 2020 Nov 30. doi:10.3389/fendo.2020.611929

7. Li P, Lin S, Li L, Cui J, Zhou S, Fan J. First-trimester fasting plasma glucose as a predictor of gestational diabetes mellitus and the association with adverse pregnancy outcomes. Pak J Med Sci. 2019 Jan-Feb;35(1):95–100. doi: 10.12669/pjms.35.1.216. PMID: 30881404; PMCID: PMC6408635

8. Riskin-Mashiah S, Younes G, Damti A, Auslender R. First-trimester fasting hyperglycemia and adverse pregnancy outcomes. Diabetes Care. 2009 Sep;32(9):1639–43. doi: 10.2337/dc09–0688. Epub 2009 Jun 23. PMID: 19549728; PMCID: PMC2732138

9. Lowe WL Jr, Scholtens DM, Kuang A, Linder B, Lawrence JM, Lebenthal Y, McCance D, Hamilton J, Nodzenski M, Talbot O, Brickman WJ, Clayton P, Ma RC, Tam WH, Dyer AR, Catalano PM, Lowe LP, Metzger BE; HAPO Follow-up Study Cooperative Research Group. Hyperglycemia and Adverse Pregnancy Outcome Follow-up Study (HAPO FUS): Maternal Gestational Diabetes Mellitus and Childhood Glucose Metabolism. Diabetes Care. 2019 Mar;42(3):372–380. doi: 10.2337/dc18–1646. Epub 2019 Jan 17. PMID: 30655380; PMCID: PMC6385693

10. Li X, Liu X, Zuo Y, Gao J, Liu Y, Zheng W. The risk factors of gestational diabetes mellitus in patients with polycystic ovary syndrome: What should we care. Medicine (Baltimore). 2021 Aug 6;100(31):e26521. doi: 10.1097/MD.0000000000026521. PMID: 34397795; PMCID: PMC8341335

11. Thau L, Gandhi J, Sharma S. Physiology, Cortisol. [Updated 2022 Aug 29]. In: StatPearls [Internet]. Treasure Island (FL): StatPearls Publishing; 2023 Jan-. www.ncbi.nlm.nih.gov/books/NBK538239

12. Sharma K, Akre S, Chakole S, Wanjari MB. Stress-Induced Diabetes: A Review. Cureus. 2022 Sep 13;14(9):e29142. doi: 10.7759/cureus.29142. PMID: 36258973; PMCID: PMC9561544

13. Eom YS, Wilson JR, Bernet VJ. Links between Thyroid Disorders and Glucose Homeostasis. Diabetes Metab J. 2022 Mar;46(2):239–256. doi: 10.4093/dmj.2022.0013. Epub 2022 Mar 24. PMID: 35385635; PMCID: PMC8987680

14. Verga Falzacappa C, Mangialardo C, Madaro L, Ranieri D, Lupoi L, Stigliano A, et al. Thyroid hormone T3 counteracts STZ-induced diabetes in mouse. PLoS One. 2011;6:e19839

15. O'Meara NM, Blackman JD, Sturis J, Polonsky KS. Alterations in the kinetics of C-peptide and insulin secretion in hyperthyroidism. J Clin Endocrinol Metab. 1993;76:79–84

16. Bhatt SP, Misra A, Gulati S, et al. Lower vitamin D levels are associated with higher blood glucose levels in Asian Indian women with pre-diabetes: a population-based cross-sectional study in North India. BMJ Open Diabetes Research and Care 2018;6:e000501. doi: 10.1136/bmjdrc-2017–000501

17. Hoseini SA, Aminorroaya A, Iraj B, Amini M. The effects of oral vitamin D on insulin resistance in pre-diabetic patients. J Res Med Sci. 2013 Jan;18(1):47–51. PMID: 23900423; PMCID: PMC3719226

18. Rad, M.G., Sharifi, M., Meamar, R. et al. The role of pancreas to improve hyperglycemia in STZ-induced diabetic rats by thiamine disulfide. Nutr. Diabetes 12, 32 (2022). doi.org/10.1038/s41387–022-00211–5

19. Pácal L, Kuricová K, Kaňková K. Evidence for altered thiamine metabolism in diabetes: Is there a potential to oppose gluco- and lipotoxicity by rational supplementation? World J Diabetes 2014; 5(3): 288–295 [PMID: 24936250 DOI: 10.4239/wjd.v5.i3.288]

20. Ge Y, Huang S, Li Y, Zhang Z, Kong M, Cui N, Tan L, Guo S, Wang S, Luo C, Hao L, Wu Y, Yang X. Pregnancy thiamine and riboflavin intake and the risk of gestational diabetes mellitus: A prospective cohort study. Am J Clin Nutr. 2023 Feb;117(2):426–435. doi: 10.1016/j.ajcnut.2022.11.014. Epub 2022 Dec 23. PMID: 36811572

21. Rees G, Brooke Z, Doyle W, Costeloe K. The nutritional status of women in the first trimester of pregnancy attending an inner-city antenatal department in the UK. J R Soc Promot Health. (2005) 125:232–8. doi: 10.1177/146642400512500516

22. Takaya J, Higashino H, Kobayashi Y. Intracellular magnesium and insulin resistance. Magnes Res. 2004 Jun;17(2):126–36. PMID: 15319146

23. Trasino SE, Gudas LJ. Vitamin A: a missing link in diabetes? Diabetes Manag (Lond). 2015;5(5):359–367. doi: 10.2217/dmt.15.30. PMID: 26535059; PMCID: PMC4623591

24. José Manuel Fernández-Real, Abel López-Bermejo, Wifredo Ricart; Cross-Talk Between Iron Metabolism and Diabetes. Diabetes 1 August 2002; 51 (8): 2348–2354. doi.org/10.2337/diabetes.51.8.2348

25. Yang HY, Hung KC, Chuang MH, Chang R, Chen RY, Wang FW, Wu JY, Chen JY. Effect of zinc supplementation on blood sugar control in the overweight and obese population: A systematic review and meta-analysis of randomized controlled trials. Obes Res Clin Pract. 2023 Jul-Aug;17(4):308–317. doi: 10.1016/j.orcp.2023.06.003. Epub 2023 Jun 27. PMID: 37385909

26. Tahir F, Majid Z. Inositol Supplementation in the Prevention of Gestational Diabetes Mellitus. Cureus. 2019 Sep 16;11(9):e5671. doi: 10.7759/cureus.5671. PMID: 31720147; PMCID: PMC6823013

27. Mashayekh-Amiri, S., Mohammad-Alizadeh-Charandabi, S., Abdolalipour, S. et al. Myo-inositol supplementation for prevention of gestational diabetes mellitus in overweight and obese pregnant women: a systematic review and meta-analysis. Diabetol Metab Syndr 14, 93 (2022). doi.org/10.1186/s13098–022-00862–5

28. Alaei Shahmiri F, Soares MJ, Zhao Y, Sherriff J. High-dose thiamine supplementation improves glucose tolerance in hyperglycemic individuals: a randomized, double-blind cross-over trial. Eur J Nutr. 2013 Oct;52(7):1821–4. doi: 10.1007/s00394–013-0534–6. Epub 2013 May 29. PMID: 23715873

29. Muley A, Fernandez R, Green H, et al. Effect of thiamine supplementation on glycaemic outcomes in adults with type 2 diabetes: a systematic review and meta-analysis. BMJ Open 2022;12:e059834. doi: 10.1136/bmjopen-2021–059834

30. Kareem O, Nisar S, Tanvir M, Muzaffer U and Bader GN (2023) Thiamine deficiency in pregnancy and lactation: implications and present perspectives. Front. Nutr. 10:1080611. doi: 10.3389/fnut.2023.1080611

31. Qu Q, Rong R, Yu J. Effect of magnesium supplementation on pregnancy outcome in gestational diabetes mellitus patients: A meta-analysis of randomized controlled trials. Food Sci Nutr. 2022 Sep 7;10(10):3193–3202. doi: 10.1002/fsn3.2561. PMID: 36249983; PMCID: PMC9548361

32. Capece U, Moffa S, Improta I, et al. Alpha-Lipoic Acid and Glucose Metabolism: A Comprehensive Update on Biochemical and Therapeutic Features. Nutrients. 2022;15(1):18. Published 2022 Dec 21. doi:10.3390/nu15010018

33. Tanaka S, Abe M, Kohno G, Kushimoto M, Ikeda J, Ogawa K, Suzuki Y, Ishihara H, Fujishiro M. A Single Episode of Hypoglycemia as a Possible Early Warning Sign of Adrenal Insufficiency. Ther Clin Risk Manag. 2020 Feb 27;16:147–153. doi: 10.2147/TCRM.S238435. PMID: 32161465; PMCID: PMC7051808

34. Kawahara T, Tsuji M, Tominaga N, Toyama N, Toda M. Frequency of Adrenal Insufficiency in Patients With Hypoglycemia in an Emergency Department: A Cross-sectional Study. J Endocr Soc. 2022 Aug 4;6(10):bvac119. doi: 10.1210/jendso/bvac119. PMID: 36042975; PMCID: PMC9419498

35. Shu Y, Zou C, Cai Y, He Q, Wu X, Zhu H, Qv M, Chao Y, Xu C, Tang L, Wu X. Vitamin C deficiency induces hypoglycemia and cognitive disorder through S-nitrosylation-mediated activation of glycogen synthase kinase 3β. Redox Biol. 2022 Oct;56:102420. doi: 10.1016/j.redox.2022.102420. Epub 2022 Aug 8. PMID: 35969998; PMCID: PMC9399387

36. Elanjian AI, Elder A, Hazin R. Hypoglycemia Induced by Zinc Supplementation for COVID-19 Prophylaxis: A Case Series. Cureus. 2023 May 10;15(5):e38828. doi: 10.7759/cureus.38828. PMID: 37303432; PMCID: PMC10252152

Glycated Hemoglobin (Hemoglobin A1c/HbA1c)

The glycated hemoglobin, or hemoglobin A1c (HbA1c), test measures the percentage of hemoglobin that is coated with glucose.

Glucose molecules in the bloodstream bind to hemoglobin, the protein in red blood cells responsible for carrying oxygen. This binding occurs randomly and spontaneously, without the need for enzymatic activity. Once glucose binds to hemoglobin, it forms a stable complex known as glycated hemoglobin or HbA1c. The extent of glycation depends on the concentration of glucose in the bloodstream and the lifespan of red blood cells. Since red blood cells have a lifespan of approximately 120 days, HbA1c reflects average blood glucose levels over the previous two or three months.

Pregnancy

Pregnancy leads to various physiological changes, including increased insulin resistance, hormonal fluctuations, and changes in blood volume. These changes can affect glucose metabolism and, consequently, HbA1c levels. In the first trimester, HbA1c levels may decrease due to increased blood volume and an expanded red blood cell mass. In the first trimester and the postpartum period, the discrepancy between average oral glucose tolerance test (OGTT) glucose and HbA1c-estimated average glucose is minimal. HbA1c decreases through the second trimester. As pregnancy progresses, insulin resistance increases, starting in the last weeks of the second trimester through the third trimester, and HbA1c levels rise. In the late second trimester, the average OGTT glucose is 13.2 mg/dL, higher than the HbA1c-estimated average glucose. Lower hemoglobin concentrations explain this discrepancy.[1]

Due to physiological reasons around discrepancies in HbA1c values, it is currently not recommended as a substitute for the OGTT.

Postpartum

After giving birth, HbA1c levels typically decrease. This can be due to the resolution of some of the physiological changes associated with pregnancy and the reduction of insulin resistance.

STANDARD LAB RANGE: 4% – 5.6%

Trimester	Standard Pregnancy Ranges	**Functional Pregnancy Ranges**
Preconception	4 - 5.6%	**5 - 5.6%**
First Trimester	4 - 6%	**4 - 5.4%**
Second Trimester	4 - 6%	**4 - 5.4%**
Third Trimester	4 - 7%	**4 - 5.7%**
Postpartum	4 - 5.6%	**5 - 5.6%**

Causes of Elevated Glycated Hemoglobin (Hemoglobin A1c/ HbA1c)

See Fasting Glucose Section.

Vitamin B12 (Cobalamin) Deficiency: Studies have shown that vitamin B12 deficiency causes falsely elevated HbA1c values.[4]

Other Possible Causes: adrenal hyperfunction, progesterone deficiency, thyroid dysfunction, vitamin D deficiency, vitamin B1 (thiamine) deficiency, zinc deficiency, iron overload/hemochromatosis, chronic infections, inflammation, excess growth hormone, sleep apnea, severe liver disease, pancreatitis, renal disease, vitamin C overdose

Elevated HbA1c is associated with maternal-fetal complications.[2]

As of the writing of this book, there is not enough evidence to support the use of the HbA1c test as a replacement for the OGTT in diagnosing gestational diabetes. Evidence does indicate that higher HbA1c in the first trimester can be used as a predictive biomarker for increased risk of GDM later in pregnancy.[3]

Treatment Strategies for Elevated Glycated Hemoglobin (Hemoglobin A1c/HbA1c)

See Fasting Glucose Section.

Diet

Several dietary strategies have been proven effective in improving blood sugar levels and reducing HbA1c. Choosing foods with a low glycemic index can help prevent rapid spikes in blood sugar levels. Low-glycemic-index foods include nonstarchy vegetables, whole grains, legumes, and most fruits. These foods are digested and absorbed more slowly, gradually increasing blood sugar levels. This is important in pregnancy when the mother still needs carbohydrates and the nutrients they contain. If patients have elevated HbA1c prior to conception, this is important for the first trimester. Fiber slows down the absorption of glucose and promotes satiety, which can help regulate blood sugar levels.

Incorporating healthy fats such as monounsaturated fats found in avocados, olive oil, nuts, seeds, and fatty fish can help improve insulin sensitivity and reduce inflammation, which may contribute to better glycemic control. Fats become important in the third trimester when maternal physiology is more catabolic. Minimize consumption of foods and beverages high in added sugars, such as sugary drinks and sweets. The Mediterranean diet emphasizes whole grains, fruits, vegetables, legumes, nuts, seeds, olive oil, fish, poultry, dairy, and processed foods. Studies have shown that adherence to the Mediterranean diet is associated with improved glycemic control, reduced risk of cardiovascular disease, and lower HbA1c levels.

Lifestyle

Exercise can have a significant impact on HbA1c levels. Regular physical activity improves insulin sensitivity, allowing the body to use insulin more effectively to regulate blood sugar levels. When cells become more sensitive to insulin, they can better uptake glucose from the bloodstream, leading to lower blood sugar levels over time. Since HbA1c is developed over time, the results of any diet or lifestyle guidelines will not have measurable effects for several months. It is best to use fasting glucose and other glucose monitoring methods to assess overall treatment effectiveness.

Supplements

Supplements depend on the underlying cause of elevated serum glucose levels.

Additional Testing

fasting insulin; complete blood count (CBC); comprehensive metabolic panel (CMP); comprehensive thyroid profile II; reverse T3 (rT3); lipid panel; vitamin D, 25-hydroxy (25-hydroxycalciferol, 25OH-D); ferritin; iron and TIBC; c-reactive protein (CRP); progesterone; oral zinc tolerance test; oral glucose tolerance test (OGTT)

Causes of Low Glycated Hemoglobin (Hemoglobin A1c/HbA1c)

See Fasting Glucose Section.

Anemia: Due to the frequency of anemia in pregnancy and low hemoglobin production as well as hemodilution, HbA1c may not be reliable. This should be considered if using the HbA1c to assess for glucose dysfunction issues.[5] This may cause the pattern of normal fasting glucose with an elevated HbA1c.

Other Possible Causes: adrenal hypofunction, vitamin C deficiency, vitamin B6 (pyridoxine) deficiency, vitamin B7 (biotin) deficiency, zinc overload, carrying multiples, low carbohydrate diet (specifically in the first trimester), genetics, secondary hypothyroidism caused by hypopituitarism, overexercising, history of bariatric surgery, alcohol use, malnutrition, certain medications (beta-blockers, antibiotics, metformin), overmanaged diabetes, infections, autoimmune disease, cancer

Treatment Strategies for Low Glycated Hemoglobin (Hemoglobin A1c/HbA1c)

See Fasting Glucose Section.

Lifestyle

Intermittent fasting has been shown to reduce hemoglobin A1c, which can be harmful for people with low levels already.

Additional Testing

fasting insulin; complete blood count (CBC); ferritin; comprehensive metabolic panel (CMP); insulin; antinuclear antibodies (ANA)

References

1. Edelson PK, James KE, Leong A, Arenas J, Cayford M, Callahan MJ, Bernstein SN, Tangren JS, Hivert MF, Higgins JM, Nathan DM, Powe CE. Longitudinal Changes in the Relationship Between Hemoglobin A1c and Glucose Tolerance Across Pregnancy and Postpartum. J Clin Endocrinol Metab. 2020 May 1;105(5):e1999–2007. doi: 10.1210/clinem/dgaa053. PMID: 32010954; PMCID: PMC7236626

2. Lemaitre M, Ternynck C, Bourry J, Baudoux F, Subtil D, Vambergue A. Association Between HbA1c Levels on Adverse Pregnancy Outcomes During Pregnancy in Patients With Type 1 Diabetes. J Clin Endocrinol Metab. 2022 Feb 17;107(3):e1117-e1125. doi: 10.1210/clinem/dgab769. PMID: 34694409; PMCID: PMC8852207

3. Valadan, M., Bahramnezhad, Z., Golshahi, F. et al. The role of first-trimester HbA1c in the early detection of gestational diabetes. BMC Pregnancy Childbirth 22, 71 (2022). doi.org/10.1186/s12884–021-04330–2

4. Aydin B, Cansu GB, Ozlu C. Relationship between glycosylated hemoglobin and vitamin B12 deficiency anemia. North Clin Istanb. 2022 Oct 21;9(5):459–463. doi: 10.14744/nci.2022.76259. PMID: 36447575; PMCID: PMC9677059

5. Alzahrani, B.A., Salamatullah, H.K., Alsharm, F.S. et al. The effect of different types of anemia on HbA1c levels in non-diabetics. BMC Endocr Disord 23, 24 (2023). doi.org/10.1186/s12902–023-01280-y

Sodium

The sodium test measures the concentration of sodium in the blood. It is an analyte found on the basic metabolic panel and comprehensive metabolic panel (CMP).

Electrolytes are substances that carry a natural positive or negative electrical charge when dissolved in water. They are required for various body processes such as conducting nerve impulses, contracting muscles, hydrating, and regulating pH levels. Electrolytes found in the body include sodium, potassium, chloride, calcium, magnesium, phosphorus, and bicarbonate.

Cations and anions are two types of electrolytes. The main difference is their electrical charge.

Cations are positively charged ions. They are formed when atoms or molecules lose one or more electrons. Common cations in the body include sodium (Na^+), potassium (K^+), calcium (Ca^{2+}), and magnesium (Mg^{2+}). These ions affect various physiological processes, such as nerve transmission, muscle contraction, and maintaining fluid balance.

Anions are negatively charged ions. They are formed when atoms or molecules gain one or more electrons. Common anions in the body include chloride (Cl^-), bicarbonate (HCO_3^-), phosphate (PO_4^{3-}), and sulfate (SO_4^{2-}). Like cations, anions also have important roles in bodily functions, such as regulating pH balance, transporting oxygen, and participating in enzyme reactions.

Sodium is the most important cation electrolyte in the body. It is used primarily for osmotic regulation and acid balance as well as renal, cardiac, and adrenal functions. Sodium is an active cation responsible for maintaining the extracellular fluid volume and regulating the membrane potential of cells. It is exchanged with potassium across cell membranes as part of active transport. Sodium regulation occurs in the kidneys, and transport occurs via sodium-chloride symporters, controlled by the hormone aldosterone.[1]

Sodium and chloride ions often move together through cell membranes in a process called cotransport. This cotransport mechanism is essential for the absorption of both ions across epithelial cells lining various tissues, such as the intestines and kidneys. Together, they regulate fluid balance by establishing osmotic gradients, influencing water movement within and between cells.

The regulation of sodium and potassium levels in the body is a complex and tightly controlled process that involves several hormones, including aldosterone and vitamin D, as well as other factors like magnesium, vasopressin (also known as antidiuretic hormone or ADH), and vasopressinase. Aldosterone is a hormone produced by the adrenal glands. Its primary function is to regulate sodium and potassium levels. When sodium levels are low in the blood, the body releases aldosterone, which acts on the kidneys to reabsorb sodium from the urine back into the bloodstream. Simultaneously, aldosterone increases the excretion of potassium in the urine. Vitamin D helps with regulating aldosterone production.

Vasopressin is produced in the hypothalamus and released by the pituitary gland. It regulates water balance and indirectly influences sodium levels. Vasopressin increases water reabsorption in the kidneys, which can dilute the blood and affect sodium concentration. When blood sodium levels rise, vasopressin secretion decreases, reducing water reabsorption. Magnesium is another mineral involved in the regulation of electrolyte balance. It helps maintain cell membrane permeability and neuromuscular function. Adequate magnesium levels are necessary for the proper functioning of sodium-potassium pumps, which transport sodium out of and potassium into cells. Vasopressinase is an enzyme produced by the placenta during pregnancy. It breaks down vasopressin in the bloodstream. This can affect water balance and blood volume, and can indirectly impact sodium and potassium levels.

Pregnancy

Sodium levels change throughout pregnancy due to increases in arginine vasopressin (AVP) and aldosterone. At the same time, as the placenta matures, it produces vasopressinase, an enzyme that degrades vasopressin. In pregnancy, it is normal for serum sodium levels to decrease by 4 to 5 mmol/L. This drop begins at conception and peaks between 8 and 12 weeks of gestation. Sodium levels increase slightly in the late third trimester. An average serum sodium level of 135 mmol/L is a normal presentation in pregnancy.

Postpartum

There are significant increases in plasma potassium and sodium concentrations in the first six weeks postpartum, when plasma chloride concentration falls.[2]

STANDARD LAB RANGE: 135 – 145 mmol/L

Trimester	Standard Pregnancy Ranges	**Functional Pregnancy Ranges**
Preconception	135-145	**135 – 142**
First Trimester	133-148	**130 – 140**
Second Trimester	129-148	**130 – 140**
Third Trimester	130-148	**130 – 140**
Postpartum	135-145	**135 – 142**

Causes of Elevated Sodium

Dehydration: Hemodilution in pregnancy naturally lowers serum electrolytes, including sodium. When expectant mothers are dehydrated, their serum electrolytes will be elevated. This may be more common in women with hyperemesis gravidarum.

Postpartum Hemorrhage: Postpartum elevated sodium can be seen in cases of Sheehan's syndrome. Sheehan's syndrome occurs when the anterior pituitary gland is damaged due to significant blood loss. Classically, this happens after delivery, when the mother loses a significant amount of blood. This blood loss results in the pituitary gland not being able to produce hormones.[3]

Renal Dysfunction: In cases of renal impairment, sodium and fluid build up in the body. This can cause swollen ankles, puffiness, a rise in blood pressure, and shortness of breath.[4] In pregnancy, the glomerular filtration rate (GFR) increases by 50%, and renal plasma flow increases by up to 80%. This causes an increased diuretic function, which leads to a reduction in serum sodium levels. In cases of kidney inflammation, this does not function correctly; sodium is not cleared from the system and instead increases in the serum.

Progesterone Deficiency: Progesterone has diuretic effects through activation of the renin-angiotensin system.[5] Blood pressure drops approximately 10 mmHg (millimeters of mercury) by the second trimester, despite a gain in intravascular volume of 30% to 50%. The drop in systemic vascular resistance is multifactorial, attributed in part to insensitivity to vasoactive hormones and activation of the renin-aldosterone-angiotensin system. A rise in serum aldosterone results in a net gain of approximately 1,000 mg of sodium.[6] Elevated progesterone levels reduce the sodium-retaining activity of aldosterone, causing clearance of sodium in the urine. A decrease in progesterone could cause elevated sodium levels.

Adrenal Hyperfunction: Aldosterone is a mineralocorticoid that regulates electrolyte balance in the body. It sends signals to the kidneys to absorb more sodium into the bloodstream and release potassium into the urine. When aldosterone is elevated, sodium is high and potassium is low. In patients with high aldosterone production and low serum vitamin D, vitamin D3 repletion decreases aldosterone.[7]

Increased Placental Vasopressinase Production: In rare cases, the placenta overproduces vasopressinase, causing an over-degradation of vasopressin. This, in turn, causes dehydration and elevated serum sodium. This is more common in women carrying multiples and those who conceived with IVF, as well as in cases of gestational diabetes. Decreased liver detoxification of vasopressin is seen in preeclampsia and liver disease. This usually presents in the third trimester and resolves within six weeks postpartum.[8]

Magnesium Deficiency: Magnesium inhibits aldosterone production, and potassium increases aldosterone production.[9] Magnesium is also important for helping to regulate the transport and balance of sodium and potassium in and out of the cells. Magnesium deficiency causes high serum sodium and low serum potassium.[10]

Water Softeners: Water softeners use sodium to soften water, and this may cause overexposure to sodium.

Other Possible Causes: preexisting diabetes, preexisting hypertension, excess sweating/hot climate, adrenal hyperfunction, metabolic alkalosis, mycotoxin exposure

Treatment Strategies for Elevated Sodium

Diet

Hydration is key. The most important step in managing elevated serum sodium is to maintain proper hydration. Staying well-hydrated helps to maintain a balance of electrolytes, including sodium. Avoid processed foods that are high in synthetic sodium. If sodium is high and potassium is low, increase magnesium-rich foods. Dark leafy greens like spinach, Swiss chard, kale, and collard greens are excellent sources of magnesium, but they need to be blanched before consuming to reduce oxalate content. Pumpkin seeds, sunflower seeds, and flaxseeds are magnesium-rich foods. Sprinkle them on salads, yogurt, or oatmeal. Other foods include avocados, legumes, and dark chocolate. A craving for chocolate may indicate a need for magnesium. Potassium-rich foods such as bananas, sweet potatoes, spinach, and yogurt can help counteract the effects of sodium on blood pressure.

Lifestyle

Intense or prolonged exercise, especially in hot and humid conditions, can lead to significant fluid loss through sweating. If adequate fluids, particularly those containing electrolytes like sodium, are not replenished during and after exercise, dehydration can occur, potentially resulting in hypernatremia. While sports drinks and electrolyte supplements can be beneficial for some, excessive consumption without adequate fluid intake can lead to elevated sodium levels in the bloodstream.

Supplements

Magnesium supplementation may help to balance elevated sodium levels. Doses of 600 mg of magnesium oxide have been used to lower elevated sodium levels outside of pregnancy. There is no data on the use of magnesium to lower hypernatremia in pregnancy at this time.

Additional Testing

complete blood count (CBC); vitamin D, 25-hydroxy (25-hydroxycalciferol, 25OH-D); progesterone; iron and TIBC; ferritin

Causes of Low Sodium

Physiological mild hyponatremia occurs during pregnancy due to increased AVP secretion caused by resetting of osmoreceptors in the hypothalamus at a lower osmolality, but values <130 mmol/L are abnormal.

Hyponatremia is the most encountered electrolyte abnormality in pregnancy. A 2021 literature review found low sodium (<130 mmol/L) associated with a significant rate of preeclampsia complications: acute kidney injury in 34.1%, HELLP syndrome in 17.1%, fetal growth restriction in 36.4%, stillbirth in 2.3%, use of magnesium sulfate in 44.2%, and postpartum maternal admission to

Adrenal Hypofunction: Hyponatremia is often seen in patients with low cortisol and aldosterone. When aldosterone is low, sodium is low but potassium and calcium are high.[13]

Antidepressant Medications: Low serum sodium is a common side effect of antidepressant medication use,[14] particularly selective serotonin reuptake inhibitors (SSRIs) and serotonin-norepinephrine reuptake inhibitors (SNRIs). SSRIs have been reported to increase the release of vasopressin. Vasopressin acts on the kidneys' collecting ducts to increase water reabsorption, allowing the body to conserve water. In the case of SSRI- or SNRI-associated vasopressin increase, excessive water reabsorption causes dilutional hyponatremia.

Hypothyroidism: Hypothyroidism can lead to decreased renal blood flow, reduced glomerular filtration rate (GFR), and tubule reabsorption dysfunction, impairing the kidneys' ability to excrete water and sodium appropriately. This can result in water retention and dilution of sodium in the bloodstream, contributing to hyponatremia. Hypothyroidism has also been associated with the excess production of vasopressin.

Other Possible Causes: low sodium in the diet, excess magnesium and/or potassium supplements, oxytocin use in childbirth, severe vomiting, severe dehydration, excess progesterone supplementation, metabolic acidosis, anemia, mycotoxin exposure

an intensive care unit in 28.7%.[11]

Sodium levels <130 mmol/L in pregnancy are associated with increased birth complications.[12]

Treatment Strategies for Low Sodium

Diet

While processed foods are often high in sodium due to added salt for flavor and preservation, several natural foods also provide significant amounts of sodium. These include vegetables like celery, carrots, and spinach as well as fruits such as tomatoes and avocados. Additionally, dairy products like milk and cheese naturally contain sodium. Incorporating these natural sodium-rich foods into the diet can help increase sodium intake in a balanced and healthful way. Furthermore, individuals can naturally increase their dietary salt intake by seasoning meals with salt or using salt-containing condiments like soy sauce or sea salt.

Supplements

Consuming electrolyte-rich sports drinks or oral rehydration solutions may help restore electrolyte balance and increase serum sodium levels in cases of mild hyponatremia. These fluids contain a combination of sodium, potassium, and other electrolytes, which can help replenish lost electrolytes and promote hydration. Reverse osmosis (RO) water filtration systems are effective at removing contaminants, but they also strip water of essential minerals. While RO water is safe to drink, replenishing lost minerals may be important for individuals who rely heavily on it for hydration.

Additional Testing

comprehensive thyroid profile II; complete blood count (CBC); progesterone

References

1. Shrimanker I, Bhattarai S. Electrolytes. [Updated 2023 Jul 24]. In: StatPearls [Internet]. Treasure Island (FL): StatPearls Publishing; Jan 2023. www.ncbi.nlm.nih.gov/books/NBK541123

2. Macdonald, H.N. and Good, W. (1971), CHANGES IN PLASMA SODIUM, POTASSIUM AND CHLORIDE CONCENTRATIONS IN PREGNANCY AND THE PUERPERIUM, WITH PLASMA AND SERUM OSMOLALITY. BJOG: An International Journal of Obstetrics & Gynaecology, 78: 798–803. doi.org/10.1111/j.1471–0528.1971.tb00341.x

3. Schury MP, Adigun R. Sheehan Syndrome. [Updated 2022 Sep 5]. In: StatPearls [Internet]. Treasure Island (FL): StatPearls Publishing; 2023 Jan-. www.ncbi.nlm.nih.gov/books/NBK459166

4. Cheung KL, Lafayette RA. Renal physiology of pregnancy. Adv Chronic Kidney Dis. 2013 May;20(3):209–14. doi: 10.1053/j.ackd.2013.01.012. PMID: 23928384; PMCID: PMC4089195

5. Paszkowski T. Renaissance of the clinical applications of a progesterone. Gin Politec Project. 2011;19:41–47

6. Cheung KL, Lafayette RA. Renal physiology of pregnancy. Adv Chronic Kidney Dis. 2013 May;20(3):209–14. doi: 10.1053/j.ackd.2013.01.012. PMID: 23928384; PMCID: PMC4089195

7. Al Refaie A, Baldassini L, De Vita M, Gonnelli S, Caffarelli C. Vitamin D and adrenal gland: Myth or reality? A systematic review. Front Endocrinol (Lausanne). 2022 Oct 13;13:1001065. doi: 10.3389/fendo.2022.1001065. PMID: 36313775; PMCID: PMC9606701

8. Ahmed A. Fetomaternal Acid-Base Balance and Electrolytes during Pregnancy. Indian J Crit Care Med. 2021 Dec;25(Suppl 3):S193-S199. doi: 10.5005/jp-journals-10071–24030. PMID: 35615608; PMCID: PMC9108779

9. Matsuoka H. [Aldosterone and magnesium]. Clin Calcium. 2005 Feb;15(2):187–91. Japanese. PMID: 15692156

10. Huang CL, Kuo E. Mechanism of hypokalemia in magnesium deficiency. J Am Soc Nephrol. 2007 Oct;18(10):2649–52. doi: 10.1681/ASN.2007070792. Epub 2007 Sep 5. PMID: 17804670

11. Morton A, Lumchee M, Kumar S, Jarvis E. Pregnancy outcomes in women with hyponatraemia and preeclampsia: Case series and literature review. Pregnancy Hypertens. 2021 Dec;26:38–41. doi: 10.1016/j.preghy.2021.08.116. Epub 2021 Sep 1. PMID: 34496324

12. Thaker S. Recognizing and Avoiding Significant Maternal Hyponatremia. J South Asian Feder Obs Gynae 2020; 12 (2):100–103

13. Jessani N, Jehangir W, Behman D, Yousif A, Spiler IJ. Secondary adrenal insufficiency: an overlooked cause of hyponatremia. J Clin Med Res. 2015 Apr;7(4):286–8. doi: 10.14740/jocmr2041w. Epub 2015 Feb 9. PMID: 25699130; PMCID: PMC4330026

14. Leth-Møller KB, Hansen AH, Torstensson M, Andersen SE, Ødum L, Gislasson G, Torp-Pedersen C, Holm EA. Antidepressants and the risk of hyponatremia: a Danish register-based population study. BMJ Open. 2016 May 18;6(5):e011200. doi: 10.1136/bmjopen-2016–011200. PMID: 27194321; PMCID: PMC4874104

Potassium

The potassium test measures the concentration of potassium in the blood. It is an analyte found on the basic metabolic panel and comprehensive metabolic panel (CMP).

Only a small amount of potassium is found in the bloodstream. Potassium levels inside red blood cells are 15 to 20 times higher than serum levels.

The sodium-potassium adenosine triphosphatase pump is responsible for regulating the homeostasis between sodium and potassium, which moves sodium out of cells in exchange for potassium, which moves into the cells. This process requires magnesium. The filtration of potassium takes place at the glomerulus of the kidneys. Aldosterone increases potassium excretion from the kidneys.[1]

Pregnancy

During the first trimester, serum potassium levels may decrease slightly. This decrease is likely due to increased renal blood flow and glomerular filtration rate (GFR), which can lead to increased potassium excretion by the kidneys. This decrease slows in the second trimester and plateaus by 28 weeks, after which levels increase, reaching their peak near the end of pregnancy.

Postpartum

There are significant increases in plasma potassium and sodium concentrations in the first six weeks postpartum when plasma chloride concentration falls.[2]

STANDARD LAB RANGE: 3.5 – 5.2 mmol/L

Trimester	Standard Pregnancy Ranges	**Functional Pregnancy Ranges**
Preconception	3.5 – 5.2	**4 – 4.5**
First Trimester	3.6 – 5	**3.6 – 5**
Second Trimester	3.6 – 5	**3.6 – 5**
Third Trimester	3.6 – 5	**3.6 – 5**
Postpartum	3.5 – 5.2	**4 – 4.5**

Causes of Elevated Potassium

Elevated potassium occurs in <1% of pregnancies.[3]

High potassium levels >5 mmol/L during the first half of pregnancy are associated with a higher risk for the development of gestational diabetes mellitus (GDM) and severe preeclampsia.[4]

Adrenal Hypofunction: When aldosterone is low, potassium is high, calcium is high, and sodium is low.

Hemolysis: When red blood cells rupture, their intracellular contents, including potassium, are released into the surrounding fluid, increasing potassium levels in the bloodstream.

Hypothyroidism: Thyroid hormones play a role in regulating kidney function, including renal blood flow and glomerular filtration rate. In hypothyroidism, decreased thyroid hormone levels can lead to reduced renal blood flow and glomerular filtration rate, impairing the kidneys' ability to excrete potassium effectively. This can result in decreased potassium excretion and potentially elevated serum potassium levels (hyperkalemia). In hypothyroidism, alterations in hormone levels, including aldosterone, can disrupt electrolyte balance and contribute to changes in serum potassium levels.

Other Possible Causes: renal issues such as kidney infections, metabolic acidosis, dehydration, hyperventilation, certain medications (potassium-sparing diuretics angiotensin-converting enzyme (ACE) inhibitors, angiotensin II receptor blockers (ARBs), NSAIDS), recent blood transfusion, anemia, mycotoxin exposure

Treatment Strategies for Elevated Potassium

Determine the underlying cause of hyperkalemia to address it accordingly.

Diet

Hydration is key. Increase fluid intake to balance out electrolytes. High potassium is less about overconsumption and more about filtration or poor utilization. It has traditionally been recommended that those with elevated potassium and renal disease avoid potassium intake. This idea is shifting, as limiting dietary potassium has not been shown to change serum potassium levels and may cause more nutritional deficiencies since most potassium-rich foods are plant-based and rich in magnesium and vitamin K as well. The idea in dietary management may be more surrounding the correction of metabolic acidosis and renal disease or supporting normal function. (See Anion Gap Section.)

Additional Testing

complete blood count (CBC); iron and TIBC; ferritin; comprehensive thyroid profile II; reverse T3 (rT3); lactate dehydrogenase (LDH)

Causes of Low Potassium

Hypokalemia occurs when serum potassium levels are under 3.6 mmol/L.

Refeeding Syndrome: In cases of severe hyperemesis gravidarum and periods of starvation, increasing food intake quickly can result in refeeding syndrome. This causes a sudden decrease in potassium, magnesium, phosphorus, and calcium. Gradual increases in food are best for those with severe HG.[5]

Adrenal Hyperfunction: When aldosterone is elevated, potassium is low.

Magnesium Deficiency: Magnesium is required for adequate transport of potassium inside and outside of the cells. Most of the potassium is found within the cells, and in cases of magnesium deficiency, potassium gets "stuck" in the cells, so the serum levels are decreased with increasing sodium levels. Elevated sodium levels with low potassium and calcium levels can indicate magnesium deficiency.[6]

Other Possible Causes: diuretic use, malnutrition, excess sweating, licorice consumption, certain herbs that affect serum potassium due to diuretic properties (dandelion), hyperthyroidism, certain medications (asthma medications, laxatives), alcohol use, genetics, metabolic alkalosis, mycotoxin exposure

Treatment Strategies for Low Potassium

Diet

Consume fruits like bananas, oranges, and melons along with vegetables such as potatoes, sweet potatoes, and spinach. Legumes like beans and lentils, nuts, seeds, and potassium-enriched foods like certain cereals and bread can also be beneficial. Try to include a source of potassium in each meal and snack, and opt for cooking methods that preserve potassium content, such as steaming vegetables.

Supplementation

Use electrolyte supplements containing potassium at around 100 to 200 mg. If serum sodium is elevated, avoid sodium electrolyte supplements. Always combine with magnesium.

Additional Testing

complete blood count (CBC); comprehensive thyroid profile II; reverse T3 (rT3); thyroid peroxidase antibodies (TPOAb); thyroglobulin antibody (TgAb); thyroid receptor antibodies (TRAb); iron and TIBC; ferritin; toxin testing

References

1. Shrimanker I, Bhattarai S. Electrolytes. [Updated 2023 Jul 24]. In: StatPearls [Internet]. Treasure Island (FL): StatPearls Publishing; Jan 2023. www.ncbi.nlm.nih.gov/books/NBK541123

2. Macdonald, H.N. and Good, W. (1971), CHANGES IN PLASMA SODIUM, POTASSIUM AND CHLORIDE CONCENTRATIONS IN PREGNANCY AND THE PUERPERIUM, WITH PLASMA AND SERUM OSMOLALITY. BJOG: An International Journal of Obstetrics & Gynaecology, 78: 798–803. doi.org/10.1111/j.1471–0528.1971.tb00341.x

3. Yang CW, Li S, Dong Y. The Prevalence and Risk Factors of Hypokalemia in Pregnancy-Related Hospitalizations: A Nationwide Population Study. Int J Nephrol. 2021 Jun 28;2021:9922245. doi: 10.1155/2021/9922245. PMID: 34258064; PMCID: PMC8261188

4. Ahmed A. Fetomaternal Acid-Base Balance and Electrolytes during Pregnancy. Indian J Crit Care Med. 2021 Dec;25(Suppl 3):S193-S199. doi: 10.5005/jp-journals-10071–24030. PMID: 35615608; PMCID: PMC9108779

5. Wolak T, Sergienko R, Wiznitzer A, Ben Shlush L, Paran E, Sheiner E. Low potassium level during the first half of pregnancy is associated with lower risk for the development of gestational diabetes mellitus and severe preeclampsia. J Matern Fetal Neonatal Med. 2010 Sep;23(9):994–8. doi: 10.3109/14767050903544736. PMID: 20059438

6. Huang CL, Kuo E. Mechanism of hypokalemia in magnesium deficiency. J Am Soc Nephrol. 2007 Oct;18(10):2649-52. doi: 10.1681/ASN.2007070792. Epub 2007 Sep 5. PMID: 17804670.

Chloride

The chloride test measures the concentration of chloride in the blood. It is an analyte found on the basic metabolic panel and comprehensive metabolic panel (CMP).

Chloride is the primary anion in the body. It is also the most abundant electrolyte outside of the cells. It helps with regulating osmotic balance and pH. Chloride is commonly found in the diet as table salt with sodium (sodium chloride). It is needed for the formation of stomach acid (HCl).[1]

Chloride and bicarbonate are inversely related. The balance between them is maintained by the chloride shift process. Carbon dioxide (CO_2) is produced in tissues as a byproduct of normal metabolism. It dissolves in the solution of blood plasma and into red blood cells (RBC), where carbonic anhydrase catalyzes its hydration to carbonic acid (H_2CO_3). Carbonic acid then spontaneously dissociates to form bicarbonate ions (HCO_3^-) and a hydrogen ion (H^+). Cell membranes are generally impermeable to charged ions (H^+, HCO_3^-), but RBCs are able to exchange bicarbonate for chloride. Thus, the rise in intracellular bicarbonate leads to bicarbonate export and chloride intake. The term *chloride shift* refers to this exchange.[2]

Chloride and sodium levels should be parallel.

Pregnancy

Plasma chloride concentration and serum osmolality rise significantly from 10 to 37 weeks, but plasma osmolality falls below the serum value as pregnancy progresses, and this difference is significant at 37 weeks gestation.[3]

Postpartum

In the six weeks postpartum, chloride levels decrease as sodium and potassium increase.

STANDARD LAB RANGE: 96 – 106 mmol/L

Trimester	Standard Pregnancy Ranges	**Functional Pregnancy Ranges**
Preconception	96 – 106	**100 – 106**
First Trimester	101 – 105	**101 – 109**
Second Trimester	97 – 109	**101 – 109**
Third Trimester	97 – 109	**97 – 109**
Postpartum	96 – 106	**96 – 106**

Causes of Elevated Chloride

See the following sections: Anion Gap and Sodium.

Sodium and chloride are often increased and decreased together to maintain balance. When they are not, this could signal dysfunction. An inverse relationship may be normal postpartum.

Metabolic Acidosis: Metabolic acidosis is a condition in which the body is too acidic. This is often due to kidney dysfunction or a loss of bicarbonate in the body. (See Anion Gap Section.)

Elevated Sodium: Causes of elevated sodium can also cause elevated chloride. (See Sodium Section.)

Other Possible Causes: excess table salt intake, adrenal hyperfunction, dehydration, diarrhea, bladder dysfunction (urinary tract infection), dehydration, hyperparathyroidism, bromide exposure, anemia, progesterone deficiency

Treatment Strategies for Elevated Chloride

See the following sections: Anion Gap and Sod See the following sections: Anion Gap and Sodium.

Sodium and chloride are often increased and decreased together to maintain balance. When they are not, this could signal dysfunction. An inverse relationship may be normal postpartum.

Additional Testing

complete blood count (CBC); iron and TIBC; ferritin; urinalysis

Causes of Low Chloride

See the following sections: Anion Gap and Sodium.

Metabolic Alkalosis: Metabolic alkalosis is a condition in which the body is too alkaline. In pregnancy, this is most often caused by a loss of chloride-rich fluids through vomiting, but it can also be caused by irritable bowel syndrome (IBS) conditions with diarrhea. This can also be caused by an increased production of aldosterone.[4]

Low Sodium: Causes of decreased sodium can also cause decreased chloride.

Other Possible Causes: hypochlorhydria, high CO_2, renal dysfunction, adrenal hypofunction, metabolic alkalosis, kidney infections, nausea and vomiting in pregnancy, bowel dysfunction (IBS), hypothyroidism, liver disease

Treatment Strategies for Low Chloride

See the following sections: Anion Gap and Sodium.

Additional Testing

comprehensive thyroid panel II; urinalysis; comprehensive stool testing

References

1. Shrimanker I, Bhattarai S. Electrolytes. [Updated 2023 Jul 24]. In: StatPearls [Internet]. Treasure Island (FL): StatPearls Publishing; 2023 Jan-. www.ncbi.nlm.nih.gov/books/NBK541123

2. Mark Feldman, Beverly Dickson, Adjusted Plasma Chloride and Bicarbonate Concentrations: An Approach to Identifying Acid–Base Disorders, The Journal of Applied Laboratory Medicine, Volume 2, Issue 6, 1 May 2018, Pages 833–840. doi.org/10.1373/jalm.2017.024794

3. Macdonald, H.N. and Good, W. (1971), CHANGES IN PLASMA SODIUM, POTASSIUM AND CHLORIDE CONCENTRATIONS IN PREGNANCY AND THE PUERPERIUM, WITH PLASMA AND SERUM OSMOLALITY. BJOG: An International Journal of Obstetrics & Gynaecology, 78: 798–803. doi.org/10.1111/j.1471–0528.1971.tb00341.x

4. Ahmed A. Fetomaternal Acid-Base Balance and Electrolytes during Pregnancy. Indian J Crit Care Med. 2021 Dec;25(Suppl 3):S193-S199. doi: 10.5005/jp-journals-10071–24030. PMID: 35615608; PMCID: PMC9108779

Carbon Dioxide Total (CO_2)

The CO_2 test measures the concentration of bicarbonate (HCO_3^-) in the blood. It is an analyte found on the basic metabolic panel and comprehensive metabolic panel (CMP).

Approximately 95% of CO_2 is in the form of bicarbonate. Therefore, the CO_2 blood test is really a measure of the blood bicarbonate level.

CO_2 is the byproduct of cellular respiration. In normal metabolic function, glucose enters the citric acid cycle to be metabolized to make adenosine triphosphate (ATP) energy. This process requires H_20 (water), O_2 (oxygen), and glucose and is catalyzed by several enzymes that rely on B vitamins for function. CO_2 is one of the byproducts of this process. CO_2 is negatively charged and works as a base in the body to regulate pH.

The chloride shift is the process by which chloride and CO_2 are exchanged in red blood cells for oxygen and CO_2 transport. When CO_2 enters the plasma as a byproduct of cellular respiration, it dissolves and degrades to become bicarbonate. Red blood cells exchange this bicarbonate for chloride. When RBCs enter the lungs, the opposite occurs to release CO_2 for exhalation, adding chloride back into the RBCs.

Pregnancy

Normal gap metabolic acidosis results due to bicarbonate losses through the gut or kidneys with subsequent gain in chloride ions.[1] During pregnancy, and especially during labor, the maternal carbon dioxide level declines considerably.

Postpartum

Renal adaptations that cause increased excretion of bicarbonate during pregnancy are reversed, leading to the reabsorption of bicarbonate and a rise in CO_2.

STANDARD LAB RANGE: 20 – 29 mmol/L

Trimester	Standard Pregnancy Ranges	**Functional Pregnancy Ranges**
Preconception	20 – 29	**25 – 30**
First Trimester	18 – 26	**18 – 26**
Second Trimester	18 – 26	**18 – 26**
Third Trimester	18 – 26	**18 – 26**
Postpartum	20 – 29	**20 – 30**

Causes of Elevated Carbon Dioxide Total (CO_2)

See Anion Gap Section.

Metabolic Alkalosis: Metabolic alkalosis is a condition in which the body is too alkaline. In pregnancy, this is most often caused by a loss of chloride-rich fluids through vomiting, but it can also be caused by irritable bowel conditions with diarrhea. This condition can also be caused by an increased production of aldosterone. Metabolic alkalosis will present with decreased chloride, decreased calcium, decreased potassium, and a normal-to-increased blood urea nitrogen (BUN).

Other Possible Causes: fever, hot tubs or hot baths, excess vomiting, adrenal hyperfunction, respiratory issues such as asthma or acute illness, sleep apnea

Treatment Strategies for Elevated Carbon Dioxide Total (CO_2)

See Anion Gap Section.

Lifestyle

Because elevated CO_2 is more associated with physiological changes, it is important to address lifestyle adjustments that may be helpful. Breathing exercises, CPAP machines, and oxygen therapy may be useful. Identifying the underlying cause is key.

Additional Testing

complete blood count (CBC); sleep study

Causes of Low Carbon Dioxide Total (CO_2)

See Anion Gap Section.

Metabolic Acidosis: Metabolic acidosis is a condition in which the body is too acidic. It is often caused by kidney dysfunction or a loss of bicarbonate.

Vitamin B1 (Thiamine) Deficiency: Anion gap is generally increased, fasting glucose levels are normal to increased, hematocrit and hemoglobin are normal to decreased, and RBC thiamine is decreased. Serum carbon dioxide levels can serve as a valuable biomarker for assessing thiamine deficiency. Thiamine is an essential nutrient that plays a crucial role in various metabolic processes, particularly in carbohydrate metabolism and energy production. Carbonic anhydrase is a ubiquitous metalloenzyme that catalyzes the reversible hydration/dehydration of carbon dioxide. Thiamine seems to regulate this enzyme.[2 3]

When thiamine deficiency occurs, it can have a direct impact on serum CO_2 levels due to its influence on multiple physiological pathways. In thiamine deficiency, the body may shift toward anaerobic metabolism, where glucose is incompletely metabolized into lactic acid. The accumulation of lactic acid can subsequently disrupt the acid-base balance in the body, leading to a condition known as metabolic acidosis. In response to this acidosis, the body attempts to compensate by increasing the exhalation of CO_2 to help regulate pH levels, further contributing to elevated serum CO_2. The presence of a significantly elevated anion gap in blood tests can be indicative of metabolic acidosis associated with thiamine deficiency.

Other Possible Causes: diabetes, dehydration, hyperemesis gravidarum

Treatment Strategies for Low Carbon Dioxide Total (CO_2)

See Anion Gap Section.

Diet

A reduced carbohydrate diet is associated with reduced CO_2 levels. For some, increasing healthy carbohydrates may be important, as well as focusing on alkalizing foods. Meats and animal products are acidic and will increase blood acidity, so limiting these foods may be beneficial for some. The primary focus, though, should be on increasing vitamin B1 (thiamine) in the diet. The best sources of dietary thiamine are legumes (lentils, black beans, pinto beans, split peas), whole grains (oats, fortified white rice, millet, wheat, sorghum, buckwheat), nuts and seeds (pistachios, chickpeas, flaxseeds, pine nuts, hemp seeds). (See Anion Gap Section.)

Supplementation

In cases of severe dehydration, IV nutrition therapy with thiamine and fluids may be beneficial. Some studies show that treatment with sodium bicarbonate can help improve metabolic acidosis.

Additional Testing

complete blood count (CBC); oral glucose tolerance test (OGTT)

References

1. Ahmed A. Fetomaternal Acid-Base Balance and Electrolytes during Pregnancy. Indian J Crit Care Med. 2021 Dec;25(Suppl 3):S193-S199. doi: 10.5005/jp-journals-10071–24030. PMID: 35615608; PMCID: PMC9108779

2. Özdemir ZÖ, Şentürk M, Ekinci D. Inhibition of mammalian carbonic anhydrase isoforms I, II and VI with thiamine and thiamine-like molecules. J Enzyme Inhib Med Chem. 2013 Apr;28(2):316–9. doi: 10.3109/14756366.2011.637200. Epub 2011 Dec 6. PMID: 22145674

3. Bager P, Hvas C, Rud C, Dahlerup J. Letter: future studies of high-dose thiamine should consider whether its effects on fatigue are related to the inhibition of carbonic anhydrase isoenzymes. Authors' reply. Aliment Pharmacol Ther. 2021 Apr;53(7):853–854. doi: 10.1111/apt.16293. PMID: 33709399

Anion Gap

The anion gap is a calculation of electrolyte balance. It is occasionally found on a comprehensive metabolic panel or calculated based on the values of electrolytes.

This calculation is used to determine whether the body is acidic or alkaline.

$(Na^+ + K^+) - (Cl^- + HCO_3^-)$ = Anion Gap

High Anion Gap = Acidosis

Low Anion Gap = Alkalosis

Pregnancy

Nausea and vomiting in the first trimester of pregnancy predispose women to a relatively low anion gap compared to the second and third trimester. There is a slight rise in the anion gap during pregnancy, as it is a natural state of acidosis.

Postpartum

The anion gap typically decreases in the postpartum period. After childbirth, these pregnancy-related physiological changes gradually resolve. The hemodilution that occurred during pregnancy starts to normalize as plasma volume returns to pre-pregnancy levels over a few weeks to months.

STANDARD LAB RANGE: 8 – 16 mmol/L

Trimester	Standard Pregnancy Ranges	**Functional Pregnancy Ranges**
Preconception	8–16	**8–16**
First Trimester	10–20	**10–20**
Second Trimester	10–18	**10–18**
Third Trimester	10–18	**10–18**
Postpartum	8–16	**8–16**

Causes of Elevated Anion Gap

Metabolic Acidosis: Metabolic acidosis is a condition in which the body is too acidic. This is often due to kidney dysfunction or a loss of bicarbonate in the body. Serum chloride increases, sodium decreases, and there is decreased calcium, increased potassium, decreased CO_2, and an increased anion gap. There may also be a decrease in RBC magnesium and RBC thiamine. You may also see a decreased alkaline phosphatase with a positive oral zinc test. BUN may also be increased.

Starvation Ketosis: In pregnancy, women are more sensitive to fasting due to the metabolic shift to insulin resistance in combination with placental lactogen and glucagon secretion. There is an increased breakdown of fatty acids that leads to the production of ketones, which increase blood acidity and the anion gap.[1] This is generally associated with women attempting intermittent fasting or not eating enough during pregnancy, especially in the third trimester, or those with vomiting episodes in the third trimester. One study found that 92% of women with prolonged labor had ketones in their urine, indicating systemic acidosis due to ketosis.[2]

Vitamin B1 (Thiamine) Deficiency: Anion gap is generally increased, fasting glucose levels are normal to increased, hematocrit and hemoglobin are normal to decreased, and RBC thiamine is decreased.

Other Possible Causes: lactic acid buildup, acute dehydration, magnesium deficiency, diabetes, thyroid dysfunction, anemia

Treatment Strategies for Elevated Anion Gap

Diet

Managing metabolic acidosis through dietary strategies involves a combination of increasing alkaline-forming foods, limiting acidic foods, and maintaining adequate hydration. Prioritizing fruits and vegetables such as leafy greens, cruciferous vegetables, citrus fruits, melons, and berries can help buffer excess acidity in the body. Increase alkaline foods such as leafy greens like spinach and kale, cruciferous vegetables such as broccoli and Brussels sprouts, and citrus fruits like lemons and oranges.

Additionally, foods like avocado, almonds, seeds, and legumes offer alkaline-forming nutrients such as healthy fats, protein, and fiber and essential minerals like potassium and magnesium. Reducing fried and processed foods will also help alkalize the body.

Supplementation

In cases of magnesium deficiency, supplementing with magnesium may help balance electrolytes and decrease anion gap. Baking soda (aka sodium bicarbonate) may help balance anion gap if lactic acid buildup is a potential factor. Studies have shown a benefit to the use of sodium bicarbonate in labor complications associated with acidosis, such as labor dystocia.[3]

Additional Testing

comprehensive thyroid profile II; complete blood count (CBC); urinalysis

Causes of Low Anion Gap

Metabolic Alkalosis: Metabolic alkalosis is a condition in which the body is too alkaline. This can also be caused by an increased production of aldosterone. Metabolic alkalosis presents with decreased chloride, increased CO_2, decreased calcium, decreased potassium, decreased anion gap, and a normal-to-increased BUN. The two primary mechanisms responsible for metabolic alkalosis are loss of chloride-rich fluid from the body through vomiting, diarrhea, or diuretic use or factors causing increased aldosterone levels.

Other Possible Causes: protein-deficient diets, low albumin, hyponatremia, excess vomiting in pregnancy, adrenal hyperfunction, excessive antacid use, hypochlorhydria

Treatment Strategies for Low Anion Gap

Diet

Staying well-hydrated is crucial for maintaining electrolyte balance. Dehydration can lead to electrolyte imbalances and may affect the anion gap. Consume a well-balanced diet that includes an appropriate mix of macronutrients (carbohydrates, proteins, and fats) and micronutrients (vitamins and minerals). This helps maintain overall health, including acid-base balance. If sodium is low, add salt to the diet and increase electrolytes. Increase protein intake. When the anion gap is low, the minimum goal should be 100 grams of protein per day.

Supplementation

Electrolyte supplements that include sodium may be helpful. If metabolic alkalosis is associated with calcium deficiency or hypocalcemia, calcium supplements may be considered.

Additional Testing

comprehensive thyroid profile II; urinalysis

References

1. Ahmed A. Fetomaternal Acid-Base Balance and Electrolytes during Pregnancy. Indian J Crit Care Med. 2021 Dec;25(Suppl 3):S193-S199. doi: 10.5005/jp-journals-10071–24030. PMID: 35615608; PMCID: PMC9108779

2. Ekanem EI, Umoiyoho A, Inyang-Otu A. Study of electrolyte changes in patients with prolonged labour in ikot ekpene, a rural community in niger delta region of Nigeria. ISRN Obstet Gynecol. 2012;2012:430265. doi: 10.5402/2012/430265

3. Wiberg-Itzel E, Wray S, Åkerud H. A randomized controlled trial of a new treatment for labor dystocia. J Matern Fetal Neonatal Med. 2018 Sep;31(17):2237–2244. doi: 10.1080/14767058.2017.1339268. Epub 2017 Jun 22. PMID: 28587493

Calcium, Total

The calcium test measures the concentration of total calcium in the blood. It is an analyte found on the basic metabolic panel and comprehensive metabolic panel (CMP).

Calcium metabolism and function are regulated by parathyroid hormones, calcitonin, and vitamin D3, as well as the bones, kidneys, and small intestines. Around 99% of all the body's calcium is stored in the bones; <1% is found in the bloodstream.

Calcitonin regulates the balance of calcium and phosphorus. Calcitonin and calcium have an inverse relationship. Calcitonin reduces calcium by blocking its breakdown and preventing the kidneys from reabsorbing it.

Parathyroid hormones (PTH) are produced when calcium levels are low. PTH raises calcium levels by releasing calcium from the bones and increases the production of calcitriol, the hormone form of vitamin D3.

Calcitriol increases small-intestine calcium absorption and decreases calcium loss through the kidneys.

Calcium is found in the bloodstream in three forms:

- Complex: calcium-bound to citrate, oxalate, carbonate, and phosphate
- Ionized: free ionic calcium
- Protein-Bound: mostly bound to albumin and some to globulin

Ionized and complex calcium are filtered by the kidneys, while protein-bound calcium is not.

Pregnancy

During pregnancy, calcium regulation changes to benefit the growth of the baby. In the first trimester, calcitonin increases and remains elevated throughout pregnancy. PTH is suppressed in the first trimester but returns to normal ranges in the third trimester. The placenta increases the production of calcitriol, which increases calcium absorption in the gut by two- or three-fold, as well as a hormone called parathyroid hormone-related peptide, which pushes calcium transfer to the baby. Serum-ionized calcium levels are unchanged in pregnancy, but there is a decrease in serum total calcium due to a decrease in serum albumin and the bound fraction of calcium, brought about by volume expansion in pregnancy.[1]

Postpartum

PTH levels increase shortly after childbirth. Despite the rise in PTH, serum calcium levels may initially drop due to the abrupt cessation of placental calcium transfer to the fetus and the loss of calcium-rich colostrum during breastfeeding. Serum calcium levels continue to decrease during the first few days postpartum, reaching their lowest point around the third or fourth day after delivery. In breastfeeding mothers, this period is often referred to as "postpartum hypocalcemia." Animal studies found that lower calcium levels are associated with better milk production. A more significant drop is associated with vitamin D deficiency. As lactation becomes established and hormonal fluctuations stabilize, serum calcium levels gradually return to normal or near-normal levels over the following weeks. For most women, serum calcium levels typically normalize by around six weeks postpartum.

STANDARD LAB RANGE: 8.7 – 10.2 mg/dL

Trimester	Standard Pregnancy Ranges	**Functional Pregnancy Ranges**
Preconception	8.7 – 10.2	**9.4 – 10**
First Trimester	8.8 – 10.6	**8.8 – 10.6**
Second Trimester	8.2 – 9	**8.2 – 9**
Third Trimester	8.2 – 9.7	**8.2 – 9.7**
Postpartum	8.7 – 10.2	**8.2 – 10**

Causes of Elevated Calcium, Total

Parathyroid Hyperfunction: Serum calcium is increased, with high PTH and phosphatase and lower serum phosphorus, chloride, magnesium, and zinc. This is a serious issue that should be addressed by a maternal-fetal medicine physician. Usually, this is due to parathyroid tumors.

Metabolic Acidosis: Acidosis reduces calcium-protein binding, increasing free calcium. Acidosis also increases the release of calcium from the bones. Assess albumin and ionized calcium levels. (See Anion Gap Section.)

Heavy Metal Exposure: With certain heavy metals, calcium will be elevated and phosphorus low.

In women with hyperparathyroidism, serum calcium levels are usually only mildly elevated during pregnancy. A significant proportion of cases go undiagnosed. Mild hypercalcemia in gestational hyperparathyroidism is generally not associated with an increased risk of obstetrical complications.[2] However, severe maternal hypercalcemia is associated with life-threatening complications for both mom and baby.

Other Possible Causes: acute dehydration, certain medications (thiazide diuretic), vitamin D overdose, hyperthyroidism

Treatment Strategies for Elevated Calcium, Total

Diet

If labs show dehydration as a cause, increase fluid intake through liquids and hydrating foods.

Supplements

If vitamin D is elevated, remove supplementation. If dehydration is the cause, IV hydration may be beneficial.

Additional Testing

parathyroid hormone (PTH); vitamin D, 25-hydroxy (25-hydroxycalciferol, 25OH-D); comprehensive thyroid panel II; reverse T3 (rT3); thyroid peroxidase antibodies (TPOAb); thyroglobulin antibody (TgAb); thyroid receptor antibodies (TRAb); heavy metal testing

Causes of Low Calcium, Total

The most common cause of hypocalcemia in pregnancy is poor oral calcium intake and vitamin D3 deficiency.

In some countries, hypocalcemia can be as high as 70% of pregnancies.[3] There is also a link between low calcium and gestational hypertension.

There is an association between ionized calcium levels and the severity of postpartum hemorrhaging.[4]

Hypothyroidism: Hypothyroidism affects calcium metabolism, and it is well documented that hypothyroidism is associated with low serum calcium and phosphorous.[5]

Low-Protein Diet/Metabolism: Low albumin can cause low serum calcium due to a decrease in protein-bound calcium and an increase in ionized and complex calcium, which is easily excreted through the kidneys. Low albumin and low calcium can go together.[6] This is generally associated with slow bone turnover and lower PTH production. If this is the case, test ionized calcium with interpretation.

Vitamin D Deficiency: Vitamin D is required for the intestinal absorption of calcium; when vitamin D is low, calcium is low.[7]

Magnesium Dysfunction: Magnesium regulates the production and release of parathyroid hormones. Both low and high levels of magnesium have been shown to affect the production of PTH and cause hypocalcemia.[8] Decreased magnesium causes impaired magnesium-dependent adenyl cyclase generation of cyclic adenosine monophosphate (cAMP), decreasing parathyroid hormone (PTH) release. Because of the drop in PTH, calcium levels also drop.[9] On the other hand, excess magnesium, in the form of magnesium sulfate found in antacids, suppresses the secretion of PTH, contributing to low calcium.[10]

Metabolic Alkalosis: Metabolic alkalosis increases calcium binding to albumin and decreases ionized calcium.

Progesterone Deficiency: Low progesterone can cause low parathyroid hormone production.

Other Possible Causes: hypoparathyroidism, hypochlorhydria, inflammatory bowel diseases, acute pancreatitis

Treatment Strategies for Low Calcium, Total

Diet

Dietary intake of calcium is often low in the prenatal diet. Proper cooking of foods can help to increase calcium absorption. Calcium-rich foods tend to be those that are high in antinutrients like phytates. Legumes should be soaked, and leafy greens like beet greens should be blanched.

Supplementation

Calcium supplementation ≥1 g/day is associated with a significant reduction in the risk of preeclampsia, particularly for women with low calcium diets. The WHO recommends 1.5 to 2 grams of calcium daily for pregnant women with low dietary calcium intake.[11] [12] Taking calcium with food in dosages of 500 mg or less increases absorption, and some studies show that 500 mg is just as effective as the higher doses of calcium. Absorption also requires adequate vitamin D3 levels. There are several forms of calcium supplements available. Calcium carbonate is the most commonly found form. It is the cheapest and contains the most elemental calcium (40%), but it requires stomach acid for absorption. Therefore, it is best taken with meals to enhance absorption. However, it may cause gastrointestinal side effects like constipation or gas in some individuals.

Calcium citrate and calcium citrate malate do not need stomach acid for absorption, making them a better option for individuals with low stomach acid or those taking acid-reducing medications. They contain less elemental calcium per dose compared to calcium carbonate (about 21%) but tend to be more easily absorbed. They can be taken with or without food.

Additional Testing

vitamin D, 25-hydroxy (25-hydroxycalciferol, 25OH-D); comprehensive thyroid profile II; ionized calcium; parathyroid hormone (PTH); progesterone; comprehensive stool testing

References

1. Ahmed A. Fetomaternal Acid-Base Balance and Electrolytes during Pregnancy. Indian J Crit Care Med. 2021 Dec;25(Suppl 3):S193-S199. doi: 10.5005/jp-journals-10071–24030. PMID: 35615608; PMCID: PMC9108779

2. Dania Hirsch, Vered Kopel, Varda Nadler, Sigal Levy, Yoel Toledano, Gloria Tsvetov, Pregnancy Outcomes in Women With Primary Hyperparathyroidism, The Journal of Clinical Endocrinology & Metabolism, Volume 100, Issue 5, 1 May 2015, Pages 2115–2122. doi.org/10.1210/jc.2015–1110

3. Almaghamsi A, Almalki MH, Buhary BM. Hypocalcemia in Pregnancy: A Clinical Review Update. Oman Med J. 2018 Nov;33(6):453–462. doi: 10.5001/omj.2018.85. PMID: 30410686; PMCID: PMC6206424

4. Epstein D, Solomon N, Korytny A, Marcusohn E, Freund Y, Avrahami R, Neuberger A, Raz A, Miller A. Association between ionised calcium and severity of postpartum haemorrhage: a retrospective cohort study. Br J Anaesth. 2021 May;126(5):1022–1028. doi: 10.1016/j.bja.2020.11.020. Epub 2020 Dec 17. PMID: 33341222

5. Jat RK, Panwar AK, Agarwal P, Sharma C, Bansal DP, Pareek A, Tyagi A, Mathur M. Assessment of Serum Minerals in Subclinical Hypothyroid and Overt Hypothyroid Patients. Cureus. 2021 Aug 6;13(8):e16944. doi: 10.7759/cureus.16944. PMID: 34513512; PMCID: PMC8418816

6. Tinawi M (January 01, 2021) Disorders of Calcium Metabolism: Hypocalcemia and Hypercalcemia. Cureus 13(1): e12420. doi:10.7759/cureus.12420

7. Manappallil RG, Krishnan R, Veetil PP, Nambiar H, Karadan U, Anil R, Josephine B. Hypocalcemic Seizure Due to Vitamin D Deficiency. Indian J Crit Care Med. 2020 Sep;24(9):882–884. doi: 10.5005/jp-journals-10071–23586. PMID: 33132579; PMCID: PMC7584818

8. Vetter T, Lohse MJ. Magnesium and the parathyroid. Curr Opin Nephrol Hypertens. 2002 Jul;11(4):403–10. doi: 10.1097/00041552–200207000-00006. PMID: 12105390

9. Gragossian A, Bashir K, Bhutta BS, et al. Hypomagnesemia. [Updated 2022 Nov 4]. In: StatPearls [Internet]. Treasure Island (FL): StatPearls Publishing; 2023 Jan-. www.ncbi.nlm.nih.gov/books/NBK500003

10. ALLEN W. ROOT, FRANK B. DIAMOND, CHAPTER 17: Disorders of Mineral Homeostasis in the Newborn, Infant, Child, and Adolescent, Editor(s): Mark A. Sperling, Pediatric Endocrinology (Third Edition), W.B. Saunders, 2008, Pages 686–769, ISBN 9781416040903, doi.org/10.1016/B978–141604090-3.50022–3. (www.sciencedirect.com/science/article/pii/B9781416040903500223)

11. Hofmeyr GJ, Lawrie TA, Atallah AN, Duley L, Torloni MR. Calcium supplementation during pregnancy for preventing hypertensive disorders and related problems. Cochrane Database Syst Rev. 2014 Jun 24;(6):CD001059. doi: 10.1002/14651858.CD001059.pub4. Update in: Cochrane Database Syst Rev. 2018 Oct 01;10:CD001059. PMID: 24960615.

12. Gomes F, Ashorn P, Askari S, Belizan JM, Boy E, Cormick G, Dickin KL, Driller-Colangelo AR, Fawzi W, Hofmeyr GJ, Humphrey J, Khadilkar A, Mandlik R, Neufeld LM, Palacios C, Roth DE, Shlisky J, Sudfeld CR, Weaver C, Bourassa MW. Calcium supplementation for the prevention of hypertensive disorders of pregnancy: current evidence and programmatic considerations. Ann N Y Acad Sci. 2022 Apr;1510(1):52–67. doi: 10.1111/nyas.14733. Epub 2022 Jan 8. PMID: 35000200; PMCID: PMC9306576.

Blood Urea Nitrogen (BUN)

Blood urea nitrogen (BUN) is a blood test that measures the amount of nitrogen in the form of urea in the bloodstream. It is an analyte found on the basic metabolic panel and comprehensive metabolic panel (CMP).

Urea is a waste product produced in the liver when the body breaks down proteins, and it is excreted by the kidneys through urine. BUN levels are used as a marker of kidney function and can provide valuable information about the health of the kidneys and other metabolic processes in the body.

The kidneys filter blood urea nitrogen (BUN) and other waste products through a complex process involving specialized structures and filtration mechanisms. The initial filtration of BUN and other waste products occurs in tiny, tuft-like clusters of capillaries known as the glomeruli. There are approximately one million glomeruli in each kidney. Blood enters the glomerulus through the afferent arteriole, which carries blood to the glomerulus. Inside the glomerulus, the blood is under high pressure due to the narrowing of the efferent arteriole (the blood vessel that exits the glomerulus). This high pressure is crucial for the filtration process.

Within the glomerulus, there is a filtration barrier that consists of three main layers: endothelium, basement membrane, and podocytes. Blood is filtered through this three-layer barrier, which selectively allows small molecules such as water and waste products like BUN to pass through while restricting the passage of larger molecules like proteins. BUN is a small waste product derived from the breakdown of proteins, so it easily passes through this filtration barrier.

As the blood is filtered in the glomerulus, a filtrate is formed in Bowman's capsule, a structure that surrounds each glomerulus. The filtrate contains water, electrolytes, waste products (including BUN), and other substances. After filtration, the filtrate flows through the renal tubules, including the proximal convoluted tubule, loop of Henle, distal convoluted tubule, and collecting duct. Throughout this journey, important substances like glucose, electrolytes (sodium, potassium), and water are actively reabsorbed into the bloodstream, while waste products may be secreted into the tubules.

The concentration of BUN in the urine can be influenced by reabsorption and secretion processes. In cases of kidney dysfunction or disease, these processes may be disrupted, leading to elevated BUN levels in the urine. The final filtrate, which now contains waste products like BUN, is excreted as urine. The urine eventually drains into the renal pelvis, enters the ureter, and is transported to the urinary bladder for storage until it is expelled from the body.

Pregnancy

The increase in glomerular filtration during pregnancy results in more efficient filtering of waste products, including BUN, from the bloodstream. Clearance increases in the first trimester and continues throughout pregnancy, only increasing again postpartum.[1] As a result, BUN levels may decrease or remain within the lower end of the normal reference range.

Postpartum

After childbirth, there is a gradual normalization of blood volume. This can lead to a concentration of blood constituents, including BUN, and result in an increase in BUN levels postpartum. The increase in BUN levels postpartum typically occurs within the first few days to a week after giving birth and normalizes by six weeks postpartum.

STANDARD LAB RANGE: 6 – 24 mg/dL

Trimester	Standard Pregnancy Ranges	**Functional Pregnancy Ranges**
Preconception	6 – 24	**10 – 15**
First Trimester	7 – 12	**7 – 9**
Second Trimester	3 – 13	**3 – 9**
Third Trimester	3 – 11	**3 – 9**
Postpartum	6 – 24	**10 – 24**

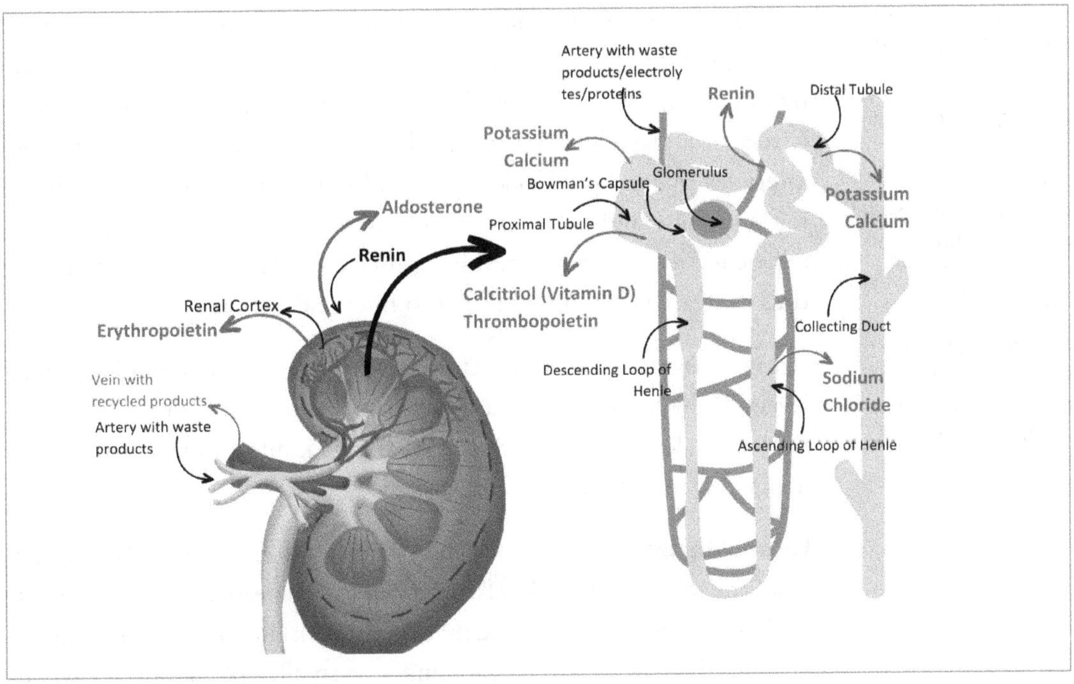

Figure 8:

Ascending Loop of Henle: reabsorption of sodium and chloride in response to aldosterone; potassium excretion; calcium regulation

Collecting Duct: Concentrates urea and regulates reabsorption of urea into loop of Henle

Descending Loop of Henle: reabsorption of water

Distal Tubule: regulates pH and electrolyte balance; stimulates production of renin and aldosterone at the macula densa

Glomerulus: filters small particles from the blood, plus urea and creatinine

Proximal Tubule: reabsorbs electrolytes, water, glucose, proteins, and nutrients, and adjusts pH; where calcitriol is produced in response to calcium levels; calcium levels regulated in both the proximal and distal tubules; thrombopoietin is produced

Causes of Elevated Blood Urea Nitrogen (BUN)

See BUN/Creatinine Ratio Section.

—

In contrast to normal pregnancy, where blood urea nitrogen (BUN) and creatinine decrease, preeclamptic women have BUN and creatinine levels like

Renal Dysfunction: An increase in BUN indicates a dysfunction in the kidneys' ability to excrete urea. Renal dysfunction may present with decreased estimated glomerular filtration rate (eGFR); elevated creatinine, albumin, calcium, sodium, and uric acid; a decrease or increase in WBC; and lower hemoglobin and hematocrit.

nonpregnant women, due to reduced GFR.[2]

BUN ≥9 mg/dL can be a biomarker of preeclampsia, generally with elevated serum creatinine and uric acid levels.[3 4]

Elevated BUN in the first trimester is associated with an increased risk of developing GDM.[5]

Progesterone Deficiency: As aldosterone increases, there is a parallel rise in progesterone, which protects the pregnant woman from hypokalemia. Progesterone has vasodilatory effects, which means it relaxes and widens blood vessels, including the renal arteries and arterioles that supply blood to the kidneys. This vasodilation reduces renal vascular resistance and increases renal blood flow. If there is a deficiency in progesterone, this can decrease glomerular filtration and thus decrease the kidneys' ability to filter and excrete urea.

Urinary Tract Infections (UTIs): UTIs can potentially affect BUN levels. Dehydration and changes in protein metabolism due to infection can elevate BUN. In severe UTIs, kidney inflammation and damage can cause renal dysfunction.

Hypochlorhydria: There is an indirect relationship between low stomach acid and BUN levels. Stomach acid is needed for the digestion of dietary proteins. It helps denature proteins and activates pepsin, an enzyme that breaks down proteins into smaller peptides. In cases of chronic low stomach acid, protein digestion may be impaired, and this can lead to undigested protein reaching the small intestine. Undigested proteins in the small intestine can serve as a source of nutrition for certain bacteria. When these bacteria metabolize undigested protein, they produce ammonia as a metabolic byproduct.

Ammonia can be absorbed into the bloodstream and transported to the liver for conversion into urea, which is then excreted by the kidneys. Increased bacterial metabolism of undigested protein can lead to higher ammonia production and subsequent increased urea production. Urea is filtered by the kidneys and excreted in the urine. If the kidneys are functioning correctly, increased urea production from bacterial metabolism of undigested protein may result in higher BUN levels, as the kidneys work to clear the excess urea from the blood.

Dehydration: Dehydration can lead to an elevated BUN level because it affects the concentration of urea in the blood. In cases of dehydration, you would typically see concentrated values on the complete blood count (CBC) as well as the CMP, including higher RBC, WBC, and platelet counts, higher electrolytes, elevated creatinine, higher alanine aminotransferase (ALT)(SGPT) and aspartate aminotransferase (AST)(SGOT), and even elevated serum fasting glucose, but with a lower CO_2.

Preeclampsia/Eclampsia (PE): Preeclampsia can cause damage to the small blood vessels (capillaries) in the glomeruli of the kidneys. When these glomerular capillaries are damaged, kidney function is impaired, leading to decreased filtration and clearance of waste products such as urea. This can result in elevated BUN levels. Preeclampsia is associated with vasoconstriction, or the narrowing of blood vessels, which reduces blood flow to various organs, including the kidneys. Reduced renal blood flow can lead to reduced glomerular filtration and less efficient waste product removal, further contributing to elevated BUN.

Hyperglycemia: There is a connection between elevated glucose levels and elevated BUN. Elevated blood glucose levels can lead to increased oxidative stress and inflammation in the glomeruli. These changes can cause thickening of the glomerular filtration basement membrane and alter its permeability, affecting the filtration process and GFR.[6]

Mycotoxin Exposure: Some mycotoxins, such as ochratoxins, have nephrotoxic effects and can impair kidney function. Elevated BUN and creatinine levels may be observed in the CMP as indicators of kidney dysfunction associated with mycotoxin exposure.

Other Possible Causes: liver damage, toxin exposure, gastrointestinal bleeding, certain medications (corticosteroids, antibiotics, nonsteroidal anti-inflammatories), infection

Treatment Strategies for Elevated Blood Urea Nitrogen (BUN)

See BUN/Creatinine Ratio Section.

Diet

In cases of impaired kidney function, reducing protein intake, particularly certain protein sources like red meat, may be necessary. In pregnancy, especially late in pregnancy, this may be difficult, as the needs for protein are increased. It may be a difficult nutrition game to increase required proteins while improving both liver metabolism of proteins as well as supporting kidney function to reduce inflammation.

Animal-based proteins, especially in organ meats and processed meats, can be high in phosphorus. High phosphorus intake is a concern in kidney disease, as impaired kidneys may struggle to excrete excess phosphorus. Plant-based proteins generally have lower phosphorus content, as the phosphorus is locked in the phytate form. Animal-based proteins can contribute to dietary acid load, as they metabolize into sulfuric and phosphoric acids. .

Supplementation

Alpha-lipoic acid is an antioxidant that may help protect kidney cells from damage and reduce oxidative stress.[7] Coenzyme Q10 (CoQ10, aka ubiquinone) has also been shown to reduce BUN and creatinine levels in cases of kidney dysfunction.[8] CoQ10 is an antioxidant that may help protect kidney cells from damage and support overall kidney function. The dose used in these studies was 50 mg/kg. N-acetyl cysteine (NAC) and silymarin (milk thistle) help patients with preeclampsia to improve kidney and hepatic dysfunction.[9] NAC is more effective at reducing BUN and creatinine levels, while milk thistle is more effective at lowering elevated liver enzymes.[10]

Additional Testing

complete blood count (CBC); urinalysis; protein and creatinine, random urine; protein, total, 24-hour urine

Causes of Low Blood Urea Nitrogen (BUN)

See BUN/Creatinine Ratio Section.

Protein-Deficient Diets: BUN is a byproduct of protein metabolism, so when an individual has a low-protein diet or is not consuming sufficient protein, BUN levels can decrease. This is more common in those with gut absorption issues. Protein requirements increase as the pregnancy progresses. The RDA for protein during the second and third trimesters is generally around 71 grams per day for most pregnant individuals. However, this can vary based on factors like pre-pregnancy weight and overall nutritional status. Most women need more than 100 grams of protein per day to meet the needs of pregnancy.

Zinc Deficiency: Zinc's role in protein metabolism can affect BUN levels indirectly.

Other Possible Causes: adrenal hypofunction, hypothyroidism, overhydration (IV fluids), liver disease, inflammatory bowel disease (celiac disease, Crohn's), vitamin B6 (pyridoxine) deficiency

Treatment Strategies for Low Blood Urea Nitrogen (BUN)

See BUN/Creatinine Ratio Section.

Diet

If low BUN is due to insufficient dietary protein, increasing protein intake may be necessary. Include high-quality protein sources in the diet such as lean meats, poultry, fish, eggs, dairy products, legumes, nuts, and seeds.

For more information, please visit my website and download my e-book *Protein Packed Pregnancy.*

Supplementation

In some cases, protein supplements or protein-rich nutritional shakes may be recommended to boost protein intake, especially if it's challenging to meet protein requirements through whole foods.

Additional Testing

comprehensive thyroid profile II; urinalysis; oral zinc tolerance test; comprehensive stool testing

References

1. Gülay Logoglu, Ufuk Bısak, Fatma Tuncay Özgünen, Tuncay Özgünen, Ayşe Doğan. Endogenous Creatinine and Blood Urea Nitrogen Clearances in Normal Pregnancy. Med J Islamic World Acad Sci. 1990; 3(4): 348–353

2. Müller-Deile J, Schiffer M. Preeclampsia from a renal point of view: Insides into disease models, biomarkers and therapy. World J Nephrol. 2014 Nov 6;3(4):169–81. doi: 10.5527/wjn.v3.i4.169. PMID: 25374810; PMCID: PMC4220349

3. Tesfa E, Munshea A, Nibret E, Mekonnen D, Sinishaw MA, Gizaw ST. Maternal serum uric acid, creatinine and blood urea levels in the prediction of preeclampsia among pregnant women attending ANC and delivery services at Bahir Dar city public hospitals, northwest Ethiopia: A case-control study. Heliyon. 2022 Oct 14;8(10):e11098. doi: 10.1016/j.heliyon.2022.e11098. PMID: 36303922; PMCID: PMC9593197

4. Ries A, Kopelman JN, Macri C. Laboratory testing for preeclampsia: result trends and screening recommendations. Mil Med. 2000 Jul;165(7):546–8. PMID: 10920656

5. Feng P, Wang G, Yu Q, Zhu W, Zhong C. First-trimester blood urea nitrogen and risk of gestational diabetes mellitus. J Cell Mol Med. 2020 Feb;24(4):2416–2422. doi: 10.1111/jcmm.14924. Epub 2020 Jan 10. PMID: 31925909; PMCID: PMC7028843

6. Ziyadeh FN. Renal tubular basement membrane and collagen type IV in diabetes mellitus. Kidney Int. 1993 Jan;43(1):114–20. doi: 10.1038/ki.1993.19. PMID: 8433550

7. Petca A, Bot M, Maru N, Calo IG, Borislavschi A, Dumitrascu MC, Petca RC, Sandru F, Zvanca ME. Benefits of α-lipoic acid in high-risk pregnancies (Review). Exp Ther Med. 2021 Nov;22(5):1232. doi: 10.3892/etm.2021.10666. Epub 2021 Aug 31. PMID: 34539828; PMCID: PMC8438679

8. Zhao, S., Wu, W., Liao, J. et al. Molecular mechanisms underlying the renal protective effects of coenzyme Q10 in acute kidney injury. Cell Mol Biol Lett 27, 57 (2022). doi.org/10.1186/s11658–022-00361–5

9. Sepideh Shabani; Fahimeh Kaveh Baghbahadorani; Farahnaz Jazaeri; Foruzan Ganji; Nayyereh Sadat Mortazavi; Leila Mahmoudnia. "The Effects of Silymarin and N-Acetylcysteine on Liver and Kidney Dysfunction in Subjects with Severe Preeclampsia." Journal of Iranian Medical Council, 4, 3, 2021, 173–182. dx.doi.org/10.18502/jimc.v4i3.7220

10. Badr A, Fouad D, Attia H. Insights Into Protective Mechanisms of Dandelion Leaf Extract Against Cisplatin-Induced Nephrotoxicity in Rats: Role of Inhibitory Effect on Inflammatory and Apoptotic Pathways. Dose Response. 2019 Sep 12;17(3):1559325819874897. doi: 10.1177/1559325819874897. PMID: 35185411; PMCID: PMC8851149

Creatinine (sCR)

The serum creatinine (sCR) test measures the concentration of creatinine in the blood. It is an analyte found on the basic metabolic panel and comprehensive metabolic panel (CMP).

It is a marker used to assess kidney function and provide information about how well the kidneys are filtering waste products from the blood.

Creatinine is a waste product generated by muscle metabolism that is released into the bloodstream. The level of creatinine in the blood is used as an indicator of how effectively the kidneys are functioning; it is considered more accurate than the estimated glomerular filtration rate (eGFR).

Creatinine is primarily filtered by the glomeruli in the initial stages of kidney function. It is not significantly reabsorbed in the renal tubules, and any excess creatinine not filtered is actively secreted. These processes allow the kidneys to efficiently clear creatinine from the bloodstream, with the majority being excreted in the urine.

Creatinine is a small, freely filtered molecule. It enters the renal system when blood is pumped into the glomerulus, a network of capillaries within the renal corpuscle. The glomerulus acts as a sieve, allowing small substances like creatinine, water, and electrolytes to pass through its filtration barrier (consisting of the endothelium, basement membrane, and podocytes) and enter Bowman's capsule, where the filtrate begins to form. Once in the renal tubules, the filtrate (which contains creatinine) flows through the renal tubular system, including the proximal convoluted tubule (PCT), loop of Henle, distal convoluted tubule (DCT), and collecting ducts.

While the renal tubules reabsorb many substances from the filtrate, creatinine is typically not reabsorbed to a significant extent. This means that most of the creatinine remains in the tubules and ultimately ends up in the urine. In addition to filtration and limited reabsorption, the renal tubules also play a role in actively secreting creatinine. The proximal convoluted tubule secretes creatinine from the blood into the tubules. This secretion process helps to ensure that any creatinine not effectively filtered in the glomerulus or reabsorbed in the tubules is efficiently removed from the body.

Pregnancy

Creatinine clearance increases approximately 50% during pregnancy. With this, there is a rapid decrease from pre-pregnancy to 24 weeks, peaking between 15 and 21 weeks of gestation with a 23.2% reduction in serum creatinine.[1] After 25 weeks of gestation, creatinine levels increase slightly.

Postpartum

Creatinine levels increase postpartum as the glomerular filtration returns to normal.

> Creatinine clearance by 24-hour urine collection is the current standard for measurement of glomerular filtration rate, or eGFR, in pregnant women to assess kidney function.[2]

STANDARD LAB RANGE: 0.57 – 1 mg/dL

Trimester	Standard Pregnancy Ranges	**Functional Pregnancy Ranges**
Preconception	0.57 – 1	**0.49 – 1**
First Trimester	0.4 – 0.7	**0.4 – 0.7**
Second Trimester	0.4 – 0.8	**0.4 – 0.66**
Third Trimester	0.4 – 0.8	**0.4 – 0.66**
Postpartum	0.57 – 1	**0.49 – 1**

Causes of Elevated Creatinine (sCR)

See BUN/Creatinine Ratio Section.

Elevations in BUN can indicate earlier kidney dysfunction in comparison to sCR. The sCR is often not affected until over half of kidney nephrons are affected by disease.

There is no discrepancy in the research on what the lower end of normal for sCR should be, but there is lots of variation in what should be the upper end of the range in pregnancy. In 2019, the UK Renal Association comprehensively reviewed the published guidelines from the National Institute for Health and Care Excellence (NICE), UK Consensus Group on Pregnancy in Renal Disease, and the National Kidney Foundation's Kidney Disease Outcomes Quality Initiative (KDOQI) and searched Ovid MEDLINE (1946 to 2018) for "Clinical practice guideline on pregnancy and renal disease." This study and another Canadian study published in the *Journal of the American Medical Association (JAMA)*, were used in a 2023 systemic review and study to assess for sCR ranges.[3,4] The general view is that

Kidney Dysfunction: Creatinine is a waste product generated by muscle metabolism. Healthy kidneys filter it out of the blood and excrete it in the urine. When the kidneys are not functioning properly, creatinine levels can rise. Inflammation, damage, or dysfunction of the kidneys is the most common cause of elevated creatinine.

Lupus: Elevated creatinine levels can be a consequence of lupus nephritis and are indicative of impaired kidney function. Lupus is characterized by an overactive immune system that mistakenly attacks healthy tissues and organs. In lupus nephritis, the immune system's inflammatory response can damage the kidneys, particularly the glomeruli. Women with lupus, especially preexisting lupus nephritis, are at a higher risk of preeclampsia.[8]

Preeclampsia: Elevated creatinine is a biomarker for preeclampsia. Abnormalities in placental development and function can lead to the release of factors into the maternal bloodstream that may contribute to kidney dysfunction. Preeclampsia can lead to vasoconstriction (narrowing of blood vessels) throughout the body, including the blood vessels supplying the kidneys. This reduced blood flow to the kidneys can impair their ability to filter waste products, including creatinine, from the bloodstream. It is also associated with endothelial dysfunction, which is a malfunction of the cells lining blood vessels (endothelial cells) and other tissues. This dysfunction can lead to increased permeability of blood vessels and damage to the glomeruli in the kidneys, where the initial filtration of blood occurs.

Hypothyroidism: In hypothyroidism, serum creatinine increases while eGFR decreases. An increase in serum creatinine is linked with an increase in TSH levels.[9] (See Thyroid-Stimulating Hormone (TSH) Section.)

Other Possible Causes: hyperglycemia, dehydration, certain medications (nonsteroidal anti-inflammatories, antibiotics), mycotoxin exposure, kidney stones, kidney infections, high-protein diets, excess protein supplements (creatine supplements), body-building and heavy weight-lifting, progesterone deficiency

levels greater than 0.8 mg/dL are indicative of kidney disease. Lower levels of 0.66 mg/dL have been found to be a protective level for pregnancy health.

Serum creatinine remains the most used biomarker of kidney function despite its known limitations: serum creatinine level is influenced by multiple factors such as age, sex, muscle mass, muscle metabolism, diet, medications, and hydration status.[5]

Serum creatinine levels can be nearly 13 times higher in preeclamptic women.[6]

Serum creatinine is usually less than 0.8 mg/dL during pregnancy; higher levels suggest intravascular volume contraction or renal involvement in preeclampsia.[7]

Treatment Strategies for Elevated Creatinine (sCR)

See BUN/Creatinine Ratio Section.

Diet

Dietary strategies should be focused on reducing the strain on the kidneys and promoting overall kidney health. This may be through improving endothelial function by strengthening the cell structure. Cell membranes are composed of a phospholipid bilayer that is highly influenced by dietary fat and phospholipid intake. Reduce processed fats, high-heat cooking, and fried foods. Increase healthy fats from fresh olive oil, coconut oil, bone-in and skin-on chicken, and fish. Cholesterol from eggs and dairy help to add structure to cells. Antioxidants help to protect the cells from oxidative stress that can cause cell death and dysfunction. Green vegetables such as Brussels sprouts, green peas, and broccoli can be natural sources of sulfur and alpha-lipoic acid. Purple and blue-colored foods contain anthocyanins, which are potent antioxidants shown to reduce cellular oxidation. Choline and betaine-rich foods may also be effective. These include liver, eggs, beets, dairy, fish, quinoa, legumes, and seafood.

Supplements

Studies have shown that treatment with alpha-lipoic acid (ALA) can decrease acute kidney injury by lowering serum blood urea nitrogen, creatinine levels, tumor necrosis factor-alpha (TNF-α), interleukin-6 (IL-6), and interleukin-1 beta (IL-1β), thereby decreasing endothelin-1 vasoconstriction, neutrophil diffusion, and inflammation in the kidneys. The dosage is generally 600 mg/day. Dandelion extract has also been shown to reduce both elevated BUN and creatinine. If both are elevated, consider adding in dandelion extract.

Additional Testing

complete blood count (CBC); antinuclear antibodies (ANA); gamma-glutamyl transpeptidase (GGT); lactate dehydrogenase (LDH); progesterone; comprehensive thyroid profile II; reverse T3 (rT3); uric acid; protein and creatinine, random urine; protein, total, 24-hour urine; urinalysis

Causes of Low Creatinine (sCR)

See BUN/Creatinine Ratio Section.

Reduced Muscle Mass: Creatinine is a waste product produced by muscle metabolism. A lack of muscle mass, which can result from conditions like muscle atrophy, malnutrition, or prolonged bed rest, may lead to lower creatinine levels.

Malnutrition: Severe malnutrition or insufficient protein intake can lead to muscle wasting and lower creatinine levels.

Advanced Maternal Age: The risk of pregnancy-related kidney disease increases with age. It is normal for creatinine levels to be lower in those of a more advanced age.

Hyperthyroidism: In hyperthyroidism, serum creatinine decreases and eGFR increases.

Sedentary Lifestyle: Regular physical activity helps maintain muscle mass and strength, whereas sedentary behavior may result in muscle wasting and decreased muscle mass over time. Since creatinine is produced from the breakdown of creatine phosphate in muscle tissue, reduced muscle mass can lead to decreased creatinine production and lower blood levels. Furthermore, sedentary individuals often have a lower metabolic rate and decreased protein turnover, which can further contribute to lower creatinine levels.

Other Possible Causes: anorexia, chronic kidney disease

Treatment Strategies for Low Creatinine (sCR)

See BUN/Creatinine Ratio Section.

Diet

Increasing protein intake can help support muscle growth and maintenance. Ensure patients are meeting caloric demands of pregnancy. Inadequate calorie intake can contribute to muscle wasting.

Supplementation

IV nutrition or meal replacement shakes may be required. Lower creatinine levels are often seen in those with a sedentary lifestyle, causing muscle wasting. It is important for those who are pregnant to balance their exercise: "Goldilocks" it (not too much, not too little—just right). For individuals who have been sedentary, it's advisable to start with low-impact exercises that are gentle on the joints and muscles. Walking, swimming, stationary cycling, and prenatal yoga are excellent options for gradually increasing physical activity levels during pregnancy. Strength-training exercises using light weights or resistance bands can help build and maintain muscle strength during pregnancy. Focus on exercises that target major muscle groups, such as squats, lunges, bicep curls, and shoulder presses. However, it's essential to use proper form and avoid heavy lifting or exercises that put excessive strain on the abdomen.

Additional Testing

comprehensive thyroid panel II; reverse T3 (rT3); thyroid peroxidase antibodies (TPOAb); thyroglobulin antibody (TgAb); thyroid receptor antibodies (TRAb); protein and creatinine, random urine; protein, total, 24-hour urine; urinalysis

References

1. Agampodi SB, Agampodi TC, Amarasinghe GS, Warnasekara JN, Hettiarachchi AU, Jayasinghe IU, Koralegedara IS, Abeyrathna P, Srimantha S, de Silva FN, Gunarathne SP, Wickramasinghe ND. Serum creatinine and estimated glomerular filtration rate (eGFR) in early pregnancy and changes during the pregnancy. PLOS Glob Public Health. 2023 Jan 26;3(1):e0000443. doi: 10.1371/journal.pgph.0000443. PMID: 36962935; PMCID: PMC10021427

2. Cheung KL, Lafayette RA. Renal physiology of pregnancy. Adv Chronic Kidney Dis. 2013 May;20(3):209–14. doi: 10.1053/j.ackd.2013.01.012. PMID: 23928384; PMCID: PMC4089195

3. Wiles K, Chappell L, Clark K, Elman L, Hall M, Lightstone L, et al. Clinical practice guideline on pregnancy and renal disease. BMC Nephrol. 2019;20(1):401. Epub 2019/11/02. doi: 10.1186/s12882–019-1560–2 ; PubMed Central PMCID: PMC6822421

4. Harel Z, McArthur E, Hladunewich M, Dirk JS, Wald R, Garg AX, et al. Serum Creatinine Levels Before, During, and After Pregnancy. Jama. 2019;321(2):205–7. Epub 2019/01/16. doi: 10.1001/jama.2018.17948; PubMed Central PMCID: PMC6439761

5. Rysz J, Gluba-Brzózka A, Franczyk B, Jabłonowski Z, Ciałkowska-Rysz A. Novel Biomarkers in the Diagnosis of Chronic Kidney Disease and the Prediction of Its Outcome. Int J Mol Sci. 2017 Aug 4;18(8):1702. doi: 10.3390/ijms18081702. PMID: 28777303; PMCID: PMC5578092

6. Tesfa E, Munshea A, Nibret E, Mekonnen D, Sinishaw MA, Gizaw ST. Maternal serum uric acid, creatinine and blood urea levels in the prediction of preeclampsia among pregnant women attending ANC and delivery services at Bahir Dar city public hospitals, northwest Ethiopia: A case-control study. Heliyon. 2022 Oct 14;8(10):e11098. doi: 10.1016/j.heliyon.2022.e11098. PMID: 36303922; PMCID: PMC9593197

7. Manaj A, Rrugia A, Manoku N. The impact of preeclampsia in pregnancy. J Prenat Med. 2011 Jan;5(1):19–22. PMID: 22439070; PMCID: PMC3279149

8. Miyamoto T, Hoshino T, Hayashi N, Oyama R, Okunomiya A, Kitamura S, Ohtake N, Suga M, Miyamoto K, Takaoka A, Aoki T, Imamura Y, Nagano S, Kita M. Preeclampsia as a Manifestation of New-Onset Systemic Lupus Erythematosus during Pregnancy: A Case-Based Literature Review. AJP Rep. 2016 Mar;6(1):e62–7. doi: 10.1055/s-0035–1566245. Epub 2015 Nov 3. PMID: 26929873; PMCID: PMC4737630

9. Naguib, R., & Elkemary, E. (2023). Thyroid Dysfunction and Renal Function: A Crucial Relationship to Recognize. Cureus, 15(2), e35242. doi.org/10.7759/cureus.35242

BUN/Creatinine Ratio

The blood urea nitrogen to creatinine ratio, often referred to as the BUN/Creatinine ratio, is a laboratory test that measures the relationship between the levels of two waste products in the blood: blood urea nitrogen and creatinine. It is an indice found on the basic metabolic panel and comprehensive metabolic panel (CMP).

The BUN/Creatinine ratio is calculated by dividing the BUN level by the creatinine level.

Pregnancy

While both BUN and creatinine decrease during pregnancy due to increasing kidney filtration rates, the BUN tends to decrease more significantly than creatinine. This can result in a lower BUN/Creatinine ratio in pregnancy compared to nonpregnant levels. A normal BUN/Creatinine ratio during pregnancy can be between 10:1 and 20:1, but it may sometimes drop below this.

Postpartum

Levels and ranges should normalize by six weeks postpartum.

> The BUN/Creatinine ratio will be abnormal and inaccurate when the BUN is high-normal and the creatine is low-normal, or when the BUN is low-normal and the creatinine is high-normal.

STANDARD LAB RANGE: 9 – 23:1

Trimester	Standard Pregnancy Ranges	**Functional Pregnancy Ranges**
Preconception	9 – 23:1	**10 – 15:1**
First Trimester	Not Established	**10 – 20:1**
Second Trimester	Not Established	**10 – 20:1**
Third Trimester	Not Established	**10 – 20:1**
Postpartum	9 – 23:1	**10 – 20:1**

Causes of Elevated BUN/Creatinine Ratio

See the following sections: Blood Urea Nitrogen (BUN) and Creatinine (sCR).

A BUN/Creatinine ratio greater than 20:1 may indicate dehydration or a condition that leads to reduced blood flow to the kidneys. This would be caused by either elevated BUN or decreased creatinine.

BUN/Creatinine ratio in pregnant women with preeclampsia is significantly increased.[1]

Dehydration: Dehydration is one of the most common causes of an elevated BUN/Creatinine ratio. When the body is dehydrated, the kidneys concentrate the urine to conserve water, which can lead to elevated BUN levels. Creatinine, however, remains relatively stable, causing an increase in the BUN/Creatinine ratio.

Reduced Blood Flow to Kidneys: Conditions that reduce blood flow to the kidneys can lead to a higher BUN/Creatinine ratio due to reduced filtration and increased reabsorption of BUN by the kidneys.

GI Bleeds: Gastrointestinal bleeding—such as from ulcers, internal hemorrhoids, or other digestive bleeds—can result in the absorption of blood proteins, leading to elevated BUN levels.

Hyperthyroidism: Serum creatinine decreases and eGFR increases in hyperthyroidism.

Other Possible Causes: high-protein diets, toxin exposure, acute muscle injury, progesterone deficiency, anemia, liver damage, pre-eclampsia/eclampsia, gastrointestinal bleeding, certain medications (corticosteroids, antibiotics, nonsteroidal anti-inflammatories), infection, age, sedentary lifestyle

Treatment Strategies for Elevated BUN/Creatinine Ratio

See the following sections: Blood Urea Nitrogen (BUN) and Creatinine (sCR).

Diet

Caffeine and alcohol can contribute to dehydration and may exacerbate kidney issues. To help maintain hydration levels, incorporate foods with high water content. Fruits and vegetables like watermelon, cantaloupe, honeydew melon, cucumber, coconut water, oranges, strawberries, and lettuce are excellent choices. If protein levels are elevated, focusing on a more pescatarian or plant-based diet may be necessary temporarily. Soda consumption is associated with both dehydration and poor kidney function.

Supplements

Alpha-lipoic acid, CoQ10, N-acetyl cysteine, and other antioxidants may be beneficial.

Additional Testing

complete blood count (CBC); iron and TIBC; ferritin; comprehensive thyroid profile II; gamma-glutamyl transpeptidase (GGT); lactate dehydrogenase (LDH); progesterone; urinalysis

Causes of Low BUN/Creatinine Ratio

See the following sections: Blood Urea Nitrogen (BUN) and Creatinine (sCR).

If the ratio is less than 10:1, it may suggest issues related to the kidneys themselves, such as acute kidney injury, chronic kidney disease, or other kidney-related problems. This would be caused by either low BUN or elevated creatinine.

Hypothyroidism: Serum creatinine increases while eGFR decreases in hypothyroidism.

Other Possible Causes: protein-deficient diet, malnutrition, low testosterone, hyperglycemia, dehydration, certain medications (nonsteroidal anti-inflammatories, antibiotics), kidney stones, kidney infections, high-protein diets, low-protein diets, progesterone deficiency, autoimmune disease, zinc deficiency, vitamin B6 (pyridoxine) deficiency

Treatment Strategies for Low BUN/Creatinine Ratio

See the following sections: Blood Urea Nitrogen (BUN) and Creatinine (sCR).

Diet

Those with signs of kidney inflammation should increase consumption of antioxidant-rich foods. Additional guidelines vary based on the underlying cause of the ratio change.

Additional Testing

complete blood count (CBC); antinuclear antibodies (ANA); gamma-glutamyl transpeptidase (GGT); lactate dehydrogenase (LDH); progesterone; comprehensive thyroid profile II; reverse T3 (rT3); protein and creatinine, random urine; protein, total, 24-hour urine; urinalysis; oral zinc tolerance test; comprehensive stool testing

References

1. Paçarizi, H., Begolli, L., Lulaj, S., & Gafurri, Z. (2012). Blood urea nitrogen/creatinine index is a predictor of prerenal damage in preeclampsia. Journal of Health Sciences, 2(1), 61–65. doi.org/10.17532/jhsci.2012.65

Estimated Glomerular Filtration Rate (eGFR)

The estimated glomerular filtration rate (eGFR) is a blood test that provides an estimate of the glomerular filtration rate (GFR), which is a key measure of kidney function. It is an indice found on the basic metabolic panel and comprehensive metabolic panel (CMP).

It is typically calculated using equations that incorporate serum creatinine levels along with other variables such as age, gender, and race.

The most commonly used equation for estimating GFR is the Modification of Diet in Renal Disease (MDRD) study equation.

$$eGFR = 175 \times (sCR / 88.4)^{-1.154} \times (Age)^{-02.203} \times (0.742 \text{ for females}) \times (1.210 \text{ if Black})$$

This is an *estimate* and is not exact. (Also note that lab results will likely indicate "African American" instead of "Black.")

"Normal" GFR is approximately 100 mL/min/1.73 m2, but it is often just documented as >90 mL/min/1.73 m2.

GFR is the rate at which the kidneys filter waste products and excess substances from the blood. The eGFR is used to assess how well the kidneys are functioning and is an important tool for diagnosing and monitoring kidney diseases. GFR is typically estimated by measuring the concentration of creatinine in the blood. Creatinine is a waste product of muscle metabolism and is freely filtered by the glomerulus. A higher concentration of creatinine in the blood indicates reduced filtration by the glomeruli.

The glomeruli are clusters of specialized capillaries in the renal cortex. Blood from the renal artery flows into these capillaries. The glomerular filtration barrier consists of three main layers: the endothelium (innermost layer), the basement membrane (middle layer), and the podocytes (outermost layer). Blood enters the glomerulus via the afferent arteriole, and it is under high pressure due to the narrower exit of the efferent arteriole. This high pressure facilitates filtration.

As blood flows through the glomerular capillaries, the filtration barrier allows small molecules like water, electrolytes, and waste products (creatinine, urea) to pass through while retaining larger molecules such as proteins (like albumin). The filtered fluid, known as the filtrate, collects within Bowman's capsule. This filtrate contains water, electrolytes, waste products, and other substances. The glomerular filtration barrier is highly selective and designed to allow the passage of essential substances while restricting the entry of larger molecules. This selectivity is crucial for maintaining the composition of the blood while eliminating waste products.

Pregnancy

In one study, GFR was increased by up to 40% or 50% in pregnancy when compared with nonpregnant values.[1] The eGFR values are the highest at approximately the twenty-fourth week. Subsequently, serum creatinine, BUN, electrolytes, serum proteins, and uric acid values decrease.[2]

Postpartum

After childbirth, many women experience diuresis, which is an increased urine production. This is partly due to the reversal of the physiological changes that occurred during pregnancy. GFR gradually returns to pre-pregnancy levels as hormonal and hemodynamic factors normalize.

> eGFR is reported as a measure of kidney function in pregnancy, even though it is acknowledged that it consistently underestimates function.[3]

STANDARD LAB RANGE: >60 mL/MIN/1.73 M2

Trimester	Standard Pregnancy Ranges	**Functional Pregnancy Ranges**
Preconception	>60	**>90**
First Trimester	131–166	**131–166**
Second Trimester	135–170	**135–170**
Third Trimester	117–182	**117–182**
Postpartum	>60	**>90**

Causes of Elevated Estimated Glomerular Filtration Rate (eGFR)

See Creatinine (sCR) Section.

Other Possible Causes: low serum creatinine, advanced maternal age, hyperfiltration, high-protein diet, hyperthyroidism, low muscle mass, anorexia, chronic kidney disease, sedentary lifestyle

Treatment Strategies for Estimated Glomerular Filtration Rate (eGFR)

See Creatinine (sCR) Section.

Additional Testing

comprehensive thyroid panel II; reverse T3 (rT3); thyroid peroxidase antibodies (TPOAb); thyroglobulin antibody (TgAb); thyroid receptor antibodies (TRAb); protein and creatinine, random urine; protein, total, 24-hour urine; urinalysis

Causes of Low Estimated Glomerular Filtration Rate (eGFR)

See Creatinine (sCR) Section.

Preeclampsia may lead to kidney disease by causing acute kidney injury, endothelial damage, and podocyte loss, which all can affect GFR.[4]

In cases of preeclampsia, the GFR and renal plasma flow decrease by between 30% and 40% compared to normal pregnancies of the same duration.[5]

Hypothyroidism: Hypothyroidism can lead to cardiovascular changes, such as bradycardia (slow heart rate) and decreased cardiac output. These changes can result in reduced blood flow to the kidneys, affecting their ability to filter blood effectively. In hypothyroidism, there may be alterations in renal hemodynamics, which can affect the glomerular filtration rate (GFR) and lead to a lower eGFR.

Hypertension: Prolonged high blood pressure can damage the blood vessels in the kidneys, leading to reduced eGFR.

Toxin Exposure: Exposure to certain toxins, chemicals, or heavy metals can damage the kidneys and reduce eGFR.

Severe Dehydration: Dehydration can lead to a temporary reduction in eGFR, as the kidneys reduce urine production to conserve water.

Obstruction: Physical blockages in the urinary tract, such as kidney or ureteral obstructions, can reduce urine flow and impair eGFR.

Oxidative Stress: Oxidative stress can contribute to reduced eGFR by causing damage to the kidneys. Oxidative stress can damage the delicate structures in the kidneys, including the glomeruli, tubules, and blood vessels. Oxidative stress can also lead to lipid peroxidation, a process in which free radicals attack lipids (fats) in cell membranes. This can damage cell membranes in the kidneys and affect their integrity and function. Oxidative stress can directly damage renal cells, including the tubular cells and podocytes in the glomeruli. As cells are damaged and lose their functionality, kidney function decreases.

Placental Dysfunction: In preeclampsia, several chemicals and substances are produced by the placenta and maternal body that can affect the kidneys and contribute to renal dysfunction. Preeclampsia is associated with an imbalance in angiogenic and anti-angiogenic factors. The placenta releases anti-angiogenic factors such as soluble FMS-like tyrosine kinase-1 (sFLT-1) and can interfere with the action of vascular endothelial growth factor (VEGF). This imbalance can lead to endothelial dysfunction and impaired kidney blood flow. Endothelin-1 is a vasoconstrictor that narrows blood vessels. In preeclampsia, there is an increase in endothelin-1 levels, which can lead to renal vasoconstriction and reduced renal blood flow.

Inflammation is a hallmark of preeclampsia. Various inflammatory cytokines, such as tumor necrosis factor-alpha (TNF-α) and interleukin-6 (IL-6), are produced during the inflammatory response. These cytokines can cause endothelial dysfunction, promote oxidative stress, and damage kidneys.

There is also a decrease in the availability of nitric oxide (NO), a vasodilator that helps regulate blood vessel tone. Reduced NO levels can lead to vasoconstriction and impaired renal perfusion.

Stress: Stress and the production of stress hormones such as cortisol and cortisone can have both direct and indirect effects on kidney function and filtration. High cortisol levels, often associated with conditions such as Cushing's syndrome or chronic stress, can impact kidney function and lead to a decrease in glomerular filtration rate (GFR). Elevated cortisol levels can lead to increased blood pressure, causing strain on renal blood vessels and reducing GFR.

Cortisol's vasoconstrictive effects narrow blood vessels, reducing renal blood flow. Dysregulation of the renin-angiotensin system and low-grade inflammation may result from high cortisol levels, potentially damaging renal function and reducing GFR. Cortisol's impact on glucose metabolism can lead to high blood sugar, potentially harming kidney blood vessels.

Furthermore, chronic stress, which elevates cortisol, can activate the sympathetic nervous system, affecting heart rate and blood pressure, ultimately influencing kidney function and GFR. Endothelial dysfunction caused by high cortisol levels can affect blood vessel dilation and constriction, further impacting renal blood flow and GFR. This rise in cortisol can be due to psychological or physical stress responses.

Vitamin D Deficiency: Vitamin D is a negative endocrine regulator of the renin-angiotensin system.[6] Renin is an enzyme produced and released by specialized cells in the kidneys in response to low blood pressure or low sodium levels. Vitamin D has been found to downregulate the production of renin. When vitamin D levels are sufficient, this can help regulate the renin-angiotensin-aldosterone system (RAAS) and prevent excessive renin release, which would otherwise lead to increased blood pressure.[7] Vitamin D can modulate aldosterone production. In conditions of vitamin D deficiency, there can be an overproduction of aldosterone, leading to sodium retention and increased blood pressure.[8]

Omega-3 Deficiency: Omega-3 fatty acids, including docosahexaenoic acid (DHA) and eicosapentaenoic acid (EPA), have been studied for their potential impact on the renin-angiotensin-aldosterone system (RAAS), hypertension, and proteinuria. Omega-3 fatty acids, particularly EPA, have been suggested to have potential antihypertensive effects by modulating the RAAS. EPA can reduce the expression and activity of components of the RAAS, such as angiotensin-converting enzyme (ACE) and angiotensin II receptors. By inhibiting these components, EPA may help lower blood pressure and mitigate the vasoconstrictive effects of angiotensin II. EPA and DHA can inhibit proteinuria development.[9]

Other Possible Causes: high serum creatinine, nonsteroidal anti-inflammatories, high homocysteine, high c-reactive protein (CRP)

Treatment Strategies for Low Estimated Glomerular Filtration Rate (eGFR)

See Creatinine (sCR) Section.

Diet

Dietary strategies for individuals with low estimated glomerular filtration rate (eGFR) aim to reduce the workload on the kidneys, manage complications, and maintain overall health. Limiting oxalate-rich foods can reduce continued inflammation and damage to the kidneys.[10] Adequate hydration is crucial, as dehydration can increase the risk of kidney stones and other kidney-related problems. Some studies have shown that regular intake of omega-3 fatty acids, especially EPA, can lead to modest reductions in blood pressure, which can be beneficial for individuals with hypertension. This effect is believed to be related to the ability of omega-3s to relax blood vessels, reduce inflammation, and inhibit the RAAS, as mentioned above.

Lifestyle

Stress management and stress-reduction techniques should be utilized. Reducing stress is especially important in the context of kidney health, as chronic stress can negatively impact kidney function. Several strategies can be beneficial for managing stress and protecting the kidneys. Regular exercise, such as low-impact activities like walking or swimming, not only reduces stress but also supports overall cardiovascular health, which is vital for kidney function. Mindfulness practices, including meditation and deep-breathing exercises, can help lower stress levels and promote relaxation, which, in turn, benefits kidney function. Lastly, seeking social support or talk therapy can be helpful.

By prioritizing good sleep hygiene practices, individuals can effectively manage stress and support their kidneys. Kidney function is regulated by the sleep-wake cycle.[11] Several studies have shown a connection between sleep patterns, decreased kidney function, and an increased risk of preeclampsia.[12]

Additional Testing

comprehensive thyroid profile II; reverse T3 (rT3); homocysteine; c-reactive protein; vitamin D, 25-hydroxy (25-hydroxycalciferol, 25OH-D); progesterone; gamma-glutamyl transpeptidase (GGT); lactate dehydrogenase (LDH); uric acid; urinalysis; protein and creatinine, random urine; protein, total, 24-hour urine; heavy metal testing

References

1. Lopes van Balen VA, van Gansewinkel TAG, de Haas S, Spaan JJ, Ghossein-Doha C, van Kuijk SMJ, van Drongelen J, Cornelis T, Spaanderman MEA. Maternal kidney function during pregnancy: systematic review and meta-analysis. Ultrasound Obstet Gynecol. 2019 Sep;54(3):297–307. doi: 10.1002/uog.20137. Epub 2019 Aug 6. PMID: 30288811; PMCID: PMC6772153

2. Cheung KL, Lafayette RA. Renal physiology of pregnancy. Adv Chronic Kidney Dis. 2013 May;20(3):209–14. doi: 10.1053/j.ackd.2013.01.012. PMID: 23928384; PMCID: PMC4089195

3. Agampodi SB, Agampodi TC, Amarasinghe GS, Warnasekara JN, Hettiarachchi AU, Jayasinghe IU, Koralegedara IS, Abeyrathna P, Srimantha S, de Silva FN, Gunarathne SP, Wickramasinghe ND. Serum creatinine and estimated glomerular filtration rate (eGFR) in early pregnancy and changes during the pregnancy. PLOS Glob Public Health. 2023 Jan 26;3(1):e0000443. doi: 10.1371/journal.pgph.0000443. PMID: 36962935; PMCID: PMC10021427

4. Kattah A. Preeclampsia and Kidney Disease: Deciphering Cause and Effect. Curr Hypertens Rep. 2020 Sep 14;22(11):91. doi: 10.1007/s11906–020-01099–1. PMID: 32926258

5. Karumanchi SA, Maynard SE, Stillman IE, Epstein FH, Sukhatme VP. Preeclampsia: a renal perspective. Kidney Int. 2005 Jun;67(6):2101–13. doi: 10.1111/j.1523–1755.2005.00316.x. PMID: 15882253

6. Li YC, Kong J, Wei M, Chen ZF, Liu SQ, Cao LP. 1,25-Dihydroxyvitamin D(3) is a negative endocrine regulator of the renin-angiotensin system. J Clin Invest. 2002;110(2):229–238

7. Malek Mahdavi A. A brief review of interplay between vitamin D and angiotensin-converting enzyme 2: Implications for a potential treatment for COVID-19. Rev Med Virol. 2020 Sep;30(5):e2119. doi: 10.1002/rmv.2119. Epub 2020 Jun 25. PMID: 32584474; PMCID: PMC7362103

8. Boxer RS, Hoit BD, Schmotzer BJ, Stefano GT, Gomes A, Negrea L. The effect of vitamin D on aldosterone and health status in patients with heart failure. J Card Fail. 2014 May;20(5):334–42. doi: 10.1016/j.cardfail.2014.01.019. Epub 2014 Feb 4. PMID: 24508026; PMCID: PMC4117205

9. Cabo, J., Alonso, R., & Mata, P. (2012). Omega-3 fatty acids and blood pressure. British Journal of Nutrition, 107(S2), S195-S200. doi:10.1017/S0007114512001584

10. Ermer T, Eckardt KU, Aronson PS, Knauf F. Oxalate, inflammasome, and progression of kidney disease. Curr Opin Nephrol Hypertens. 2016 Jul;25(4):363–71. doi: 10.1097/MNH.0000000000000229. PMID: 27191349; PMCID: PMC4891250

11. Calero K, Anderson WM. Can poor sleep cause kidney disease? Another step closer to the answer. J Clin Sleep Med. 2019;15(3):371–372

12. Georgiou N, Fasoulakis Z, Theodora M, Pappas VA, Papamanolis V, Kalagasidou S, Blontzos N, Kambas NJ, Kontomanolis EN. Association of Pregestational Maternal Sleeping Disorders and Preeclampsia: A Retrospective Cohort Study and Review of the Literature. Cureus. 2019 Mar 28;11(3):e4338. doi: 10.7759/cureus.4338. PMID: 31187003; PMCID: PMC6541156

Uric Acid

The uric acid blood test measures the concentration of uric acid in the bloodstream. It is an individual analyte, not part of a panel.

Uric acid is a heterocyclic compound and organic acid that plays a crucial role in the human body as a waste product of the metabolic breakdown of purines, nucleic acid, and nucleoprotein metabolism. Purines are a type of chemical compound found in many foods and cells of the body, and they are essential for various biological processes. Nucleic acids, including DNA and RNA, contain purine bases, and purines are released when nucleic acids are broken down during normal cellular processes. Uric acid is a natural component of urine and is primarily excreted from the body through the kidneys.

Pregnancy

During early pregnancy, uric acid levels fall, frequently to 3 mg/dL or below. This is usually due to the uricosuric effects from estrogen, hemodilution, and the increase in glomerular filtration rate. Uric acid levels increase during the third trimester, reaching levels of up to 4 or 5 mg/dL by term.[1]

Postpartum

In the immediate postpartum period (within the first hours to days), uric acid levels may rise slightly due to factors such as dehydration and the stress associated with labor and delivery. This is often temporary and tends to return to normal within a day or two as the body rehydrates and stress decreases. Within the first few weeks after childbirth, uric acid levels usually decrease and return to the pre-pregnancy baseline. This decrease is related to the reversal of the physiological changes that occurred during pregnancy, such as the reduction in blood volume (as hemodilution is resolved) and the normalization of kidney function. If a woman is breastfeeding, uric acid levels may remain slightly lower than her pre-pregnancy baseline. Prolactin can influence uric acid metabolism and increase uric acid excretion in breast milk.

STANDARD LAB RANGE: 8 – 16 mg/dL

Trimester	Standard Pregnancy Ranges	**Functional Pregnancy Ranges**
Preconception	8 – 16	**3 – 5**
First Trimester	2 – 4.1	**2 – 4.1**
Second Trimester	2.4 – 4.9	**2.4 – 4.9**
Third Trimester	3.1 – 6.3	**3.1 – 6.3**
Postpartum	8 – 16	**3 – 5**

Causes of Elevated Uric Acid

See the following sections: Estimated Glomular Filtration Rate (eGFR) and Creatinine (sCR).

Early onset preeclampsia has been linked to higher uric acid concentration.[2] Currently, scientific evidence does not recommend using uric acid as a predictive biomarker for preeclampsia.[3]

Decreased GFR: One of the primary functions of the kidneys is to filter waste products, including uric acid, from the blood and excrete them in the urine. When the glomerular filtration rate is decreased, the kidneys are less effective at filtering and excreting uric acid. This can result in reduced uric acid clearance from the bloodstream.

Preeclampsia: High uric acid levels have been associated with an increased risk of preeclampsia during pregnancy. Preeclampsia is characterized by widespread dysfunction of the endothelium, which is the lining of blood vessels. High uric acid levels have been linked to endothelial dysfunction in various studies. Endothelial dysfunction can lead to vasoconstriction (narrowing of blood vessels) and reduced blood flow, contributing to the high blood pressure and organ damage seen in preeclampsia.

Oxidative Stress: Elevated uric acid levels can also contribute to oxidative stress, which is an imbalance between the production of reactive oxygen species (ROS) and the body's ability to neutralize them. Oxidative stress can damage cells, including endothelial cells, and may play a role in preeclampsia.

Placental Hypoxia: Hypoxia in tissues such as the placenta can cause an increase in uric acid.

Other Possible Causes: rheumatoid arthritis, psoriasis, thyroid dysfunction, liver disease, high purine diet, alcohol use, certain medications (aspirin in doses less than 1g/day), diuretics, dehydration, genetics

Treatment Strategies for Elevated Uric Acid

See the following sections: Estimated Glomular Filtration Rate (eGFR) and Creatinine (sCR).

Diet

The primary dietary strategy used to reduce uric acid is to remove purines from the diet. Purines are naturally occurring compounds found in certain foods that can be metabolized into uric acid. Reducing the intake of foods high in purines can help lower uric acid levels. Some purine-rich foods include organ meats (liver, kidney), certain seafood (anchovies, sardines, mackerel), and some types of meat (beef, pork). While it's important to limit purine-rich foods, it's also crucial to maintain a healthy intake of protein during pregnancy. Switching to poultry, tofu, and dairy products will help keep protein intake adequate while reducing purine-rich foods.

Vitamin C has been shown to reduce uric acid production and improve uric acid excretion.[4] Foods that are rich in vitamin C, like citrus fruits, strawberries, and kiwi, may help lower uric acid levels. Some studies suggest that consuming cherries or cherry extract may help lower uric acid levels.[5] High intake of fructose, especially from sugary drinks and foods, has been linked to an increase in uric acid.[6] Reducing the consumption of high-fructose corn syrup and sugary beverages can be beneficial.

Lifestyle

Encourage moderate-intensity aerobic exercise such as brisk walking and swimming, aiming for at least 150 minutes of exercise per week.

Supplementation

Studies show that vitamin C in dosages of about 500 mg/day helped lower uric acid levels.[7] The benefit plateaued in dosages greater than this. These studies were done primarily on non-pregnant men with gout, so the dosage in pregnancy may be different.

Additional Testing

complete blood count (CBC); comprehensive metabolic panel (CMP); c-reactive protein (CRP); antinuclear antibodies (ANA); comprehensive thyroid profile II; reverse T3 (rT3); homocysteine; vitamin D, 25-hydroxy (25-hydroxycalciferol, 25OH-D); progesterone; gamma-glutamyl transpeptidase (GGT); lactate dehydrogenase (LDH); urinalysis; protein and creatinine, random urine; protein, total, 24-hour urine; heavy metal testing

Causes of Low Uric Acid

See the following sections: Estimated Glomular Filtration Rate (eGFR) and Creatinine (sCR).

Molybdenum Insufficiency/Deficiency: Xanthine oxidase is an enzyme that catalyzes the conversion of purines, such as xanthine and hypoxanthine, into uric acid. This enzymatic reaction involves the transfer of electrons and oxygen to the purine compounds, ultimately producing uric acid as the end product. Molybdenum serves as a cofactor for xanthine oxidase, which means that it is an essential component for the enzyme to function properly. Without molybdenum, xanthine oxidase cannot efficiently convert purines into uric acid.

Excess Calcium: Calcium competes with uric acid for reabsorption in the renal tubules of the kidneys. When there is an increased intake of dietary calcium or when blood calcium levels are elevated, it can lead to increased excretion of uric acid in the urine. This competition for reabsorption can result in lower serum uric acid levels.

Vitamin B12 (Cobalamin) Deficiency: Vitamin B12 is involved in the metabolism of purines. Vitamin B12 deficiency may disrupt purine metabolism, potentially leading to alterations in uric acid levels.

Other Possible Causes: certain medications (aspirin in doses greater than 2g/day), metabolic acidosis, anorexia or fasting, vitamin D deficiency, genetics, liver disease, advanced maternal age, hyperfiltration, hyperthyroidism, chronic kidney disease, sedentary lifestyle, inflammatory bowel disease, excess copper, excess coffee consumption

Treatment Strategies for Low Uric Acid

See the following sections: Estimated Glomular Filtration Rate (eGFR) and Creatinine (sCR).

Diet

Dietary strategies to maintain or promote low serum uric acid levels may include molybdenum-rich foods. Legumes such as lentils, beans, and peas are good sources of molybdenum. They can be included in soups, salads, stews, and other dishes. Whole grains like oats, barley, and buckwheat contain molybdenum and can be included in the diet through grain-based side dishes.

Additional Testing

complete blood count (CBC); vitamin B12 (cobalamin); methylmalonic acid; vitamin D, 25-hydroxy (25-hydroxycalciferol, 25OH-D); comprehensive metabolic panel (CMP); gamma-glutamyl transpeptidase (GGT); lactate dehydrogenase (LDH)

References

1. Niyonzima FN, Dusabimana A, Mutijima JB. Pregnancy Induced Hypertension and Uric Acid Levels among Pregnant Women Attending Ruhengeri Referral Hospital, in Rwanda. East Afr Health Res J. 2021;5(1):44–49. doi: 10.24248/eahrj.v5i1.650. Epub 2021 Jun 11. PMID: 34308244; PMCID: PMC8291203

2. Bellos I, Pergialiotis V, Loutradis D, Daskalakis G. The prognostic role of serum uric acid levels in preeclampsia: A meta-analysis. J Clin Hypertens (Greenwich). 2020 May;22(5):826–834. doi: 10.1111/jch.13865. Epub 2020 Apr 27. PMID: 32338457; PMCID: PMC8030030

3. Pecoraro V, Trenti T. Predictive value of serum uric acid levels for adverse maternal and perinatal outcomes in pregnant women with high blood pressure. A systematic review and meta-analysis. Eur J Obstet Gynecol Reprod Biol. 2020 Sep;252:447–454. doi: 10.1016/j.ejogrb.2020.07.042. Epub 2020 Jul 22. PMID: 32736271

4. Juraschek SP, Miller ER 3rd, Gelber AC. Effect of oral vitamin C supplementation on serum uric acid: a meta-analysis of randomized controlled trials. Arthritis Care Res (Hoboken). 2011 Sep;63(9):1295–306. doi: 10.1002/acr.20519. PMID: 21671418; PMCID: PMC3169708

5. Chen PE, Liu CY, Chien WH, Chien CW, Tung TH. Effectiveness of Cherries in Reducing Uric Acid and Gout: A Systematic Review. Evid Based Complement Alternat Med. 2019 Dec 4;2019:9896757. doi: 10.1155/2019/9896757. PMID: 31885677; PMCID: PMC6914931

6. Russo E, Leoncini G, Esposito P, Garibotto G, Pontremoli R, Viazzi F. Fructose and Uric Acid: Major Mediators of Cardiovascular Disease Risk Starting at Pediatric Age. Int J Mol Sci. 2020 Jun 24;21(12):4479. doi: 10.3390/ijms21124479. PMID: 32599713; PMCID: PMC7352635

7. Brzezińska O, Styrzyński F, Makowska J, Walczak K. Role of Vitamin C in Prophylaxis and Treatment of Gout-A Literature Review. Nutrients. 2021 Feb 22;13(2):701. doi: 10.3390/nu13020701. PMID: 33671646; PMCID: PMC7926958

Protein

Total serum protein is a measure of the total amount of protein in the blood, and it includes both albumin and globulin. It is an analyte found on the comprehensive metabolic panel (CMP).

The amount of albumin and globulin in the bloodstream will affect the total protein value.

Protein metabolism is the complex process by which the body synthesizes, breaks down, and regulates the levels of proteins within the cells and tissues. Proteins, including albumin and globulins, are essential macromolecules made up of amino acids. Protein metabolism is tightly regulated to maintain a balance between protein synthesis and degradation. The balance is influenced by various factors, including dietary intake of protein, hormonal signals (insulin, growth hormone, thyroid hormones), nutrient cofactors, and the body's overall protein needs.

Protein absorption begins in the stomach and requires hydrochloric acid and pepsin. Hydrochloric acid (HCl) denatures proteins, unfolding their complex structure, and pepsin breaks proteins into smaller polypeptides. The pancreas releases protease enzymes, such as trypsin and chymotrypsin, which further break down polypeptides into smaller peptides. The final stage of protein digestion occurs in the brush border of the small intestine, where peptidases (enzymes) break down peptides into individual amino acids. Amino acids are absorbed through the small intestine into the bloodstream. Once absorbed, amino acids are transported to the liver or to other tissues in the body to be synthesized.

Amino acid transporters are highly selective, meaning they only allow specific amino acids to enter the cells. Different transporters are responsible for the uptake of different amino acids.

ASC1 transporters handle both neutral and cationic amino acids, such as serine and arginine. ASC1 is sodium-dependent.

PEPT1 is responsible for di- and tripeptides, which are composed of multiple amino acids linked together. Once inside the enterocytes, these peptides are further broken down to release individual amino acids.

SLC6A19 is responsible for transporting neutral amino acids, such as phenylalanine, leucine, and isoleucine. This transporter is stimulated by several other enzymes, including ACE2. SLC6A19 is sodium-dependent.

Transporters work in a few ways. Some use active transport, which requires ATP; some need sodium in combination with the amino acids to cross; and others exchange amino acids for hydrogen.

Protein filtration in the kidneys occurs in the glomeruli. Blood pressure in the glomerulus is significantly higher than in regular capillaries. High pressure forces plasma to be pushed into the Bowman's capsule. Small substances like water, electrolytes, and waste products can easily pass through, but larger proteins such as albumin are usually retained within the bloodstream because they are too large to pass through the small gaps between the podocyte foot processes (pedicles). After filtration, the glomerular filtrate moves through the renal tubules, where reabsorption and secretion processes occur. Damage to the podocytes can cause a "leaking" of proteins into the urine.

The liver can break down amino acids through deamination, a process that removes the amino group from an amino acid, leaving behind the carbon skeleton. The amino group is converted into ammonia (NH_3) and eventually converted into urea in the liver.

Amino acids are the building blocks of proteins. They are organic compounds composed of carbon, hydrogen, oxygen, and nitrogen, with some containing sulfur. There are 21 amino acids in total but 20 common amino acids that make up proteins, and they can be classified into two main categories: essential and nonessential.

Essential amino acids are ones that the human body cannot synthesize on its own, and therefore, they must be obtained from diet. These include histidine, isoleucine, leucine, lysine, methionine, phenylalanine, threonine, tryptophan, and valine. These amino acids are essential for the synthesis of new proteins, enzymes, hormones, and various other molecules in the body.

Nonessential amino acids are ones that the human body can synthesize from other sources, such as intermediates in metabolic pathways and other amino acids. There is controversy over these amino acids being termed "nonessential," as evidence also points to the need for these in the diet. These include alanine, arginine, asparagine, aspartic acid, cysteine, glutamic acid, glutamine, glycine, proline, serine, and tyrosine.

Some amino acids may become conditionally essential under certain circumstances. This means that although the body can usually synthesize them, there are conditions or situations where the body's ability to produce these amino acids may be insufficient. In pregnancy, glycine is a "conditionally essential" amino acid, meaning it must be consumed in the diet during pregnancy.

Pregnancy

During pregnancy, serum total protein levels undergo significant changes due to a combination of factors. Hemodilution begins in the first trimester and decreases protein concentrations in the bloodstream. However, the maternal body responds by increasing protein synthesis, with approximately 15% higher serum total protein levels in the second trimester and a further 25% increase in the third trimester, primarily due to elevated albumin and globulin levels. This synthesis balances the hemodilution effect and maintains essential functions. As pregnancy progresses into the third trimester, serum total protein levels tend to plateau as the rate of protein synthesis balances the hemodilution. Some studies show increased total protein just before the onset of labor.

An important factor in the etiology of protein changes is the effect of hormones, especially estrogen, on the synthesis and degradation of these proteins.[1]

Postpartum

The hemodilution effect that occurred during pregnancy is rapidly reversed, resulting in a reduction in blood plasma volume. Because of this decrease in plasma volume, serum protein levels start to rise, reflecting a concentration of proteins in the bloodstream.

STANDARD LAB RANGE: 6 – 8.5 g/dL

Trimester	Standard Pregnancy Ranges	**Functional Pregnancy Ranges**
Preconception	6 – 8.5	**6 – 8.5**
First Trimester	6.2 – 7.6	**6.2 – 7.6**
Second Trimester	5.7 – 6.9	**5.7 – 6.9**
Third Trimester	5.6 – 6.7	**5.6 – 6.7**
Postpartum	6 – 8.5	**6 – 8.5**

Causes of Elevated Protein

Dehydration: When a person is dehydrated, you will usually see elevated albumin, chloride, creatinine, hemoglobin, hematocrit, BUN, and sometimes MCV/MCH. In some cases, dehydration can cause an apparent increase in serum protein levels during pregnancy. Dehydration may result from insufficient fluid intake, vomiting (common in early pregnancy), or other factors that lead to fluid loss. This is common in women with hyperemesis gravidarum. In these cases, serum globulins will be elevated with a lower albumin to globulin (A/G) ratio.

Infections/Inflammation: Infections or inflammatory conditions can lead to elevated levels of acute-phase proteins, which are part of the globulin fraction of serum proteins. Infections such as UTIs or other inflammatory processes might cause transient increases in serum protein levels.

Cholestasis of Pregnancy: Cholestasis of pregnancy, also known as intrahepatic cholestasis of pregnancy (ICP), is a liver disorder that is characterized by impaired bile flow. This condition can lead to elevated serum protein levels, as well as increased levels of total serum bile acid, alanine aminotransferase (ALT)(SGPT), and alkaline phosphatase (ALP).

Other Possible Causes: adrenal hypofunction, liver dysfunction, rheumatoid arthritis, certain types of cancer, hypertension/preeclampsia, hyperthyroidism, high sodium diet, dehydration

Treatment Strategies for Elevated Protein

Diet

If inflammation is the cause of the elevated protein, encourage them to increase antioxidant-rich foods and to "eat hydration"—that is, prioritize foods that not only nourish the body but also contribute to overall hydration such as watermelon, cucumber, and oranges or hydrating soups and broths. These foods provide a dual benefit of increasing hydration while offering valuable nutrients.

Supplementation

In cases of inflammation, antioxidant supplementation may be useful. Supplementation will depend on identifying the underlying cause.

Additional Testing

complete blood count (CBC); c-reactive protein (CRP); comprehensive thyroid profile II; reverse T3 (rT3); thyroid peroxidase antibodies (TPOAb); thyroglobulin antibody (TgAb); thyroid receptor antibodies (TRAb); iron and TIBC; ferritin; bile acid, serum; gamma-glutamyl transpeptidase (GGT); lactate dehydrogenase (LDH); antinuclear antibodies (ANA)

Causes of Low Protein

Gut Inflammation/Poor Absorption: Inflammatory bowel diseases (IBDs) such as Crohn's disease, can lead to the erosion of the intestinal lining, reducing the surface area available for nutrient absorption. The small intestine, where most protein absorption occurs, may become inflamed, resulting in damaged or ulcerated areas. This can impair the uptake of amino acids and other nutrients from digested protein. Inflammation can also lead to the downregulation or dysfunction of transporters, making it more difficult for the body to absorb amino acids from the diet.

Kidney Dysfunction: Kidney inflammation, like that seen in preeclampsia, can cause a decrease in albumin through urine protein loss. Since serum total protein includes both albumin and globulin (among other proteins), a decrease in albumin levels due to kidney dysfunction can contribute to a decrease in serum total protein levels.

Thyroid Dysfunction: Thyroid hormones stimulate the synthesis as well as the degradation of proteins.[2] Hypothyroidism can slow down protein absorption and synthesis in the body. This is partly due to a decrease in the metabolic rate and the body's reduced ability to build and repair tissues. There is also a slowdown in the production of digestive enzymes, which can affect the digestion and absorption of dietary proteins.

Hyperthyroidism, on the other hand, accelerates the breakdown of proteins. Elevated thyroid hormone levels can lead to increased proteolysis, resulting in a higher rate of protein catabolism.

Vitamin B6 (Pyridoxine) Deficiency: Vitamin B6 is essential for the conversion of amino acids into the precursor molecules required for protein synthesis.[3] Its active form, pyridoxine-5'-phosphate, also known as P5P or pyridoxal-5'-phosphate (PLP) is the coenzyme that interacts with various enzymes to facilitate specific reactions in the body. Aminotransferase enzymes are responsible for transferring amino groups (NH2) between amino acids. Certain decarboxylase enzymes, which remove carboxyl groups from amino acids, also require vitamin B6 as a cofactor. These enzymes play a role in amino acid metabolism and neurotransmitter synthesis. Serine hydroxymethyltransferase is an enzyme that is part of the serine-glycine interconversion pathway and affects the metabolism of the amino acids serine and glycine. Vitamin B6 is necessary for its activity.

Zinc Deficiency: Zinc is a cofactor for many enzymes involved in various stages of protein synthesis, including pepsin activity. It is also involved in maintaining the structural stability of proteins.[4] Aminoacyl-tRNA synthetases, which rely on zinc, ensure that the correct amino acid is attached to the corresponding tRNA molecule. This is essential for ensuring the accuracy of protein synthesis. Zinc-dependent metalloproteinases are needed for breaking down proteins, and zinc plays a role in various post-translational modifications of proteins, including phosphorylation and acetylation.

Selenium Deficiency: Selenium is a cofactor for certain enzymes involved in protein synthesis. It is incorporated into selenoproteins, a class of proteins that contain the amino acid selenocysteine (Sec) and have diverse functions in the body. These selenoproteins are involved in various steps of protein synthesis and metabolism.

Vitamin B3 (Niacin) Deficiency: Niacin is involved in the synthesis of HCl, which converts pepsinogen to pepsin, both of which are needed for protein digestion.

Chloride Deficiency: Chloride is a structural component of HCl, which breaks down proteins. (See Chloride Section.)

Magnesium Deficiency: Magnesium deficiency has been associated with decreased HCl production. Magnesium is involved in various enzymatic reactions, including those related to protein synthesis. Elevated sodium levels with low potassium and calcium levels can indicate magnesium deficiency.

Other Possible Causes: protein-deficient diets, low albumin, low globulin, hyponatremia, vitamin B1 (thiamine) deficiency

Treatment Strategies for Low Protein

Diet

Consuming 100 or more grams of protein per day should be the goal in pregnancy. This can be achieved by incorporating different protein sources, which will ensure that the patient gets a well-rounded mix of essential amino acids. Different protein sources have different amino acid profiles, so incorporating a range of foods can be beneficial.

Please visit my website www.FunctionalMaternity.com to download my e-book *Protein Packed Pregnancy*.

Supplementation

Studies have shown that supplementing with selenium, vitamin C, and vitamin E significantly increases total protein, albumin, and globulin levels, although it does not have an effect on A/G ratio in animal models.[5]

Additional Testing

comprehensive thyroid profile II; reverse T3 (rT3); thyroid peroxidase antibodies (TPOAb); thyroglobulin antibody (TgAb); thyroid receptor antibodies (TRAb); urinalysis; 24-hour urinary protein; complete blood count (CBC); vitamin B12 (cobalamin); homocysteine; oral zinc tolerance test; comprehensive stool testing

References

1. Joseph JC, Baker C, Sprang ML, Bermes EW. Changes in plasma proteins during pregnancy. Ann Clin Lab Sci. 1978 Mar-Apr;8(2):130–41. PMID: 76457

2. Müller, M.J., Seitz, H.J. Thyroid hormone action on intermediary metabolism. Klin Wochenschr 62, 97–102 (1984). doi.org/10.1007/BF01738699

3. Sampson, D A, Kretsch, M J, Young, L A, & Jansen, G R. Marginal B-6 intake affects protein synthesis in rat tissues. United States

4. Bates J, McClain CJ. The effect of severe zinc deficiency on serum levels of albumin, transferrin, and prealbumin in man. Am J Clin Nutr. 1981 Sep;34(9):1655–60. doi: 10.1093/ajcn/34.9.1655. PMID: 6792896

5. Mehta, Jitendra & Purohit, Govind Narayan & Kumar, Ashok & Kumar, Harvindra & Kumar, Amit & Narula, Harvindra. (2019). Effects of non enzymatic antioxidants on serum total proteins and its fractions in Magra rams in arid region of Rajasthan. 8. 542–547

Albumin

Serum albumin is the measure of how much albumin is in a blood sample. It is an analyte found on the comprehensive metabolic panel (CMP).

The majority of albumin is produced in the liver, and liver function affects albumin production. Therefore, albumin levels can be an indicator of liver function. Albumin is the most abundant serum protein in the body. Changes in serum protein levels often are related to changes in albumin levels.

Albumin is primarily synthesized in liver hepatocytes. Various nutrients and cofactors are needed for albumin synthesis. For example, vitamin B6 (pyridoxine) is essential for transaminase enzymes, which are involved in amino acid metabolism. Zinc is also involved in protein synthesis, including albumin.

Edema is the accumulation of excess fluid in the interstitial spaces, leading to swelling and tissue enlargement. Disruptions in the normal osmotic regulation between tissues and blood can result in edema. Albumin exerts an osmotic pull on water molecules, preventing them from leaving the blood vessels. In fact, albumin is responsible for 80% of the fluid balance between the blood and tissues. This is especially important in the capillaries. A common cause of edema is hypoalbuminemia.

Albumin also acts as a carrier protein, binding to various substances like hormones (thyroid hormones, steroids), fatty acids, bilirubin, and drugs. It transports these substances through the blood. It also has antioxidant properties and can bind to and neutralize harmful molecules, contributing to the body's defense against oxidative stress.

Pregnancy

In the early stages of pregnancy, hemodilution leads to decreased serum albumin levels beginning in the first trimester, which becomes more accentuated with advanced gestation.[1] Serum albumin levels decrease during pregnancy while the concentration of most other maternal serum proteins of hepatic origin remains stable or increases.[2] As pregnancy progresses, the liver adapts by increasing albumin synthesis to compensate for the initial decrease, but serum levels stay in the low/normal ranges.

Postpartum

Serum albumin concentrations rapidly increase after delivery and stabilize after 15 weeks postpartum.[3] The resolution of hemodilution starts shortly after delivery. As plasma volume decreases, albumin concentrations in the blood increase, effectively raising serum albumin levels.

Serum albumin levels are inversely related to oxidative stress.[4]

STANDARD LAB RANGE: 3.9 – 5 g/dL

Trimester	Standard Pregnancy Ranges	**Functional Pregnancy Ranges**
Preconception	3.9 – 5	**4 – 4.8**
First Trimester	3.1 – 5.1	**3.1 – 5.1**
Second Trimester	2.6 – 4.5	**3.3 – 4.5**
Third Trimester	2.3 – 4.2	**3.3 – 4.5**
Postpartum	3.9 – 5	**3.9 – 5**

Causes of Elevated Albumin

Dehydration: Dehydration can cause elevated albumin, chloride, creatinine, hemoglobin, hematocrit, BUN, and sometimes MCV/MCH.

Infections/Inflammation: Infections or inflammatory conditions can lead to elevated levels of albumin. This can be a common finding in those with rheumatoid arthritis, autoimmune disease, or other chronic inflammatory diseases. Acute trauma can also be associated with elevated albumin.

Low Estrogen: Studies show that estrogen supplementation decreases serum albumin levels. Estrogen therapy, specifically oral contraceptive use, can cause higher transferrin production and lower albumin production. There are no studies on estrogen and albumin production/levels in pregnancy. In theory, a decrease in estrogen production by the placenta may cause a reverse of this pattern, with elevated albumin and decreased transferrin production.

Thyroid Dysfunction: Both hypothyroidism and hypothyroidism can affect serum albumin in various ways. Hypothyroidism can present with either elevated or decreased albumin. Thyroid hormones are needed for albumin synthesis as well as degradation. There can be either a decrease in serum albumin due to a decrease in production, or an increase due to a decrease in degradation. The relationship between thyroid hormones and albumin are more pronounced with total T3 values.

Other Possible Causes: high-protein diet, adrenal hypofunction, acute liver dysfunction, genetics, cancer

Treatment Strategies for Elevated Albumin

See Total Serum Protein Section.

Diet

Ensuring adequate hydration is crucial for maintaining proper fluid balance and electrolyte levels in the body. If dehydration is a contributing factor, drinking plenty of fluids, including water and electrolyte-rich beverages, can help address dehydration and lower serum albumin levels. Antioxidants such as vitamin C, vitamin E, selenium, and flavonoids have anti-inflammatory and antioxidant properties that may help reduce oxidative stress and inflammation.

Supplements

Identifying the underlying cause is important for correct supplementation.

Additional Testing

complete blood count (CBC); c-reactive protein (CRP); antinuclear antibodies (ANA); comprehensive thyroid profile II; gamma-glutamyl transpeptidase (GGT); lactate dehydrogenase (LDH)

Causes of Low Albumin

Albuminemia <3.3 g/dL at 32 weeks is associated with a higher risk of preeclampsia/eclampsia, lower birth weight, and lower gestational age.[5]

Preeclampsia: Hypoalbuminemia is a comorbidity of preeclampsia (PE) but not gestational hypertension (GH), and it results from serum albumin leaking from the maternal body via urine. Hypoalbuminemia occurs mainly due to systemic small-vessel spasm, increased secretion of angiotensin, and damaged and increased permeability of vascular endothelial cells, thereby leading to clearance and a loss of many plasma proteins (especially serum albumin), causing intravascular

Studies have found that patients with more severe preeclampsia often have a serum albumin level <3 g/dL.[6] Levels below 3 g/dL are found in pregnant women with imminent eclampsia, preeclampsia, pulmonary edema, HELLP syndrome, and an IUD, but not in intrauterine growth restriction (IUGR), placental abruption, severe oligohydramnios, or uncontrolled hypertension.[7]

Serum albumin ≤3 g/dL is highly associated with severe proteinuria (>2 g/day).[8]

In hypoalbuminemia, it is important to determine whether the cause is due to a decrease in production, hemodilution, or increased loss via the urine.

dehydration. Low albumin is a primary cause of edema in pregnancy, specifically pitting edema, which is associated with preeclampsia.[9]

Inflammation/Oxidative Stress: Severe decreases in albumin are more likely to be associated with inflammation than malnutrition.[10]

Vitamin B6 (Pyridoxine) Deficiency: Vitamin B6 plays a role in albumin synthesis by participating in enzymatic reactions related to amino acid metabolism and transamination. Transamination involves the transfer of amino groups between molecules and is catalyzed by transaminase enzymes. These enzymes require coenzymes like pyridoxine-5'-phosphate, also known as P5P or pyridoxal-5'-phosphate (PLP), the active form of vitamin B6, to facilitate the transfer of amino groups during the conversion of amino acids.

Zinc Deficiency: Zinc acts as a cofactor for transcription factors that regulate gene expression, enabling the activation of genes responsible for albumin production. Additionally, it serves as a cofactor for enzymes involved in amino acid metabolism and transamination, specifically those required for albumin production. Moreover, zinc stabilizes the structural integrity of certain proteins, including albumin, ensuring their proper functioning in the bloodstream.

Thyroid Dysfunction: Thyroid hormones stimulate albumin synthesis by enhancing gene transcription and protein translation in hepatocytes. Thyroid hormones also increase the rate of albumin degradation, thereby regulating serum albumin levels. Elevated thyroid hormone levels may accelerate albumin catabolism, leading to lower serum albumin concentrations. Studies have shown both high and low albumin concentrations with thyroid dysfunction patterns, depending on whether synthesis or degradation is affected.

Low free T4 levels have also been linked to low albumin levels.[11] T3, specifically, exerts its effects by binding to thyroid hormone receptors (TRs) in the nucleus of target cells. When T3 binds to TRs, it acts as a transcription factor, regulating the expression of various genes. This includes genes involved in the synthesis of thyroxine-binding globulin (TBG) and other plasma proteins, such as albumin and globulins. Low albumin and low globulin may indicate T3 syndrome. Severe hypoalbuminemia can be seen in postpartum thyrotoxicosis. This is often associated with elevated bilirubin.

Adrenal Hyperfunction: Cortisol can have complex effects on albumin synthesis. In some situations, particularly during chronic stress or illness, cortisol may promote the breakdown of muscle proteins and contribute to amino acid availability for albumin synthesis. Elevated cortisol levels can also increase protein catabolism, including albumin, leading to a decrease in serum albumin levels. Like thyroid hormones, depending on the mechanism of action, cortisol may cause increased synthesis or increased breakdown.

Calcium Deficiency: Calcium acts as an activator for various enzymes and coenzymes essential for metabolic pathways related to protein synthesis. Disruptions in calcium metabolism, whether due to excessive or insufficient levels, can potentially influence albumin synthesis.

Environmental Toxin Exposure: Exposure to environmental chemicals, including pesticides, bisphenol A (BPA), and organophosphates, can potentially impact serum albumin levels. Polychlorinated bisphenols have been found to decrease serum albumin levels.[12]

Other Possible Causes: protein-deficient diets, vitamin C deficiency, inflammatory bowel diseases, hypochlorhydria, vitamin B12 (cobalamin) deficiency, vitamin B9 (folate) deficiency, selenium deficiency, vitamin B3 (niacin) deficiency, chloride deficiency, vitamin B1 (thiamine) deficiency, magnesium deficiency, progesterone deficiency

Treatment Strategies for Low Albumin

See Total Serum Protein Section.

Diet

For those with lower albumin levels, the Brewer Diet helps to increase a variety of nutrients, including calcium, protein, zinc, and vitamin B6 (pyridoxine), as well as an array of amino acids. Omega-3 fatty acids have an inverse relationship with the urine albumin/creatinine ratio. Omega-3 fatty acids, found in fatty fish (such as salmon, mackerel, and sardines), flaxseeds, chia seeds, and walnuts, have anti-inflammatory properties and may help reduce kidney inflammation associated with certain conditions. Foods that are high in naturally occurring albumin include eggs and dairy. Modified citrus pectin is a soluble dietary fiber derived from the peel and pulp of citrus fruits. Some research suggests that modified citrus pectin may bind BPA and other heavy metals in the gastrointestinal tract and facilitate their excretion from the body. Because supplementation has not been researched in pregnancy, add citrus rinds to water instead.

Lifestyle

Polychlorinated biphenyls (PCBs) and bisphenol compounds such as BPA are common in plastics. Many companies have moved away from BPA but have replaced it with other PCBs, such as bisphenol S. BPA is commonly found in plastic products, including food and beverage containers, plastic wraps, and water bottles. Whenever possible, choose BPA-free alternatives such as glass, stainless steel, or BPA-free plastics labeled with recycling codes #1, #2, #4, or #5.

To reduce exposure to BPA from canned foods, opt for fresh, frozen, or dried foods whenever possible. If using canned foods, choose products labeled as "BPA-free" or those packaged in alternative materials. Avoid microwaving food or beverages in plastic containers, as heat can cause BPA and other chemicals to leach into the food.

Use a water filtration system certified to remove contaminants such as PCBs, BPA, and other chemicals. PCBs and BPA can also be found in certain household products, including some paints, sealants, adhesives, and thermal paper receipts. Have patients choose products labeled as "BPA-free" or "low-VOC" (volatile organic compound) whenever possible.

Supplementation

Protein supplements may be recommended in some cases. Additional supplements will vary based on the identified causes.

Additional Testing

complete blood count (CBC); vitamin B12 (cobalamin); methylmalonic acid; homocysteine; urinalysis; 24-hour urinary protein; c-reactive protein (CRP); gamma-glutamyl transpeptidase (GGT); lactate dehydrogenase (LDH); progesterone; oral zinc tolerance test

References

1. Yagur, Y., Ribak, R., Ben Ezry, E. et al. Do maternal albumin levels affect post-operative complications after cesarean delivery? BMC Pregnancy Childbirth 22, 909 (2022). doi.org/10.1186/s12884–022-05215–8

2. Maher JE, Goldenberg RL, Tamura T, Cliver SP, Hoffman HJ, Davis RO, Boots L. Albumin levels in pregnancy: a hypothesis—decreased levels of albumin are related to increased levels of alpha-fetoprotein. Early Hum Dev. 1993 Oct;34(3):209–15. doi: 10.1016/0378–3782(93)90178-w. PMID: 7507040

3. Zhao S, Gockenbach M, Grimstein M, Sachs HC, Mirochnick M, Struble K, Belew Y, Wang J, Capparelli EV, Best BM, Johnson T, Momper JD, Maharaj AR. Characterization of Plasma Protein Alterations in Pregnant and Postpartum Individuals Living With HIV to Support Physiologically-Based Pharmacokinetic Model Development. Front Pediatr. 2021 Oct 13;9:721059. doi: 10.3389/fped.2021.721059. PMID: 34722417; PMCID: PMC8550258

4. Saitou T, Watanabe K, Kinoshita H, Iwasaki A, Owaki Y, Matsushita H, Wakatsuki A. Hypoalbuminemia is related to endothelial dysfunction resulting from oxidative stress in parturients with preeclampsia. Nagoya J Med Sci. 2021 Nov;83(4):741–748. doi: 10.18999/nagjms.83.4.741. PMID: 34916718; PMCID: PMC8648536

5. Martell-Claros, N.1; Abad-Cardiel, M.1; García-Donaire, J.1; De Los Santos, C.2; Gonzalez, V.2; Fuentes, M.1; De La Fuente, J.A.3; Perez-Perez, N.3; Sosa, L.2. HYPOALBUMINEMIA AS A RISK FACTOR OF PREECLAMPSIA- ECLAMPSIA IN HIGH-RISK PREGNANCY. Journal of Hypertension 37():p e240, July 2019. | DOI: 10.1097/01.hjh.0000573076.28399.b1

6. Gojnic M, Petkovic S, Papic M, Mostic T, Jeremic K, Vilendecic Z, Djordjevic S. Plasma albumin level as an indicator of severity of preeclampsia. Clin Exp Obstet Gynecol. 2004;31(3):209–10. PMID: 15491066

7. Chen H, Tao F, Fang X, Wang X. Association of hypoproteinemia in preeclampsia with maternal and perinatal outcomes: A retrospective analysis of high-risk women. J Res Med Sci. 2016 Nov 2;21:98. doi: 10.4103/1735–1995.193170. PMID: 28163744; PMCID: PMC5244641

8. Seong WJ, Chong GO, Hong DG, Lee TH, Lee YS, Cho YL, Chun SS, Park IS. Clinical significance of serum albumin level in pregnancy-related hypertension. J Obstet Gynaecol Res. 2010 Dec;36(6):1165–73. doi: 10.1111/j.1447–0756.2010.01296.x. Epub 2010 Oct 11. PMID: 21040199

9. Sufrin S, Nessa A, Islam MT, Das RK, Rahman MH. Study on Serum Albumin in Third Trimester of Pregnancy. Mymensingh Med J. 2015 Jul;24(3):464–6. PMID: 26329940

10. Soeters PB, Wolfe RR, Shenkin A. Hypoalbuminemia: Pathogenesis and Clinical Significance. JPEN J Parenter Enteral Nutr. 2019 Feb;43(2):181–193. doi: 10.1002/jpen.1451. Epub 2018 Oct 4. PMID: 30288759; PMCID: PMC7379941

11. Lisowska-Myjak, B., Strawa, A., Zborowska, H. et al. Associations between the thyroid panel and serum protein concentrations across pregnancy. Sci Rep 11, 15970 (2021). doi.org/10.1038/s41598–021-94358–3

12. Cave, M., C. Pinkston, S. Rai, B. Wahlang, K. Head, G. Carswell, L. Birnbaum, AND B. Chorley. Persistent organic pollutant exposures are associated with liver toxicity and decreased albumin in a highly exposed human cohort. American Association for the Study of Liver Disease (AASLD) The Liver Meeting, Washington, DC, November 04 – 08, 2022. doi.org/10.23645/epacomptox.21717740

Globulin

The serum globulin blood test measures the total concentration of globulin proteins in the serum. It is an analyte found on the comprehensive metabolic panel (CMP).

Globulins are one of the two major categories of proteins found in the blood, with the other category being albumin. Approximately 40% of total proteins are composed of globulins.

Globulins = Total Protein - Albumin

Globulins can be further divided into different subclasse: alpha-globulins, beta-globulins, and gamma-globulins.

Alpha-Globulins

Alpha-globulins have various functions including transport and enzyme regulation.

- Ceruloplasmin is the major copper-carrying protein in the blood, which also plays a role in iron metabolism.
- Haptoglobin binds to free hemoglobin released from red blood cells when they break down. This prevents the loss of iron through urine and protects the kidneys from potential damage caused by free hemoglobin.
- Thyroxine-binding globulin (TBG) binds and transports thyroxine (T4) in the blood.

Beta-Globulins

Beta-globulins have various functions, including the transport of substances and contributing to immune responses.

- C-reactive protein (CRP) is an acute-phase protein that increases concentration in response to inflammation, infection, or tissue injury.
- Complement components C3, C4, and C5 are involved in various immune responses, including inflammation, opsonization (marking pathogens for destruction), and the formation of the membrane attack complex (MAC) to destroy pathogens.

- Low-density lipoprotein (LDL) contains a mixture of lipids and proteins and carries cholesterol to cells.
- Transferrin binds and transports iron in the blood.

Gamma-Globulins

Gamma-globulins, also known as immunoglobulins (Ig), are part of the immune system. There are several classes of immunoglobulins with distinct functions. Some examples include:

- *IgA (Immunoglobulin A)*: Primarily found in mucosal secretions, such as saliva, tears, and mucous membranes, IgA protects the body's mucosal surfaces from pathogens.
- *IgD (Immunoglobulin D)*: This is found on the surface of β cells and is involved in the initiation of the immune response.
- *IgE (Immunoglobulin E)*: This is primarily associated with allergic and hypersensitivity reactions. It binds to mast cells and basophils, triggering the release of histamines in response to allergens.
- *IgG (Immunoglobulin G)*: As an adaptive immune response, IgG provides long-term protection against infections and can cross the placenta to provide passive immunity to newborns.
- *IgM (Immunoglobulin M)*: This is the first antibody produced in response to an infection or exposure to an antigen.

Pregnancy

Serum globulin increases through the later second and third trimesters. This increase helps to offset the decrease in albumin and to maintain serum protein at a constant level.[1] Alpha- and beta-globulins begin to increase in the first trimester then increase more significantly in the second and third trimesters.

Postpartum

In the immediate postpartum period, serum globulin levels may remain relatively stable. If the individual is breastfeeding, they may experience changes in their globulin levels, particularly regarding immunoglobulins. Breast milk contains immunoglobulins that are transferred from the mother to the infant to provide passive immunity. This transfer can lead to a temporary decrease in the mother's immunoglobulin levels.

> More research has been done on the individual globulin fractions as biomarkers of pregnancy disease than on total serum globulin.

STANDARD LAB RANGE: 1.5 – 4.5 g/dL

Trimester	Standard Pregnancy Ranges	**Functional Pregnancy Ranges**
Preconception	1.5 – 4.5	**2.4 – 2.7**
First Trimester	1.5 – 4.5	**2.5 – 4.5**
Second Trimester	1.5 – 4.5	**2.5 – 4.5**
Third Trimester	1.5 – 4.5	**2.5 – 4.5**
Postpartum	1.5 – 4.5	**2.4 – 2.7**

Causes of Elevated Globulin

See Total Serum Protein Section.

High serum globulin levels are seen in women with hyperemesis gravidarum (HG).[2]

True identification of the underlying cause may require additional testing of individual globulin subtypes based on other labs and symptoms.

Dehydration: Dehydration leads to a decrease in the volume of blood plasma. As a result, the concentration of all blood components, including globulins, may appear higher in the blood sample because there is less fluid to dilute them.

Liver Disease: This can include cirrhosis, nonalcoholic fatty liver disease (NAFLD), hepatitis, or other diseases of the liver. Preeclampsia is characterized by high blood pressure and damage to multiple organ systems, including the liver. Preeclampsia can trigger an inflammatory response and increased oxidative stress in the body, which can affect liver function. As a result, the liver may respond by producing acute-phase reactants and immunoglobulins as part of the body's response to inflammation and tissue damage. Liver enzymes and markers, including globulins, may become elevated in response to liver inflammation and damage.

Inflammatory Bowel Disease (IBD): IBD conditions such as Crohn's disease and ulcerative colitis are characterized by chronic inflammation in the gastrointestinal tract. This chronic inflammation can contribute to an increase in serum globulin levels, primarily by elevating the levels of immunoglobulins. In addition to immunoglobulins, other acute-phase reactants such as c-reactive protein (CRP) can also increase in response to chronic inflammation. These proteins can further contribute to elevated serum globulin levels.

Adrenal Dysfunction: Cortisol's effects on LDL production are complex and can be influenced by both high and low cortisol levels. Cholesterol is an essential precursor in the synthesis of steroid hormones, including cortisol, and it is a key component of cell membranes. When cortisol levels are elevated, such as during periods of stress, it can lead to an increase in LDL production. On the other hand, if cortisol levels are insufficient, there may be an increase in the production of LDL to facilitate the need for cholesterol in cortisol synthesis.

Inflammation: CRP production is part of the body's defense mechanism to detect and respond to infection, injury, or inflammatory processes. As CRP is synthesized and released into the bloodstream, it contributes to elevated serum globulin levels.

Other Possible Causes: oxidative stress, parasitic infections, acute viral or bacterial infections, autoimmune disease, zinc deficiency, vitamin D deficiency, thyroid dysfunction

Treatment Strategies for Elevated Globulin

See Total Serum Protein Section.

Diet

Reducing elevated globulin levels through dietary strategies involves an anti-inflammatory approach that prioritizes foods rich in antioxidants. An anti-inflammatory diet includes a colorful array of fruits and vegetables, especially berries, leafy greens, spices like turmeric and ginger, omega-3 fatty acids from sources like fatty fish, and flaxseeds. Incorporating nuts, seeds, whole-meat proteins, and probiotic-rich foods like full-fat yogurt can provide healthy fats. Green tea may offer antioxidant benefits. Avoid processed and sugary foods, and minimize caffeine consumption. Beet juice and the Mediterranean diet have shown promise in the treatment of liver diseases, including NAFLD.

Lifestyle

Sleep deprivation (sleep duration ≤5 hours) is associated with higher serum IgA, IgG, and IgM and higher C3 and C4 levels.[3] Improve sleep habits and hygiene to reduce immune responses and inflammation.

Supplementation

Zinc is essential for immune function and may help modulate immune responses. Some studies have explored its potential to reduce immunoglobulin production in specific situations.

Zinc lozenges are a safe supplement option in pregnancy that can help prevent overdosing on zinc and suppressing copper. N-acetyl cysteine has been shown to reduce CRP levels.[4] Selenium supplementation has also been shown to decrease CRP levels, as well as reduce immunoglobulin production.[5]

Additional Testing

complete blood count (CBC); c-reactive protein (CRP); antinuclear antibodies (ANA); ceruloplasmin; copper, total; vitamin D, 25-hydroxy (25-hydroxycalciferol, 25OH-D); comprehensive thyroid profile II; serum protein electrophoresis (SPEP); gamma-glutamyl transpeptidase (GGT); lactate dehydrogenase (LDH); urinalysis; comprehensive stool testing; oral zinc tolerance test

Causes of Low Globulin

See Total Serum Protein Section.

True identification of underlying causes may require additional testing of individual globulin subtypes based on other labs and symptoms.

Preeclampsia: Kidney damage in preeclampsia can result from elevated blood pressure and reduced blood flow to the kidneys, leading to impaired function. The damaged kidneys may allow the escape of various proteins, including globulins, into the urine. Consequently, proteinuria can contribute to a decrease in serum globulin levels.

Vitamin B6 (Pyridoxine) Deficiency: Vitamin B6 is a cofactor in enzymatic reactions that are needed for proper protein synthesis. It also modulates inflammation and immune responses. Deficiencies disrupt the balance of pro-inflammatory and anti-inflammatory proteins.

Hypothyroidism: The liver is the primary site of TBG synthesis. Thyroid hormones, primarily T4, stimulate the liver to produce more TBG. When thyroid hormone levels rise, the liver increases TBG production to accommodate the higher thyroid hormone concentrations. The production of thyroid hormones T4 and T3 is regulated by the hypothalamic-pituitary-thyroid (HPT) axis. When thyroid hormone levels in the blood are low, the hypothalamus releases thyrotropin-releasing hormone (TRH), which stimulates the pituitary gland to release thyroid-stimulating hormone (TSH). TSH, in turn, prompts the thyroid gland to produce more T4 and T3. When thyroid hormone levels are adequate, the HPT axis reduces the production of TRH and TSH, leading to a decrease in thyroid hormone production and TBG synthesis.

Other Possible Causes: protein-deficient diets, chronic infections, vitamin D deficiency, copper deficiency, selenium deficiency, autoimmune disease, chronic infections

Treatment Strategies for Low Globulin

See Total Serum Protein Section.

Diet

Ensure an adequate intake of high-quality protein sources. Ensuring an adequate intake of vitamin B6 through a balanced diet or supplementation will help support proper protein synthesis. Identifying the underlying cause of low serum globulin may require knowing the individual deficiency of globulin production.

Supplementation

Bovine colostrum has shown some benefit in increasing globulin levels in some studies. Bovine colostrum contains various antimicrobial compounds, including lactoferrin, lactoperoxidase, and lysozyme, which help protect against infections and inhibit the growth of bacteria, viruses, and fungi. Overall, it is considered a safe supplement in humans, but there is limited data available for safety in pregnancy.

Additional Testing

complete blood count (CBC); urinalysis; 24-hour urinary protein; c-reactive protein (CRP); antinuclear antibodies (ANA); oral zinc tolerance test; vitamin D, 25-hydroxy (25-hydroxycalciferol, 25OH-D); comprehensive thyroid profile II; serum protein electrophoresis (SPEP); transferrin; lipid panel; copper, total; ceruloplasmin

References

1. Haram K, Augensen K, Elsayed S. Serum protein pattern in normal pregnancy with special reference to acute-phase reactants. Br J Obstet Gynaecol. 1983 Feb;90(2):139–45. doi: 10.1111/j.1471–0528.1983.tb08898.x. PMID: 6600623

2. Begum, JA & Sultana, R & Naher, S. (2010). Serum Levels of Total Protein, Albumin and Globulin in Woman with Hyperemesis Gravidarum. Journal of Dhaka Medical College. 19. 10.3329/jdmc.v19i1.6254

3. Hui L, Hua F, Diandong H, Hong Y. Effects of sleep and sleep deprivation on immunoglobulins and complement in humans. Brain Behav Immun. 2007 Mar;21(3):308–10. doi: 10.1016/j.bbi.2006.09.005. Epub 2006 Oct 27. Erratum in: Brain Behav Immun. 2010 May;24(4):678–9. PMID: 17070668

4. Askari M, Faryabi R, Mozaffari H, Darooghegi Mofrad M. The effects of N-Acetylcysteine on serum level of inflammatory biomarkers in adults. Findings from a systematic review and meta-analysis of randomized clinical trials. Cytokine. 2020 Nov;135:155239. doi: 10.1016/j.cyto.2020.155239. Epub 2020 Aug 12. PMID: 32799012

5. Djalalinia S, Hasani M, Asayesh H, Ejtahed HS, Malmir H, Kasaeian A, Zarei M, Baygi F, Rastad H, Mahdavi Gorabi A, Qorbani M. The effects of dietary selenium supplementation on inflammatory markers among patients with metabolic diseases: a systematic review and meta-analysis of randomized controlled trials. J Diabetes Metab Disord. 2021 Jun 9;20(1):1051–1062. doi: 10.1007/s40200–021-00821–3. PMID: 34222098; PMCID: PMC8212246

Albumin to Globulin Ratio (A/G Ratio)

The albumin-globulin ratio (A/G ratio) is a calculated value derived from the results of blood tests that measure the levels of albumin and globulins in the bloodstream. It is an analyte found on the comprehensive metabolic panel (CMP).

The A/G ratio is used to assess the ratio of albumin to globulin. The liver is a vital organ responsible for the synthesis of many blood proteins. In some cases, the A/G ratio can be used as an indicator of kidney function, as albumin is lost through the urine in kidney inflammation and damage.

> Albumin/Globulin = A/G ratio

Its accuracy is limited, and it should not be use as a single analyte, especially in pregnancy.

Pregnancy

Since albumin concentration decreases and the alpha and beta-globulin concentrations increase, there is a sharp decline in the A/G ratio during pregnancy. A/G ratio is significantly reduced in the first and second trimesters, and either plateaus or decreases slightly more in the third trimester.[1 2]

Postpartum

In the immediate postpartum period, the body starts to shed excess fluid, leading to a more concentrated blood composition. This can result in a transient increase in albumin levels, potentially leading to a higher A/G ratio.

STANDARD LAB RANGE: 1.2 – 2.2:1

Trimester	Standard Pregnancy Ranges	**Functional Pregnancy Ranges**
Preconception	1.2 – 2.2:1	**1.5 – 2.0:1**
First Trimester	1.2 – 2.2:1	**1.0 – 2.0:1**
Second Trimester	1.2 – 2.2:1	**1.0 – 2.0:1**
Third Trimester	1.2 – 2.2:1	**1.0 – 2.0:1**
Postpartum	1.2 – 2.2:1	**1.5 – 2.0:1**

Causes of Elevated Albumin to Globulin Ratio (A/G Ratio)

See the following sections: Total Serum Protein, Serum Albumin, and Serum Globulin.

Other Possible Causes: thyroid dysfunction, low estrogen, infections, inflammation, high-protein diet, adrenal hypofunction, acute liver dysfunction, vitamin B6 (pyridoxine) deficiency, vitamin D deficiency, selenium deficiency, autoimmune disease, genetics, cancer

Treatment Strategies for Elevated Albumin to Globulin Ratio (A/G Ratio)

See the following sections: Total Serum Protein, Serum Albumin, and Serum Globulin.

Additional Testing

complete blood count (CBC); c-reactive protein (CRP); vitamin D, 25-hydroxy (25-hydroxycalciferol, 25OH-D); comprehensive thyroid profile II; reverse T3 (rT3); serum protein electrophoresis (SPEP); urinalysis; antinuclear antibodies (ANA)

Causes of Low Albumin to Globulin Ratio (A/G Ratio)

See the following sections: Total Serum Protein, Serum Albumin, and Serum Globulin.

Other Possible Causes: dehydration, liver disease, protein-deficient diets, vitamin C deficiency, inflammatory bowel diseases, parasitic infections, acute viral or bacterial infections, autoimmune disease, hypochlorhydria, inflammation, oxidative stress, thyroid dysfunction, adrenal hyperfunction, vitamin D deficiency, vitamin B6 (pyridoxine) deficiency, vitamin B12 (cobalamin) deficiency, vitamin B9 (folate) deficiency, selenium deficiency, vitamin B3 (niacin) deficiency, zinc deficiency, chloride deficiency, vitamin B1 (thiamine) deficiency, magnesium deficiency, calcium deficiency, progesterone deficiency, environmental toxin exposure

Treatment Strategies for Low Albumin to Globulin Ratio (A/G Ratio)

See the following sections: Total Serum Protein, Serum Albumin, and Serum Globulin.

Additional Testing

complete blood count (CBC); c-reactive protein (CRP); oral zinc tolerance test; vitamin D, 25-hydroxy (25-hydroxycalciferol, 25OH-D); vitamin B12 (cobalamin); methylmalonic acid; homocysteine; comprehensive thyroid profile II; reverse T3 (rT3); serum protein electrophoresis (SPEP); urinalysis; 24-hour urinary protein; comprehensive stool testing; gamma-glutamyl transpeptidase (GGT); lactate dehydrogenase (LDH); progesterone; antinuclear antibodies (ANA); heavy metal testing

References

1. Das A, Teli A.B, Borkotoki S. Study of Liver Function Tests in Normal Pregnancy: A Hospital-Based Study. International Journal of Health Sciences and Research. 2016(6);156–160

2. Joseph JC, Baker C, Sprang ML, Bermes EW. Changes in plasma proteins during pregnancy. Ann Clin Lab Sci. 1978 Mar-Apr;8(2):130–41. PMID: 76457

Bilirubin, Total

Total bilirubin measures the total amount of both conjugated and unconjugated bilirubin in the blood sample. It is an analyte found on the comprehensive metabolic panel (CMP).

Approximately 80% of bilirubin is made from the breakdown of hemoglobin in old red blood cells and prematurely destroyed erythroid cells in the bone marrow. The remainder comes from the turnover of various heme-containing proteins found in other tissues, primarily the liver and muscles.[1]

Red blood cells have a lifespan of about 120 days. When they reach the end of their lifespan, they are removed from circulation and broken down through hemolysis. Hemolysis releases hemoglobin from the red blood cells.

Hemoglobin is a protein that carries oxygen in the blood. During hemolysis, hemoglobin is released from the red blood cell and broken down into its heme and globin components.

The heme part is further converted into biliverdin by an enzyme called heme oxygenase. Biliverdin is green in color. An enzyme called biliverdin reductase then converts biliverdin into bilirubin, a yellow pigment. Bilirubin is initially insoluble in water, so it binds to albumin in the blood. This form of bilirubin is called unconjugated bilirubin and is transported to the liver.

Unconjugated bilirubin is combined with glucuronic acid inside the liver, making it water-soluble. This form of bilirubin is called conjugated bilirubin. Conjugated bilirubin is excreted into the bile, which is released into the small intestine to aid in the digestion and absorption of fats.

In the small intestine, conjugated bilirubin is further modified by gut bacteria. This process transforms it into urobilinogen, some of which is reabsorbed and excreted in the urine, while the rest is eliminated in feces. The urobilinogen that is not reabsorbed in the intestines is further transformed into stercobilin, which gives feces its characteristic brown color.

Bilirubin is a natural antioxidant that scavenges free radicals. Experimental findings suggest that all forms of bilirubin—unconjugated, conjugated, free, and albumin-bound—possess significant antioxidant properties. Bilirubin is believed to hinder the creation of advanced glycation end products, inhibit protein kinase C activity, and play a role in mitigating inflammatory responses.[2] Other studies have shown that elevations in bilirubin may be protective against hemochromatosis.[3]

Pregnancy

Total bilirubin concentrations are decreased during all three trimesters of pregnancy.[4] Increased RBC production increases hemoglobin breakdown, but hemodilution causes a net decrease in serum levels. Unconjugated bilirubin levels remain stable from preconception through pregnancy, with a slight drop in the second and third trimesters. Conjugated bilirubin levels decrease throughout pregnancy, starting in early pregnancy.

Postpartum

Maternal bilirubin levels may rise slightly due to the elimination of excess red blood cells that were required during pregnancy. However, these levels typically return to normal within a few days after childbirth. In some cases, postpartum complications such as hemorrhage during delivery or hemolysis can lead to elevated bilirubin levels in the immediate postpartum period.

STANDARD LAB RANGE: 0.0 – 1.2 mg/dL

Trimester	Standard Pregnancy Ranges	**Functional Pregnancy Ranges**
Preconception	0.0 – 1.2	**0.0 – 1.9**
First Trimester	0.1 – 0.4	**0.1 – 0.4**
Second Trimester	0.1 – 0.8	**0.1 – 0.8**
Third Trimester	0.1 – 1.1	**0.1 – 1.1**
Postpartum	0.0 – 1.2	**0.0 – 1.9**

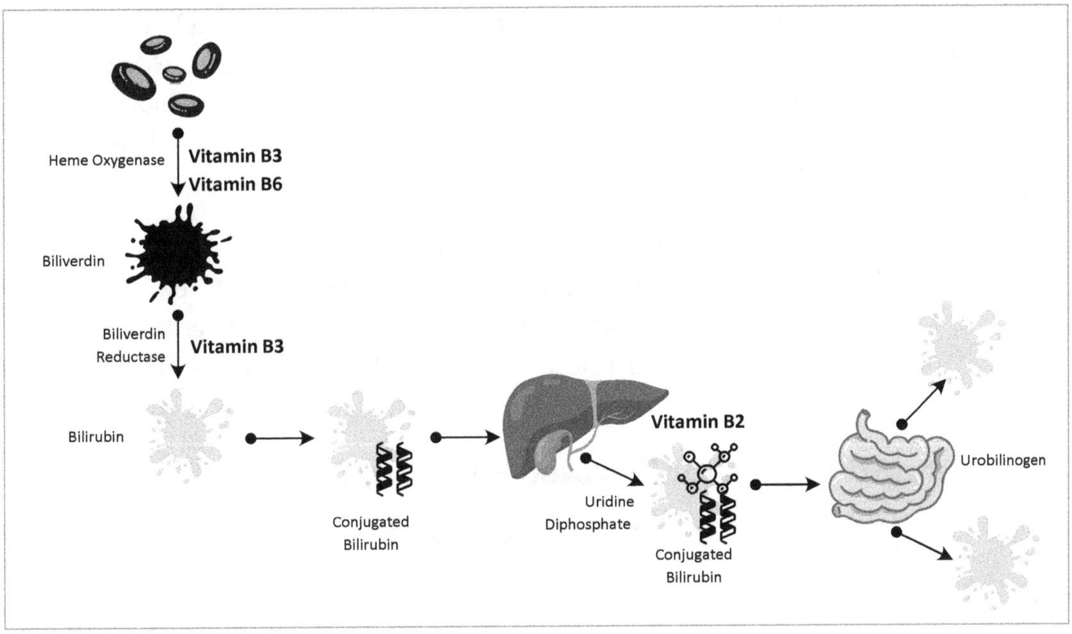

Figure 9: Bilirubin Metabolism

Hemoglobin is broken down into heme and globin components. Vitamin B6 (pyridoxine) is needed for the breakdown of heme. The heme part is further converted into biliverdin through the action of an enzyme called heme oxygenase. Biliverdin is then converted into bilirubin by an enzyme called biliverdin reductase. Bilirubin is initially insoluble in water, so it binds to albumin in the blood. This form of bilirubin is called unconjugated bilirubin and is transported to the liver. Inside the liver, it is conjugated (combined) with glucuronic acid. This requires UDP, a coenzyme used in the reaction catalyzed by the UDP-glucanosyltransferase (UGT) enzymes, which conjugate bilirubin with glucuronic acid to form conjugated bilirubin. This is riboflavin-dependent. Conjugated bilirubin is excreted into the bile, which is further modified by gut bacteria. This process transforms it into urobilinogen. Urobilinogen is either reabsorbed and excreted in the urine or excreted with the stools.

Causes of Elevated Total Bilirubin, Total

See the following sections: Serum Iron (Iron), Hemoglobin (HB), and Bile Acid.

Any increase in serum alanine aminotransferase (ALT) (SGPT), aspartate aminotransferase (AST)(SGOT), serum gamma-glutamyl transpeptidase (GGT), serum bilirubin, or fasting total bile acid concentrations

Hemolysis: Oxidative stress occurs when there is an imbalance between the production of ROS and the body's ability to detoxify them, leading to cellular damage. Oxidative stress reduces the lifespan of red blood cells and increases the rate of hemolysis.

Intrahepatic Cholestasis of Pregnancy (ICP): Intrahepatic cholestasis of pregnancy (ICP) is a liver disorder that can occur in the second or third trimester. It is characterized by impaired bile flow within the liver and the buildup of bile acid in the bloodstream. The accumulated bile acid in the blood can disrupt the normal function-

should always be considered pathologic in pregnancy.

ing of hepatocytes. As a result, the liver may struggle to conjugate bilirubin with glucuronic acid effectively, leading to elevated levels of unconjugated bilirubin. As a result, bilirubin accumulates in the blood, causing hyperbilirubinemia. Elevated bilirubin only presents in approximately 25% of ICP cases.[5]

Other Possible Causes: Gilbert's syndrome, mycotoxin exposure, toxin exposure, preeclampsia, selenium deficiency, manganese deficiency, thyroid dysfunction, thalassemia, sickle cell anemia, iron overload, zinc deficiency, vitamin B12 (cobalamin) deficiency

Treatment Strategies for Elevated Bilirubin, Total

See the following sections: Serum Iron (Iron), Hemoglobin (HB), and Bile Acid.

Diet

Antioxidant-rich foods such as berries and leafy greens can further reduce inflammation and oxidative stress. Additionally, the patient should limit processed foods and avoid rancid oils. Ginger has traditionally been used to aid digestion and support liver health. It may help stimulate bile production and improve bilirubin excretion. Beets contain betaine, which supports liver function and may aid in the excretion of bilirubin.

Supplements

Dandelion root has been used in traditional medicine to support liver health and aid in the management of jaundice. A typical dosage range is between 500 and 2,000 milligrams per day, divided into two or three doses.

Additional Testing

complete blood count (CBC); vitamin B12 (cobalamin); methylmalonic acid; homocysteine; ferritin; iron and TIBC; bile acid, serum; gamma-glutamyl transpeptidase (GGT); comprehensive thyroid profile II; c-reactive protein (CRP)

Causes of Low Bilirubin, Total

See the following sections: Serum Iron (Iron) and Hemoglobin (HB).

Zinc Overload: Supplementation of zinc sulfate increases bilirubin excretion and decreases its serum level.

Other Possible Causes: severe hemolytic anemia, certain medications (antibiotics, antivirals), autoimmune disease, vitamin B6 (pyridoxine) deficiency, iron deficiency

Treatment Strategies for Low Bilirubin, Total

See the following sections: Serum Iron (Iron) and Hemoglobin (HB).

Additional Testing

complete blood count (CBC); ferritin; iron and TIBC; gamma-glutamyl transpeptidase (GGT); comprehensive thyroid profile II; c-reactive protein (CRP); oral zinc tolerance test; antinuclear antibodies (ANA)

References

1. Kalakonda A, Jenkins BA, John S. Physiology, Bilirubin. [Updated 2022 Sep 12]. In: StatPearls [Internet]. Treasure Island (FL): StatPearls Publishing; Jan 2023. www.ncbi.nlm.nih.gov/books/NBK470290

2. Chung JO, Park SY, Chung DJ, Chung MY. Relationship between anemia, serum bilirubin concentrations, and diabetic retinopathy in individuals with type 2 diabetes. Medicine (Baltimore). 2019;98(43):e17693. doi:10.1097/MD.0000000000017693

3. Alizadeh BZ, Njajou OT, Houwing-Duistermaat JJ, et al. Does bilirubin protect against hemochromatosis gene (HFE) related mortality? Am J Med Genet A. 2004;129A(1):39–43. doi:10.1002/ajmg.a.30163

4. Bacq Y. The Liver in Normal Pregnancy. In: Madame Curie Bioscience Database [Internet]. Austin (TX): Landes Bioscience; 2000–2013. www.ncbi.nlm.nih.gov/books/NBK6005

5. Pillarisetty LS, Sharma A. Pregnancy Intrahepatic Cholestasis. [Updated 2023 Jun 4]. In: StatPearls [Internet]. Treasure Island (FL): StatPearls Publishing; Jan 2023. www.ncbi.nlm.nih.gov/books/NBK551503

Alkaline Phosphatase (ALP)

Alkaline phosphatase (ALP) measures the total ALP from all isotopes in the blood sample. It is an analyte found on the comprehensive metabolic panel (CMP).

Alkaline phosphatase is a zinc metalloprotein enzyme found in various tissues throughout the body, including the liver, bones, kidney, intestine, and placenta. It is called "alkaline" because it works optimally at a slightly basic or alkaline pH. Thyroid hormones are required to synthesize alkaline phosphatase, and it can be a biomarker of thyroid function.

It primarily acts as a dephosphorylating enzyme, removing phosphate groups from various molecules, influencing metabolic and signaling pathways. In bone tissue, ALP plays a key role in bone mineralization by facilitating the formation of hydroxyapatite crystals, which are essential for the structural integrity of bones. In the gut, it aids in nutrient absorption by breaking down phosphate-containing compounds from the diet. ALP also contributes to cell growth and differentiation in tissues like the liver and bone, potentially modulates immune responses, and is produced by the placenta during pregnancy.

ALP isozymes are variants of the ALP enzyme found in different tissues throughout the body. Each isozyme has slightly different properties and is associated with specific functions. Here are the four main ALP isozymes.

Bone ALP (BAP): This isozyme is primarily found in bone tissue and is produced by osteoblasts, the bone-forming cells. It is essential for bone mineralization, as it helps create the optimal environment for the formation of hydroxyapatite crystals, which give bones their structural strength. Elevated levels of bone ALP can be seen in conditions involving increased bone turnover, such as bone growth, fracture healing, or certain bone diseases. Newer research shows that it may also help with the production of calcitriol from the kidneys due to its relation in studies to parathyroid hormones, calcium, and bone turnover.[1]

Intestinal ALP (IAP): This isozyme is primarily found in the small intestine, particularly in the brush border of the intestinal mucosa. Its primary role is in dephosphorylating dietary compounds, such as phosphate-containing molecules, facilitating nutrient absorption. Elevated levels of IAP in the blood may be associated with conditions affecting the intestine, such as celiac disease or other gastrointestinal disorders.

Liver ALP (LAP): Liver ALP is produced by hepatocytes in the liver. It is released into the bloodstream when liver cells are damaged, making it a common marker for liver health.

Elevated levels of liver ALP can be indicative of liver diseases, including hepatitis, cirrhosis, or biliary obstruction. It is also involved in lipid metabolism within the liver.

Placental ALP (PLAP): Placental ALP is produced by the placenta during pregnancy. It contributes to the formation of the maternal-fetal barrier, which separates maternal blood from fetal blood within the placenta. This barrier is essential for regulating the exchange of nutrients, gases, and waste products between the maternal and fetal circulations. Elevated levels of placental ALP are normal during pregnancy.

Pregnancy

During pregnancy, alkaline phosphatase may reach three times the upper normal limit.[2] This increase begins at the end of the first trimester and continues through the third trimester.[3] Total ALP levels in the blood increase during pregnancy, with placental ALP being a key contributor. Placental ALP levels progressively rise throughout pregnancy, peaking in the third trimester and contributing to the elevated total ALP levels observed in pregnant women.

Postpartum

Over the following weeks, typically within the first few weeks after childbirth, ALP levels should gradually return to nonpregnant or baseline levels.

> Over 1,000 drugs, herbs, and physiological conditions affecting ALP activity have been documented; therefore, as a single analyte, it is not reliable.

STANDARD LAB RANGE: 44 – 121 IU/L

Trimester	Standard Pregnancy Ranges	**Functional Pregnancy Ranges**
Preconception	44 – 121	**50 – 121**
First Trimester	17 – 88	**45 – 120**
Second Trimester	25 – 126	**100 – 320**
Third Trimester	38 – 229	**100 – 320**
Postpartum	44 – 121	**50 – 121**

Causes of Elevated Alkaline Phosphatase (ALP)

Bone Loss: ALP bone isoenzyme will increase when there is a breakdown of bone. In this case, there may also be a decrease in serum calcium and vitamin D.

Placental Dysfunction: Placental dysfunction, which can result from various factors like preeclampsia, gestational diabetes, or placental insufficiency, can cause the placenta to release placental ALP into the maternal bloodstream at higher levels than usual. This increase in placental ALP contributes to the overall ALP elevation seen in pregnant women. These values are often extreme.

Intrahepatic Cholestasis of Pregnancy (ICP): ALP is elevated in ICP up to fourfold, but this is not helpful for diagnosis of the disorder since ALP is already elevated in pregnancy due to production by the placenta.[4]

Liver Disease: Elevated bilirubin, alanine aminotransferase (ALT) (SGPT), aspartate aminotransferase (AST)(SGOT), alkaline phosphatase (ALP), and gamma-glutamyl transpeptidase (GGT) would indicate liver inflammation or disease.

Hyperthyroidism: In hyperthyroidism, ALP and ALT are often elevated.[5] Thyroid hormones in excess accelerate bone turnover, increasing bone resorption and decreasing bone formation. This heightened bone activity causes the release of ALP from bone tissue into the bloodstream. Additionally, hyperthyroidism may impact liver function, prompting hepatocytes to produce and release ALP. The result is an increase in ALP levels in the blood, a phenomenon attributed to both liver and bone ALP isoenzymes. In pregnancy, this same mechanism can cause an increase in placental ALP isoenzymes. The frequency of abnormal levels of each liver function test in hyperthyroidism is 33% for ALT, 23% for AST, 44% for ALP, 12% for total bilirubin, and 24% for GGT.[6]

Other Possible Causes: Gilbert's syndrome, gallstones, adrenal hyperfunction, inflammatory bowel diseases (celiac disease), hyperparathyroidism, renal dysfunction, vitamin D deficiency, calcium deficiency, bone trauma/fracture, cancer

Treatment Strategies for Elevated Alkaline Phosphatase (ALP)

Extreme elevations in ALP are a serious complication that needs medical management. Slight elevations are normal in pregnancy.

Supplements

Accurate supplement treatment may depend on the underlying cause of the elevated ALP and which isoform is contributing to increased levels. Studies have suggested that milk thistle and ginger supplementation may help reduce ALP levels in individuals with liver conditions. Supplementing with vitamin D may be beneficial if elevated ALP levels are due to bone disorders or vitamin D deficiency.

Additional Testing

alkaline phosphatase isoenzymes; complete blood count (CBC); comprehensive thyroid profile II; thyroid peroxidase antibodies (TPOAb); thyroglobulin antibody (TgAb); thyroid receptor antibodies (TRAb); c-reactive protein (CRP); gamma-glutamyl transpeptidase (GGT); vitamin D, 25-hydroxy (25-hydroxycalciferol, 25OH-D); bile acid, serum; parathyroid hormone; comprehensive stool testing

Causes of Low Alkaline Phosphatase (ALP)

Zinc Deficiency: Low ALP is a biomarker of zinc deficiency.[10 11] Zinc is not only in the structure of ALP but also affects overall function. It can act as a cofactor for some forms of alkaline phosphatase. In this role, zinc ions can bind to the enzyme's active site and help catalyze the dephosphorylation reactions carried out by ALP. Zinc's presence can enhance the enzyme's activity, making it more effective at removing phosphate groups from its substrates. Decreased RBC zinc, low-normal WBC, and a decreased lymphocyte percentage may indicate zinc deficiency.

Magnesium Deficiency: Magnesium affects ALP function, but less so the production. Studies show that low ALP is often associated with low magnesium. Magnesium supplementation helps improve enzyme function but not production.[12]

Hypothyroidism: Hypothyroidism typically presents with a lower ALP and higher AST. Thyroid hormones regulate metabolism and tissue growth. Reduced thyroid hormone activity can result in decreased bone resorption and decreased ALP release from bone tissue.

Low ALP in pregnancy has been shown to predict IUGR of the fetus and a high-risk pregnancy.[7]

The low ALP during pregnancy probably reflects a reduced placental size or decreased ability to produce ALP.[8]

According to a 2023 study published in *The Lancet*, serum ALP levels (≤116 IU/L) in late pregnancy increase the risk of venous thromboembolism.[9]

Furthermore, liver function may be impaired in hypothyroidism, affecting the production and release of ALP by hepatocytes. The combined effect is often a decrease in ALP levels in the bloodstream, which can be observed in individuals with hypothyroidism. It is also important to address both zinc and magnesium in these cases.[13]

Progesterone Deficiency: Progesterone has also been shown to stimulate the expression of ALP.[14]

Other Possible Causes: low-protein diet, malnutrition, estrogen dominance, vitamin D deficiency

Treatment Strategies for Low Alkaline Phosphatase (ALP)

Diet

Consuming zinc-rich foods is essential for maintaining proper zinc levels in the body. These include lean meats, poultry, seafood (such as oysters), dairy products, nuts, seeds, and whole grains.

Supplements

Around 50 mg of zinc has been shown to increase ALP levels over the course of 12 weeks of treatment. Caution should be taken with high doses at this level, as they can impair iron absorption and decrease serum copper levels, both of which are important in pregnancy. Dosage should be limited to <20 mg a day. Zinc taste testing, also known as the zinc sulfate taste test or zinc tally test, is used to assess zinc status in the body. The test involves administering a small amount of zinc sulfate solution orally and evaluating the taste perception. The taste reaction is thought to be related to the body's zinc status, as individuals with zinc insufficiencies or deficiencies typically report a neutral or slightly metallic taste, while those with adequate zinc may perceive a stronger, unpleasant taste. Additional supplementation will depend on the underlying etiology of decreased ALP production. Zinc lozenges can be used similarly, and when taste is present, supplementation is stopped to reduce the risk of zinc overload.

Additional Testing

oral zinc tolerance test; complete blood count (CBC); comprehensive thyroid profile II; c-reactive protein (CRP); vitamin D, 25-hydroxy (25-hydroxycalciferol, 25OH-D); progesterone

References

1. Bellastella G, Scappaticcio L, Longo M, Carotenuto R, Carbone C, Caruso P, Maio A, Paglionico VA, Vietri MT, Maiorino MI, Esposito K. New insights into vitamin D regulation: is there a role for alkaline phosphatase? J Endocrinol Invest. 2021 Sep;44(9):1891–1896. doi: 10.1007/s40618–021-01503-w. Epub 2021 Jan 25. PMID: 33492600; PMCID: PMC8357672

2. McErlean S, King C. Does an abnormally elevated maternal alkaline phosphatase pose problems for the fetus? BMJ Case Rep. 2019 Apr 30;12(4):e229109. doi: 10.1136/bcr-2018–229109. PMID: 31040142; PMCID: PMC6506124

3. Nissim Arbib, Kira Nahum Sacks, Lina Salman, Orly Sneh-Arbib, Alexandra Berezowsky, Eyal Krispin, Eran Hadar. Normal distribution of alkaline phosphatase levels during pregnancy. Clin. Exp. Obstet. Gynecol. 2021, 48(6), 1393–1399. doi.org/10.31083/j.ceog4806220

4. Singh G, Sidhu K. Cholestasis of Pregnancy: A Prospective Study. Med J Armed Forces India. 2008 Oct;64(4):343–5. doi: 10.1016/S0377–1237(08)80017–2. Epub 2011 Jul 21. PMID: 27688573; PMCID: PMC5035245

5. Huang MJ, Liaw YF. Clinical associations between thyroid and liver diseases. J Gastroenterol Hepatol. 1995 May–Jun;10(3):344–50. doi: 10.1111/j.1440–1746.1995.tb01106.x. PMID: 7548816

6. Scappaticcio L et al 2020. Abnormal liver blood tests in patients with hyperthyroidism: Systematic review and meta-analysis. Thyroid. Epub 2020 Dec 16. PMID: 33327837

7. Holmgren PA, Stigbrand T, Damber MG, von Schoultz B. Serum levels of placental alkaline phosphatase in high-risk pregnancies. Obstet Gynecol 1979;54:631–4

8. Ranganath L, Taylor W, John L, Alfirevic Z. Biochemical diagnosis of placental infarction/damage: acutely rising alkaline phosphatase. Annals of Clinical Biochemistry. 2008;45(3):335–338. doi:10.1258/acb.2007.007098

9. Li Q, Wang H, Wang H, Deng J, Cheng Z, Lin W, Zhu R, Chen S, Guo J, Tang LV, Hu Y. Association between serum alkaline phosphatase levels in late pregnancy and the incidence of venous thromboembolism postpartum: a retrospective cohort study. EClinicalMedicine. 2023 Jul 20;62:102088. doi: 10.1016/j.eclinm.2023.102088. PMID: 37533415; PMCID: PMC10393549

10. Weismann K, Høyer H. Serum alkaline phosphatase and serum zinc levels in the diagnosis and exclusion of zinc deficiency in man. Am J Clin Nutr. 1985 Jun;41(6):1214–9. doi: 10.1093/ajcn/41.6.1214. PMID: 4003329

11. Cho YE, Lomeda RA, Ryu SH, Sohn HY, Shin HI, Beattie JH, Kwun IS. Zinc deficiency negatively affects alkaline phosphatase and the concentration of Ca, Mg and P in rats. Nutr Res Pract. 2007 Summer;1(2):113–9. doi: 10.4162/nrp.2007.1.2.113. Epub 2007 Jun 30. PMID: 20535396; PMCID: PMC2882585

12. Heaton, F. Effect of Magnesium Deficiency on Plasma Alkaline Phosphatase Activity. Nature 207, 1292–1293 (1965). doi.org/10.1038/2071292b0

13. Al-Janabi G, Hassan HN, Al-Fahham A. Biochemical changes in patients during hypothyroid phase after thyroidectomy. J Med Life. 2022 Jan;15(1):104–108. doi: 10.25122/jml-2021–0297. PMID: 35186143; PMCID: PMC8852639

14. Di Lorenzo D, Giannì M, Savoldi GF, Ferrari F, Albertini A, Garattini E. Progesterone-induced expression of alkaline phosphatase is associated with a secretory phenotype in T47D breast cancer cells. Biochem Biophys Res Commun. 1993 May 14;192(3):1066–72. doi: 10.1006/bbrc.1993.1525. PMID: 8507182

Aspartate Aminotransferase (AST) (SGOT)

Aspartate aminotransferase (AST), also known as serum glutamic oxaloacetic transminase (SGOT), measures total AST in a blood sample and is an analyte found on the comprehensive metabolic panel (CMP).

AST is an enzyme found in the body's cells, particularly in the heart, liver, and kidneys but also in the muscles, RBCs, and brain. AST testing provides a total AST count from all sources. It can be elevated in cardiac, liver, or kidney damage but is more specific for cardiovascular inflammation.

Aspartate transaminase catalyzes the interconversion of aspartate and α-ketoglutarate to oxaloacetate and glutamate.

L-Aspartate + α-Ketoglutarate ↔ Oxaloacetate + L-Glutamate

AST is a pyridoxine-5'-phosphate, also known as P5P or pyridoxal-5'-phosphate (PLP).[1]

There are two isoenzymes of AST found in humans.

Cytoplasmic AST (cAST or GOT1): This isoenzyme is primarily found in the cytoplasm of cells, including liver cells. It is involved in the transamination reactions of aspartate and α-ketoglutarate to produce oxaloacetate and glutamate. The cytoplasmic AST is coded for by the GOT1 gene.

Mitochondrial AST (mAST or GOT2): This isoenzyme is found in the mitochondria of cells, including heart and skeletal muscle cells. It participates in transamination reactions and is particularly abundant in tissues with high energy requirements. The GOT2 gene codes for it.

AST participates in energy production by helping to maintain the citric acid cycle (Krebs cycle) and the proper functioning of the tricarboxylic acid cycle. Elevated levels of AST in the bloodstream are often used as a marker of tissue damage, especially in the liver and heart, and the placenta in pregnancy. When these organs are damaged, AST is released into the bloodstream, and its levels increase.

Pregnancy

The effects of pregnancy in serum ALT and AST activity levels are somewhat controversial. A slight increase in ALT and/or AST activity during the third trimester has been found in a few studies. Most studies, however, show that serum ALT and AST activity levels do not change during pregnancy or remain within the normal limits established in nonpregnant women.[2] Physiologically, a slight increase before the onset of labor may be a normal finding as mild contractions increase. This should not cause AST levels to increase past healthy ranges.

Postpartum

AST levels can increase during childbirth and increase 88% within the first five days of postpartum. This is increased further in cesarean delivery and anesthesia use during labor.[3] During labor and delivery, the body can undergo various physiological stressors, including muscle contractions, increased cardiac output, and changes in blood volume. These factors may temporarily elevate AST levels. Certain medications and anesthesia used during childbirth can affect liver function and influence AST levels. Any temporary elevation of AST due to the stress of childbirth and hormonal changes typically returns to normal levels within a few weeks as the body recovers.

STANDARD LAB RANGE: 0 – 40 IU/L

Trimester	Standard Pregnancy Ranges	**Functional Pregnancy Ranges**
Preconception	0–40	**10 – 30**
First Trimester	3–23	**10 – 30**
Second Trimester	3–33	**10 – 30**
Third Trimester	4–32	**10 – 30**
Postpartum	0–40	**10 – 40**

Causes of Elevated Aspartate Aminotransferase (AST)(SGOT)

Hyperemesis Gravidarum (HG): HG is not a liver disease in the strict sense, but it leads to liver dysfunction in 50% of cases.[5] There are mild (>50 IU/L) to up to twentyfold elevations in AST and ALT and, rarely, mild jaundice. Liver function abnormalities typically resolve upon resolution of vomiting. This would also be accompanied by low potassium, low sodium, and ketones in the urine.

Elevated AST is more of a marker for cardiovascular inflammation and tissue damage but can also be elevated in cases where damage is in other tissues. When the AST is higher than

ALT, a non-liver cause should be considered.

Higher ALT/AST in early pregnancy, even within the normal range, is an independent risk factor of GDM.[4]

HELLP Syndrome: In mild cases of preeclampsia, there is a mild elevation of serum AST/ALT/alkaline phosphatase as well as minor signs of coagulation issues and thrombocytopenia.[6] In HELLP syndrome, the ongoing destruction of red blood cells and platelets, along with the constriction of small blood vessels, can lead to ischemia and inflammation in the liver. This contributes to elevated AST levels. These elevated levels of AST serve as a clinical marker for the severity of cardiovascular and liver involvement in HELLP syndrome and are an important part of diagnosing and monitoring the condition.

Cardiovascular Inflammation: The body may experience widespread inflammatory responses and cellular damage in conditions marked by cardiovascular inflammation and oxidative stress. This can, in turn, trigger stress responses in various organs, including the liver and the heart. Elevated AST levels can result from this physiological stress as the enzymes are released into the bloodstream when the liver and heart cells are affected.[7]

Insulin Resistance: Studies show that insulin resistance without diabetes can be associated with elevated AST levels.[8] In insulin resistance, the body's cells become less responsive to the effects of insulin, resulting in elevated blood glucose levels. Chronic hyperglycemia can lead to fat accumulation in the liver, a condition known as nonalcoholic fatty liver disease (NAFLD). As NAFLD progresses, it can cause inflammation and injury to liver cells, which, in turn, may release AST into the bloodstream, elevating AST levels. This elevation in AST levels serves as an indirect marker of liver damage resulting from insulin resistance.

Hypothyroidism: This is usually associated with lower ALP and higher AST levels. Studies have reported a significant positive association between aspartate aminotransferase (AST) levels and elevated mean levels of thyroid-stimulating hormone (TSH) in patients with liver cirrhosis compared with healthy controls.[9] Subclinical hypothyroidism, characterized by an elevated serum TSH level and normal thyroxine (T4) level, is considered benign in most cases. However, its effect on the liver is like that of overt hypothyroidism.[10]

Hemolysis: Hemolysis releases AST as the RBCs are destroyed, which can increase serum AST levels.

Other Possible Causes: oxidative stress, myocarditis, hepatitis, biliary dysfunction, gut dysbiosis, iron overload/hemochromatosis, rheumatoid arthritis, overexercising, certain medications (acetaminophen), embolisms, trauma, acute illness, Wilson disease (excess copper), environmental chemical exposure

Treatment Strategies for Elevated Aspartate Aminotransferase (AST)(SGOT)

Diet

Reducing the consumption of added sugars, including high-fructose corn syrup, can be beneficial. Processed foods are notorious for their high synthetic sodium content and rancid fats. Excess sodium in this form can lead to high blood pressure, increasing the risk of heart disease and contributing to fluid retention and liver stress. The combination of unhealthy fats, high sugar content, and chemical additives in processed foods can lead to chronic inflammation and oxidative stress, both of which are associated with cardiovascular and liver tissue damage.

Fatty fish like salmon, mackerel, and sardines are rich in omega-3 fatty acids, which have anti-inflammatory effects and can help reduce inflammation in blood vessels. Berries such as blueberries, strawberries, and raspberries are high in antioxidants, including anthocyanins, which have anti-inflammatory properties and can protect blood vessels. High-quality dark chocolate with a high cocoa content is rich in flavonoids that can improve vascular function and reduce inflammation. Foods like broccoli, cauliflower, and Brussels sprouts contain compounds that support liver detoxification and reduce inflammation. Herbs and spices like ginger, cinnamon, and cilantro have anti-inflammatory and liver-protective properties.

Dietary vitamin E intake is as effective, if not more so, than supplemental vitamin E intake at lowering AST levels. The aim would be 800 IU of vitamin E per day in dietary form. Beet kvass is a fermented beet juice that has been shown to reduce markers of liver inflammation and damage. Have patients consume between 1 and 2 tablespoons per day.

Supplements

Zinc supplementation has been shown to decrease AST levels. Most studies use high doses of zinc that are contraindicated in pregnancy. If ALP is low and AST and ALT are elevated, zinc supplementation in lozenge form may be warranted.[11] Omega-3 fish oils have also been shown to improve AST levels, generally given at approximately 2,000 mg of total omega.[12] And 500 mg of alpha-lipoic acid has been shown to decrease AST levels.[13] Some studies suggest that milk thistle supplementation may help reduce AST levels in individuals with liver diseases.

Probiotics are beneficial bacteria that support gut health. They may also indirectly help reduce inflammation and improve liver function. Some studies suggest that probiotic supplementation may help reduce AST levels in some individuals.

Additional Testing

oral zinc tolerance test; complete blood count (CBC); comprehensive thyroid profile II; c-reactive protein (CRP); homocysteine; gamma-glutamyl transpeptidase (GGT); lactate dehydrogenase (LDH); bile acid, serum; comprehensive stool testing

Causes of Low Aspartate Aminotransferase (AST)(SGOT)

AST <10 IU/L is a biomarker of vitamin B6 (pyridoxine) deficiency.

Vitamin B6 (Pyridoxine) Deficiency: A deficiency in vitamin B6 can lead to a reduction of AST in the bloodstream, as well as reduced function. PLP is the active form of vitamin B6. It serves as a coenzyme for AST and other aminotransferases.[14] Lower vitamin B6 levels have also been shown to falsely decrease or normalize AST levels when damage and disease are present. This is important because the correction of vitamin B6 levels may cause an increase in AST when damage is present.

Other Possible Causes: low-protein diet, hypothyroidism, hemolytic anemia, mitochondrial dysfunction, genetics

Treatment Strategies for Low Aspartate Aminotransferase (AST) (SGOT)

Diet

Increasing protein-rich foods and those high in vitamin B6 can be beneficial for supporting and optimizing AST levels. Protein-rich foods such as red meats, poultry, and fish, and plant-based sources like legumes and tofu, provide the necessary amino acids involved in AST metabolism.

Supplements

Supplements of vitamin B6 may be helpful in some cases. In these cases, typical doses of supplemental vitamin B6 range from 10 mg to 25 mg, taken two to three times per day. Pyridoxine hydrochloride is the most common and widely available form of vitamin B6 supplement. It is water-soluble and easily absorbed by the body. Pyridoxine-5'-phosphate, also known as P5P or pyridoxal-5'-phosphate (PLP), is the active coenzyme form of vitamin B6 that is directly involved in numerous enzymatic reactions in the body. PLP supplements are often preferred by individuals with difficulty converting pyridoxine hydrochloride into its active form. PLP supplements are thought to have higher bioavailability and may be particularly useful for individuals with certain genetic variations affecting vitamin B6 metabolism.

Additional Testing

complete blood count (CBC); comprehensive thyroid profile II; reverse T3 (rT3)

References

1. Kirsch JF, Eichele G, Ford GC, Vincent MG, Jansonius JN, Gehring H, Christen P. Mechanism of action of aspartate aminotransferase proposed on the basis of its spatial structure. J Mol Biol. 1984 Apr 15;174(3):497–525. doi: 10.1016/0022–2836(84)90333–4. PMID: 6143829

2. Bacq Y. The Liver in Normal Pregnancy. In: Madame Curie Bioscience Database [Internet]. Austin (TX): Landes Bioscience; 2000–2013. www.ncbi.nlm.nih.gov/books/NBK6005

3. David AL, Kotecha M, Girling JC. Factors influencing postnatal liver function tests. BJOG. 2000 Nov;107(11):1421–6. doi: 10.1111/j.1471–0528.2000.tb11659.x. PMID: 11117773

4. Song S, Zhang Y, Qiao X, Duo Y, Xu J, Peng Z, Zhang J, Chen Y, Nie X, Sun Q, Yang X, Wang A, Lu Z, Sun W, Fu Y, Dong Y, Yuan T, Zhao W. ALT/AST as an Independent Risk Factor of Gestational Diabetes Mellitus Compared with TG/HDL-C. Int J Gen Med. 2022 Jan 5;15:115–121. doi: 10.2147/IJGM.S332946. PMID: 35023950; PMCID: PMC8743491

5. Shekhar S, Diddi G. Liver disease in pregnancy. Taiwanese Journal of Obstetrics and Gynecology. 2015(54):5;475–482. ISSN 1028–4559. doi.org/10.1016/j.tjog.2015.01.004. (www.sciencedirect.com/science/article/pii/S1028455915001503)

6. Sharma AV, John S. Liver Disease in Pregnancy. [Updated 2023 Jun 12]. In: StatPearls [Internet]. Treasure Island (FL): StatPearls Publishing; Jan 2023. www.ncbi.nlm.nih.gov/books/NBK482201

7. Ndrepepa, Gjin. Aspartate aminotransferase and cardiovascular disease—a narrative review. J Lab Precis Med 2021;6:6. doi: 10.21037/jlpm-20–93

8. Liu C, Shao M, Lu L, Zhao C, Qiu L, Liu Z. Obesity, insulin resistance and their interaction on liver enzymes. PLoS One. 2021 Apr 21;16(4):e0249299. doi: 10.1371/journal.pone.0249299. PMID: 33882064; PMCID: PMC8059853

9. Kim, Hyun Jin. "Importance of thyroid-stimulating hormone levels in liver disease." Journal of Pediatric Endocrinology and Metabolism, vol. 33, no. 9, 2020, pp. 1133–1137. doi.org/10.1515/jpem-2020–0031

10. Vos MB, Abrams SH, Barlow SE, Caprio S, Daniels SR, Kohli R, Mouzaki M, Sathya P, Schwimmer JB, Sundaram SS, Xanthakos SA. NASPGHAN Clinical Practice Guideline for the Diagnosis and Treatment of Nonalcoholic Fatty Liver Disease in Children: Recommendations from the Expert Committee on NAFLD (ECON) and the North American Society of Pediatric Gastroenterology, Hepatology and Nutrition (NASPGHAN). J Pediatr Gastroenterol Nutr. 2017 Feb;64(2):319–334. doi: 10.1097/MPG.0000000000001482. PMID: 28107283; PMCID: PMC5413933

11. Hanje AJ, Fortune B, Song M, Hill D, McClain C. The use of selected nutrition supplements and complementary and alternative medicine in liver disease. Nutr Clin Pract. 2006 Jun;21(3):255–72. doi: 10.1177/0115426506021003255. PMID: 16772543; PMCID: PMC4239999

12. Lu W, Li S, Li J, Wang J, Zhang R, Zhou Y, Yin Q, Zheng Y, Wang F, Xia Y, Chen K, Liu T, Lu J, Zhou Y, Guo C. Effects of Omega-3 Fatty Acid in Nonalcoholic Fatty Liver Disease: A Meta-Analysis. Gastroenterol Res Pract. 2016;2016:1459790. doi: 10.1155/2016/1459790. Epub 2016 Aug 29. PMID: 27651787; PMCID: PMC5019889

13. Salehi B, Berkay Yılmaz Y, Antika G, Boyunegmez Tumer T, Fawzi Mahomoodally M, Lobine D, Akram M, Riaz M, Capanoglu E, Sharopov F, Martins N, Cho WC, Sharifi-Rad J. Insights on the Use of α-Lipoic Acid for Therapeutic Purposes. Biomolecules. 2019 Aug 9;9(8):356. doi: 10.3390/biom9080356. PMID: 31405030; PMCID: PMC6723188

14. Ueland PM, Ulvik A, Rios-Avila L, Midttun Ø, Gregory JF. Direct and Functional Biomarkers of Vitamin B6 Status. Annu Rev Nutr. 2015;35:33–70. doi: 10.1146/annurev-nutr-071714–034330. Epub 2015 May 13. PMID: 25974692; PMCID: PMC5988249

Alanine Aminotransferase (ALT)(SGPT)

Alanine aminotransferase (ALT), also known as serum glutamic pyruvic transaminase (SGPT), measures total AST in a blood sample and is an analyte found on the comprehensive metabolic panel (CMP).

While ALT is predominantly found in the liver, smaller amounts of the enzyme are also present in other tissues such as the heart, skeletal muscles, kidneys, and placenta. Its presence in the liver makes it a marker for liver function and damage.

The synthesis and activity of ALT are tightly regulated in response to the body's metabolic needs. Various factors, including hormonal signals, substrate availability (amino acids), and the overall energy state of the cell, can influence ALT production and activity. Hormones like insulin and glucagon play a role in regulating ALT in the liver.

ALT catalyzes the conversion of L-alanine and 2-oxoglutarate into pyruvate and L-glutamate.

L-Alanine + 2-Oxoglutarate ↔ Pyruvate + L-Glutamate

This transamination reaction is fundamental for the interconversion of amino acids and contributes to the synthesis of proteins, as well as to the regulation of the body's nitrogen balance. ALT requires pyridoxine-5'-phosphate, also known as P5P or pyridoxal-5'-phosphate (PLP), as a cofactor.

Pregnancy

The effects of pregnancy on serum ALT and AST activity levels are somewhat controversial. In a few studies, a slight increase in ALT and/or AST activity has been found during the third trimester. Most studies, however, show that serum ALT and AST activity levels do not change during pregnancy or remain within the normal limits established in nonpregnant women.[1]

Postpartum

ALT can increase up to 147% within the first five days postpartum.[2] This should return to normal by six weeks postpartum. Those with preeclampsia or traumatic births may have elevated ALT that takes longer to return to normal.

STANDARD LAB RANGE: 0 – 32 IU/L

Trimester	Standard Pregnancy Ranges	**Functional Pregnancy Ranges**
Preconception	0-32	**10 – 30**
First Trimester	3-30	**10 – 20**
Second Trimester	2-33	**10 – 20**
Third Trimester	2-25	**10 – 25**
Postpartum	0-32	**10 – 40**

Causes of Elevated Alanine Aminotransferase (ALT)(SGPT)

ALT >25 IU/L in the third trimester is associated with liver disease in pregnancy, including ICP and preeclampsia.[3]

High-normal ALT in the first trimester is associated with an increased risk of gestational hypertension and preeclampsia.[4]

ALT >20 IU/L between 8 and 18 weeks gestation is associated with gestational diabetes.[5]

HELLP Syndrome: In mild cases of preeclampsia, there is only a slight elevation of serum AST, ALT, and alkaline phosphatase. HELLP syndrome is characterized by liver involvement, including hepatocellular injury and impaired liver function. The elevation in ALT levels seen in HELLP syndrome is primarily due to liver cell damage or necrosis caused by ischemia (reduced blood flow), inflammation, and oxidative stress.

Environmental Chemical Exposure: Mercury, dioxins, and PCBs are significantly associated with acute elevations in ALT.

Mycotoxin Exposure: Mycotoxin exposure, particularly to hepatotoxic mycotoxins such as aflatoxins and ochratoxins, can cause liver damage and elevate liver enzyme levels, including ALT, AST, and ALP.

Vitamin D Deficiency: Vitamin D deficiency has been linked to liver dysfunction and elevated ALT levels. In individuals with underlying liver conditions, vitamin D deficiency may exacerbate liver inflammation and injury.

Excess Exercise: While ALT is primarily found in the liver, small amounts are also present in skeletal muscle tissue. During intense physical activity or strenuous exercise, muscle breakdown and injury can occur, releasing ALT into the bloodstream.

Other Possible Causes: oxidative stress, insulin resistance, autoimmune disease, thyroid dysfunction, hepatitis, biliary dysfunction, iron overload/hemochromatosis, rheumatoid arthritis, certain medications (acetaminophen, antidepressants), trauma, acute illness, Wilson disease (excess copper)

Treatment Strategies for Elevated Alanine Aminotransferase (ALT)(SGPT)

Diet

Berries such as strawberries, blueberries, raspberries, and blackberries are rich in antioxidants, including flavonoids and polyphenols, which have anti-inflammatory and liver-protective properties. These compounds may help reduce liver inflammation and oxidative stress, potentially supporting ALT levels.

Citrus fruits like oranges, lemons, limes, and grapefruits are high in vitamin C and other antioxidants. Vitamin C has been shown to support liver detoxification processes and may help reduce liver inflammation. Citrus fruits also contain flavonoids such as naringenin, which has been studied for its potential liver-protective effects. Apples are rich in fiber, antioxidants, and phytochemicals, including flavonoids and polyphenols, which have been associated with liver health benefits. Consuming apples and their skins may help promote bile production, support liver detoxification, and reduce inflammation in the liver.

Beets are a good source of betalains, which are pigments with antioxidant and anti-inflammatory properties. Betalains may help protect liver cells from damage and support liver detoxification processes. Beets also contain nitrates, which can help improve blood flow to the liver. Cruciferous vegetables like broccoli, Brussels sprouts, cauliflower, and cabbage contain compounds called glucosinolates, which have been studied for their potential anti-cancer and liver-protective effects. These vegetables also contain sulfur compounds that support liver detoxification pathways. Artichokes are rich in antioxidants, fiber, and compounds such as cynarin and silymarin, which have been shown to support liver health. Artichoke extract has been studied for its potential to reduce liver inflammation and improve liver function tests, including ALT levels.

In cases of elevated ALT, it is also important to focus on fatty acid balance and protein intake. Fatty acid balance means including fat sources from polyunsaturated fats (PUFAs), monounsaturated fats (MUFAs), saturated fats, and cholesterol. Everything in nutrient needs to be "Goldilocks," as in not too hot, not too cold, just right. This goes for dietary fats as well.

Often when liver disease is present, the conventional nutrition protocol is to remove saturated fats and cholesterol. Unfortunately, updated research does not support this antiquated thought process. Cooking PUFAs can render them rancid and increase oxidative stress, cell damage, and pregnancy disease.

Cholesterol needs increase throughout pregnancy, so adequate dietary intake should also increase. Cook with more solid fats such as beef tallow, butter, ghee, pork lard, and coconut oil. Reduce liquid oils such as canola. Use fresh-pressed olive oil as a drizzle or dressing but not in high-heat cooking.

Lifestyle

Chronic stress can contribute to liver inflammation and worsen liver function. In those who are doing strenuous exercises, or even those who are just emotionally stressed, incorporating stress-reducing techniques such as deep breathing, meditation, yoga, and mindfulness can help them manage both physical and emotional stress levels.

Supplements

Research suggests that n-acetyl cysteine (NAC) supplementation may help improve liver function and reduce ALT levels in individuals with liver diseases or acetaminophen toxicity in pregnancy. NAC doses are usually between 600 and 1,200 mg twice daily. The half-life of NAC ranges from approximately 5.6 to 6.25 hours after oral administration. Silymarin, the active ingredient found in milk thistle, has antioxidant and anti-inflammatory properties and has been studied for its potential liver-protective effects. Some research suggests that milk thistle may help reduce ALT levels in individuals with liver conditions.

Additional Testing

complete blood count (CBC); iron and TIBC; ferritin; antinuclear antibodies (ANA); comprehensive thyroid profile II; c-reactive protein (CRP); homocysteine; gamma-glutamyl transpeptidase (GGT); lactate dehydrogenase (LDH); bile acid, serum; vitamin D; 25-hydroxy (25-hydroxycalciferol, 25OH-D); heavy metal testing

Causes of Low Alanine Aminotransferase (ALT)(SGPT)

ALT <10 IU/L is a biomarker of vitamin B6 (pyridoxine) deficiency.[6] There is more research on the use of low ALT as a biomarker of vitamin B6 deficiency than AST.

Vitamin B6 (Pyridoxine) Deficiency: ALT, like other aminotransferases, requires a coenzyme to perform its enzymatic function. Specifically, ALT uses the active form of vitamin B6 as a cofactor. Pyridoxine-5'-phosphate, also known as P5P or pyridoxal-5'-phosphate (PLP), serves as a coenzyme by facilitating the transfer of amino groups between amino acids and 2-oxo acids, which is the central activity of ALT. Without an adequate supply of vitamin B6, ALT cannot function properly. Low ALT is a biomarker of vitamin B6 deficiency. If vitamin B6 is deficient, either AST or ALT will be 10 IU/L or below.

Gluconeogenesis Dysfunction: ALT is an important enzyme for amino acid metabolism and gluconeogenesis; low levels can be associated with dysfunction in these metabolic pathways.

Other Possible Causes: low-protein diet, low muscle mass, hypothyroidism, genetics

Treatment Strategies for Low Alanine Aminotransferase (ALT) (SGPT)

Diet

Incorporate foods rich in vitamin B6—such as organ meats, fish, beans, legumes, nuts, seeds, dairy products, eggs, and dark leafy greens—into meals. Protein sources like poultry can provide both vitamin B6 and essential amino acids.

Supplements

In some cases, PLP vitamin B6 supplements may be helpful. Protein supplements may also be an option.

Additional Testing

complete blood count (CBC); comprehensive thyroid profile II

References

1. Bacq Y. The Liver in Normal Pregnancy. In: Madame Curie Bioscience Database [Internet]. Austin (TX): Landes Bioscience; 2000–2013. www.ncbi.nlm.nih.gov/books/NBK6005

2. David AL, Kotecha M, Girling JC. Factors influencing postnatal liver function tests. BJOG. 2000 Nov;107(11):1421–6. doi: 10.1111/j.1471–0528.2000.tb11659.x. PMID: 11117773

3. Kushner T, Park C, Masand D, Rosenbluth E, Carroll C, Grace M, Rodriguez-Rivas C, De La Cruz H, Overbey J, Sperling R. Prevalence of elevated alanine aminotransferase (ALT) in pregnancy: A cross-sectional labor and delivery-based assessment. Medicine (Baltimore). 2022 Oct 7;101(40):e30408. doi: 10.1097/MD.0000000000030408. PMID: 36221350; PMCID: PMC9542988

4. Zhang Y, Sheng C, Wang D, Chen X, Jiang Y, Dou Y, Wang Y, Li M, Chen H, He W, Yan W, Huang G. High-normal liver enzyme levels in early pregnancy predispose the risk of gestational hypertension and preeclampsia: A prospective cohort study. Front Cardiovasc Med. 2022 Sep 12;9:963957. doi: 10.3389/fcvm.2022.963957. PMID: 36172586; PMCID: PMC9510982

5. Song S, Zhang Y, Qiao X, et al. ALT/AST as an Independent Risk Factor of Gestational Diabetes Mellitus Compared with TG/HDL-C. Int J Gen Med. 2022;15:115-121. Published 2022 Jan 5. doi:10.2147/IJGM.S332946

6. Yamazaki H, Kamitani T, Matsui T, Yamamoto Y, Fukuhara S. Association of low alanine aminotransferase with loss of independence or death: A 5-year population-based cohort study. J Gastroenterol Hepatol. 2019 Oct;34(10):1793–1799. doi: 10.1111/jgh.14631. Epub 2019 Feb 27. PMID: 30761612

Lactate Dehydrogenase (LDH)

Lactate dehydrogenase (LDH), also known as lactic dehydrogenase, is a critical enzyme found in various cells throughout the human body. This is a single analyte that is not found in a specific panel.

There are several LDH isoforms; the serum LDH measures the total.

LDH plays a pivotal role in anaerobic metabolism by catalyzing the interconversion of pyruvate and lactate, a process essential for energy production when oxygen supply is limited.

$$\text{Pyruvate} + \text{NADH} + H^{+} \rightarrow \text{Lactate} + \text{NAD}^{+}$$

Vitamin B3 (niacin) works as a cofactor.

LDH is found in specific tissues, including the heart, liver, skeletal muscles, and red blood cells. There are five main LDH isoforms, designated as LDH-1, LDH-2, LDH-3, LDH-4, and LDH-5. These isoforms differ in their composition and tissue distribution. The designation LDH-1 represents the LDH isoform with the highest concentration of LDH-1 subunits, and LDH-5 represents the isoform with the highest concentration of LDH-5 subunits.

- LDH-1 is predominantly found in the heart and red blood cells.
- LDH-2 is mainly found in the reticuloendothelial system (spleen and liver) and red blood cells.
- LDH-3 is present in the lungs.
- LDH-4 is found in the kidneys and the placenta.
- LDH-5 is mainly found in the skeletal muscles.

LDH activity is dependent on the metabolic switch to anaerobic respiration. The enzyme becomes more active during extreme muscular activity, like in childbirth.[1]

Tissue damage causes a release of LDH into the bloodstream.

Pregnancy

LDH levels tend to increase slightly throughout pregnancy, with the most significant increases occurring in the third trimester. This rise in LDH levels is thought to result from increased metabolic demands on the body during pregnancy and the expansion of blood volume. LDH levels may exhibit a temporary increase during labor and childbirth. This elevation is often attributed to the physical stress, muscle exertion, and metabolic demands associated with the process of giving birth. It can also result from tissue damage, including muscle damage, that may occur during labor.

Postpartum

LDH levels may remain elevated due to the ongoing physiological processes related to labor. The magnitude of the increase can vary among individuals. LDH levels typically start to return to baseline levels in the days and weeks following childbirth.

STANDARD LAB RANGE: 121 – 224 IU/L

Trimester	Standard Pregnancy Ranges	**Functional Pregnancy Ranges**
Preconception	121 – 224	**140 – 210**
First Trimester	78 – 443	**120 – 200**
Second Trimester	80 – 447	**120 – 200**
Third Trimester	82 – 524	**150 – 400**
Postpartum	121 – 224	**140 – 400**

Causes of Elevated Lactate Dehydrogenase (LDH)

LDH levels >400 IU/L are associated with hypertension and preeclampsia. The higher the number, the more severe the symptomology.[23]

Hypoxia/Placental Damage: Genetic expression of LDH and activity increases in preeclamptic placentas. This is primarily seen in placental hypoxia due to various causes. Decreased oxygen levels increase the synthesis and activity of LDH. LDH is vulnerable to hypoxia, and it is the most prevalent in placental tissues. Elevated LDH is a sign of placental cellular damage.

Hemolysis: Only two of the five isoforms (LDH-1 and LDH-2) are released from ruptured red blood cells. As a result, the extra LDH in the plasma contributes to higher LDH levels in blood tests. Hemolysis can occur for various reasons such as oxidative stress, autoimmune conditions, infections, or exposure to certain toxins.

Vitamin B12 (Cobalamin) & Vitamin B9 (Folate) Deficiency: LDH-1 and LDH-2 are often increased in vitamin B12 and folate deficiencies. This is predominantly due to changes in RBC function and health, causing shortened lifespan or hemolysis and a release in LDH.

Asthma: In cases of lung inflammation or asthma, LDH-3 and LDH-5 are elevated. Generally, there is also an increase in WBC count, as well as eosinophils and globulin.

Other Possible Causes: oxidative stress, chemical exposure, liver and gallbladder dysfunction, anemia, cardiovascular inflammation, overexercising, birth control use, active infections

Treatment Strategies for Elevated Lactate Dehydrogenase (LDH)

Diet

Focus on antioxidants in the diet, which would include a variety of fruits, vegetables, and herbs that are known for their high antioxidant content. Foods such as blueberries, strawberries, spinach, kale, and broccoli are packed with antioxidants like vitamins C and E, as well as phytochemicals such as flavonoids and carotenoids. Additionally, herbs like turmeric, ginger, and oregano are well-regarded for their antioxidant properties. Nuts, seeds, and whole grains also contribute to an antioxidant-rich diet. Incorporating these nutrient-dense foods can potentially reduce oxidative damage at the cellular level.

Various conditions can cause damage to the cells of the placenta and induce hypoxia. The cells are sensitive to oxidative stress, particularly lipid peroxidation. While increasing antioxidants in the diet is important for reducing the oxidative stress, supporting healthy cell membranes is also important. Cell membranes are made of phospholipids, fatty acids, and cholesterol. Everything in functional medicine and nutrition is about balance.

Dietary fats affect the cell membranes based on their structure. Polyunsaturated fats (PUFAs) that are liquid at room and body temperature give the membranes flexibility. Saturated fats and cholesterol that are solid at room temperature give the membranes structure and stability. Too much one way or the other and we have cell membrane dysfunction. Dietary intake of fatty acids should also be balanced to support this need. Avoiding high-heat exposure to seed oils such as sunflower and canola can keep them from going rancid and increasing trans-fat production, which can also damage cell membranes. Cooking with more solid fats such as beef tallow, lard, butter, ghee, and coconut oil provides a balance of fatty acids and protects against rancid oils. Use fresh olive oil as a drizzle or dressing.

Supplements

Vitamin E supplementation has been shown to reduce LDH levels in runners.[4] There is no similar research in pregnancy, but studies have shown a protective effect of vitamin A and vitamin E supplements in pregnancy against preeclampsia.[5] Other supplemental treatment strategies may depend on other mechanisms of action. If hemolysis is suspected, superoxide dismutase enzyme (SOD) may also be beneficial. Vitamin C has also been shown to decrease LDH levels. In elevated LDH cases, address hypoxia causes.

Additional Testing

complete blood count (CBC); vitamin B12 (cobalamin); methylmalonic acid; homocysteine; iron and TIBC; ferritin; comprehensive metabolic panel (CMP); c-reactive protein (CRP); gamma-glutamyl transpeptidase (GGT); lactate dehydrogenase isoenzyme test

Causes of Low Lactate Dehydrogenase (LDH)

Low LDH can cause hypoglycemia.

Heavy Metal Exposure: Certain heavy metals such as lead (Pb), mercury (Hg), and cadmium (Cd) have been reported to inhibit LDH activity. These metals can bind to the enzyme's active site or disrupt its cofactor binding, thereby interfering with LDH catalytic function.

Pesticide Exposure: Some pesticides, including organophosphates and carbamates, have been shown to inhibit LDH activity. These pesticides may exert their inhibitory effects through various mechanisms, such as altering enzyme structure or interfering with enzyme-substrate interactions.

Antioxidant Therapy: Excess supplementation with high-dose vitamin C or vitamin E can cause low test results. If results are low, remove vitamin C and vitamin E supplements and retest.

Vitamin B1 (Thiamine) Deficiency: Thiamine is a cofactor for several enzymes involved in carbohydrate metabolism, including LDH. Adequate thiamine levels are necessary for optimal LDH activity.

Iron Deficiency: LDH-1 and LDH-2 contain heme, and an iron deficiency will cause a decrease in the synthesis of these two isoenzymes, which causes anemia.

Other Possible Causes: low-protein diet, genetic disorders, malnutrition, hypothyroidism

Treatment Strategies for Low Lactate Dehydrogenase (LDH)

Additional Testing

lactate dehydrogenase isoenzyme test; comprehensive thyroid profile II; reverse T3 (rT3); iron and TIBC; ferritin; heavy metal testing

References

1. Farhana A, Lappin SL. Biochemistry, Lactate Dehydrogenase. [Updated 2023 May 1]. In: StatPearls [Internet]. Treasure Island (FL): StatPearls Publishing; Jan 2023. www.ncbi.nlm.nih.gov/books/NBK557536

2. Reddy Eleti M, Agrawal M, Dewani D, Goyal N. Serum LDH Levels in Normotensive and Preeclamptic-Eclamptic Pregnant Women and Its Correlation With Fetomaternal Outcome. Cureus. 2023 Apr 6;15(4):e37220. doi: 10.7759/cureus.37220. PMID: 37159784; PMCID: PMC10163943

3. Jyoti Hak, Nayar-Un-Nisa, Swarn Gupta. LDH Levels in Pregnancy and its Association with Severity of the Disease and Feto-maternal Outcome in Preeclampsia and Eclampsia. JK Science Journal of Medical Education and Research. 2015 Jul-Sept. 17(3): 110–113

4. Itoh H, Ohkuwa T, Yamazaki Y, Shimoda T, Wakayama A, Tamura S, Yamamoto T, Sato Y, Miyamura M. Vitamin E supplementation attenuates leakage of enzymes following 6 successive days of running training. Int J Sports Med. 2000 Jul;21(5):369–74. doi: 10.1055/s-2000–3777. PMID: 10950448

5. Li N, Yang Y, Yue X, Zhang X. Predictive value of vitamin A and E levels in preeclampsia and postpartum kidney injury. Am J Transl Res. 2021 Apr 15;13(4):3427–3434. PMID: 34017518; PMCID: PMC8129214

Gamma-Glutamyl Transpeptidase (GGT)

A gamma-glutamyl transpeptidase (GGT) test measures the levels of GGT enzyme in the blood. It is a single analyte that is not found in a specific panel.

GGT is primarily found in the liver, bile ducts, and kidneys, with smaller amounts in other tissues and the highest concentrations in the liver. It is responsible for the breakdown and metabolism of glutathione, a tripeptide composed of three amino acids: glutamate, cysteine, and glycine. Glutathione is an important antioxidant that helps protect cells from oxidative damage caused by free radicals and reactive oxygen species (ROS). The breakdown of glutathione is essential for maintaining its balance within the cell and ensuring its proper function.

GGT cleaves the gamma-glutamyl bond in glutathione, releasing the amino acid cysteine. GGT's breakdown of glutathione contributes to the recycling of its constituent amino acids (glutamate, cysteine, and glycine). This recycling process ensures the availability of these amino acids for the synthesis of new glutathione molecules.

GGT is synthesized within cells through a process involving gene expression and protein synthesis. The GGT enzyme is encoded by the GGT1 gene.

GGT is often used as a marker of liver function along with aspartate aminotransferase (AST) (SGOT), alanine aminotransferase (ALT)(SGPT), and lactate dehydrogenase (LDH). GGT levels can also be elevated in non-liver conditions, such as pancreatic diseases and certain cardiovascular diseases.

While GGT is involved in glutathione metabolism, it is not considered a direct biomarker of glutathione levels in the body. GGT activity may indirectly influence glutathione levels by altering its turnover rate.

Pregnancy

GGT levels decrease throughout pregnancy, often masking liver damage or only slightly elevating in cases of liver damage. The decrease in GGT is more pronounced in the second and third trimesters.[1] This decrease may be more pronounced in those who took oral contraceptives prior to pregnancy or had more severe morning sickness in the first trimester.

Postpartum

In the weeks following childbirth, GGT levels typically start to normalize and return to pre-pregnancy baseline levels. Breastfeeding has been suggested to influence liver function, and GGT levels may be influenced during the breastfeeding period. Some studies suggest that breastfeeding may be associated with lower GGT levels, possibly due to hormonal and metabolic factors. There is an increase in GGT status in the breast milk through increased GGT production in the breast tissues.[2] The rate at which GGT levels return to normal can vary among individuals, and factors such as overall health, the presence of any liver conditions, and lifestyle choices may play a role.

STANDARD LAB RANGE: 0 – 65 IU/L

Trimester	Standard Pregnancy Ranges	**Functional Pregnancy Ranges**
Preconception	0-65	**10 – 30**
First Trimester	2-23	**2 – 23**
Second Trimester	4-22	**4 – 22**
Third Trimester	3-26	**3 – 26**
Postpartum	0-65	**10 – 30**

Causes of Elevated Gamma-Glutamyl Transpeptidase (GGT)

A GGT level >26.9 IU/L in the early second trimester may indicate an increased risk of developing GDM.[3]

Oxidative Stress: The association between elevated GGT and oxidative stress is related to the involvement of GGT in the breakdown and recycling of glutathione. Elevated GGT levels are considered a marker of oxidative stress and increased cellular turnover. When cells are under stress, such as exposure to oxidative damage or inflammation, GGT is released into the bloodstream. Studies have shown a direct correlation between elevated GGT levels and oxidative stress in the β cells of the pancreas, causing a decrease in insulin production, and thus an increase in blood sugar levels and higher risk of gestational diabetes diagnosis.[4] [5] Elevated GGT has been associated with several diseases that are characterized by oxidative stress patterns, including preeclampsia.[6]

Hyperthyroidism: Rises in alkaline phosphatase (ALP) and GGT are seen in about 64% and up to 62% of thyrotoxicosis cases, respectively.[7] Elevations in the postpartum period may indicate postpartum thyrotoxicosis and a need for deeper thyroid analysis.

Iron Overload/Hemochromatosis: Elevated GGT levels can serve as a marker of liver dysfunction in the context of iron overload. GGT is involved in the metabolism of glutathione, an essential antioxidant, and its release may reflect the liver's attempt to manage oxidative stress. Additionally, iron overload can contribute to liver damage and inflammation, further influencing GGT levels. The interaction between iron overload and elevated GGT underscores the intricate relationship between oxidative stress, liver function, and enzymatic responses.[8] (See Iron Section.)

Environmental Chemical Exposure: Several different heavy metals, pesticides, and other environmental chemicals have been associated with elevations in liver enzymes, including GGT.[9] Glyphosates have been shown to upregulate multiple enzymes involved in glutathione metabolism, including GGT, as well as cause the depletion of glutathione levels.[10]

Selenium Deficiency: Selenium is an essential component of the active site of glutathione peroxidase, serving as a cofactor necessary for its enzymatic activity. Glutathione peroxidase uses glutathione to neutralize ROS and lipid peroxides. During this process, the selenium-containing enzyme reduces glutathione disulfide (GSSG) back to its active form, glutathione (GSH). Selenium deficiency can compromise the activity of glutathione peroxidase, leading to reduced efficiency in recycling glutathione. Serum selenium levels are inversely related to risk of liver disease.[11]

Other Possible Causes: oxidative stress, liver and gallbladder dysfunction, gallstones or impaired bile flow, intrahepatic cholestasis of pregnancy (ICP), alcohol use, certain medications (nonsteroidal anti-inflammatory drugs/NSAIDs), antibiotics, antiepileptic medications), viral infections (such as Epstein-Barr virus or cytomegalovirus), hyperthyroidism

Treatment Strategies for Elevated Gamma-Glutamyl Transpeptidase (GGT)

Diet

Dietary factors and specific nutrients are important for supporting and potentially treating conditions associated with oxidative stress. Antioxidant-rich foods such as fruits and vegetables are valuable for their high content of vitamins C and E, as well as other phytochemicals with antioxidant properties. These compounds neutralize free radicals and ROS, reducing oxidative stress. Omega-3 fatty acids, found in fatty fish, flaxseeds, and walnuts, possess anti-inflammatory properties and may contribute to the management of oxidative stress-related diseases.

Additionally, incorporating foods rich in coenzyme Q10, zinc, and selenium can enhance the body's antioxidant defenses. Beet kvass is a fermented drink that offers the benefits of beet juice and probiotics.

Lifestyle

Chronic sleep deprivation has been linked to increased oxidative stress and inflammation. Establishing consistent and sufficient sleep patterns can help the body's natural repair mechanisms and reduce stress on the liver. Regular exercise is another important lifestyle factor. Physical activity has been shown to have anti-inflammatory effects and can enhance the body's antioxidant defenses. The key to exercise is to make sure it is not too strenuous and to focus on activities such as walking, yoga, and Pilates.

Supplements

Studies have shown that between 100 and 500 mg/day of alpha-lipoic acid had beneficial effects on metabolic conditions, liver function, and gestational diabetes.[12] [13] Silymarin, the active ingredient found in milk thistle, has also been shown to decrease elevated liver enzymes, including GGT.[14] Probiotic supplements contain beneficial bacteria that support gut health and may help improve liver function indirectly by reducing gut inflammation and improving intestinal barrier function. Some research suggests that probiotic supplementation may help lower liver enzyme levels in individuals with liver diseases.

Additional Testing

complete blood count (CBC); comprehensive metabolic panel (CMP); c-reactive protein (CRP); lactate dehydrogenase (LDH); comprehensive thyroid profile II; thyroid peroxidase antibodies (TPOAb); thyroglobulin antibody (TgAb); thyroid receptor antibodies (TRAb); iron and TIBC; ferritin; bile acid, serum

Causes of Low Gamma-Glutamyl Transpeptidase (GGT)

Hypothyroidism: GGT activity is frequently increased in patients with hyperthyroidism and may be decreased in patients with hypothyroidism.[15]

Vitamin B6 (Pyridoxine) Deficiency: The synthesis of glutathione involves several enzymatic reactions, and one of these enzymes, gamma-glutamylcysteine synthetase (GCS), is dependent on vitamin B6. GCS catalyzes the conversion of glutamate and cysteine into gamma-glutamylcysteine, a precursor in the synthesis of glutathione. Vitamin B6 is a cofactor for the enzyme GCS, meaning it is essential for the proper functioning of GCS during this step of glutathione synthesis.

Other Possible Causes: low-protein diet, magnesium deficiency, zinc deficiency, hemodilution, genetics

Treatment Strategies for Low Gamma-Glutamyl Transpeptidase (GGT)

Additional Testing

complete blood count (CBC); comprehensive metabolic panel (CMP); comprehensive thyroid profile II; thyroid peroxidase antibodies (TPOAb); thyroglobulin antibody (TgAb); reverse T3 (rT3); oral zinc tolerance test

References

1. Bacq Y. The Liver in Normal Pregnancy. In: Madame Curie Bioscience Database [Internet]. Austin (TX): Landes Bioscience; 2000–2013. www.ncbi.nlm.nih.gov/books/NBK6005

2. Dorothy B Colagiovanni, Dennis J Meyer, Julie M Wolf, Karen Hart, Elizabeth Abbott, Corrie Santos, High γ-Glutamyltransferase (GGT) Activity in Human Breast Milk Confounds Interpretation of High Serum GGT Activity in a Nursing Infant with Liver Disease, Clinical Chemistry, Volume 51, Issue 9, 1 September 2005, Pages 1750–1751, doi.org/10.1373/clinchem.2005.053819

3. Kong M, Liu C, Guo Y, et al. Higher level of GGT during mid-pregnancy is associated with increased risk of gestational diabetes mellitus. Clin Endocrinol (Oxf). 2018;88(5):700–705. doi:10.1111/cen.13558

4. Haghighi S, Amini M, Pournaghshband Z, Amini P, Hovsepian S. Relationship between gamma-glutamyl transferase and glucose intolerance in first degree relatives of type 2 diabetics patients. J Res Med Sci. 2011;16(2):123–129

5. Tan PC, Mubarak S, Omar SZ. Gamma-glutamyltransferase level in pregnancy is an independent risk factor for gestational diabetes mellitus. J Obstet Gynaecol Res. 2008;34(4):512–517. doi:10.1111/j.1447-0756.2008.00815.x

6. Bai C, Zhang M, Zhang Y, et al. Gamma-Glutamyltransferase Activity (GGT) Is a Long-Sought Biomarker of Redox Status in Blood Circulation: A Retrospective Clinical Study of 44 Types of Human Diseases. Oxid Med Cell Longev. 2022;2022:8494076. Published 2022 Jun 6. doi:10.1155/2022/8494076

7. Yorke E. Hyperthyroidism and Liver Dysfunction: A Review of a Common Comorbidity. Clin Med Insights Endocrinol Diabetes. 2022;15:11795514221074672. Published 2022 Feb 7. doi:10.1177/11795514221074672

8. Mohapatra E, Priya R, Nanda R, Patel S. Serum GGT and serum ferritin as early markers for metabolic syndrome. J Family Med Prim Care. 2020;9(7):3458–3463. Published 2020 Jul 30. doi:10.4103/jfmpc.jfmpc_570_20

9. Yorita Christensen KL, Carrico CK, Sanyal AJ, Gennings C. Multiple classes of environmental chemicals are associated with liver disease: NHANES 2003–2004. Int J Hyg Environ Health. 2013;216(6):703–709. doi:10.1016/j.ijheh.2013.01.005

10. Gunatilake S, Seneff S, Orlando L. Glyphosate's Synergistic Toxicity in Combination with Other Factors as a Cause of Chronic Kidney Disease of Unknown Origin. Int J Environ Res Public Health. 2019;16(15):2734. Published 2019 Jul 31. doi:10.3390/ijerph16152734

11. Xu L, Lu Y, Wang N, Feng Y. The Role and Mechanisms of Selenium Supplementation on Fatty Liver-Associated Disorder. Antioxidants (Basel). 2022;11(5):922. Published 2022 May 8. doi:10.3390/antiox11050922

12. Aslfalah H, Jamilian M, Rafiei F, Khosrowbeygi A. Reduction in maternal serum values of glucose and gamma-glutamyltransferase after supplementation with alpha-lipoic acid in women with gestational diabetes mellitus. J Obstet Gynaecol Res. 2019;45(2):313–317. doi:10.1111/jog.13842

13. Petca A, Bot M, Maru N, et al. Benefits of α-lipoic acid in high-risk pregnancies (Review). Exp Ther Med. 2021;22(5):1232. doi:10.3892/etm.2021.10666

14. Jamalian M, Mahmodiyeh B, Saveiee S, Solhi H. Investigating the impact of silymarin on liver oxidative injury. J Family Med Prim Care. 2020;9(3):1707–1711. Published 2020 Mar 26. doi:10.4103/jfmpc.jfmpc_929_19

15. Azizi F. Gamma-Glutamyl transpeptidase levels in thyroid disease. Arch Intern Med. 1982;142(1):79–81

Bile Acid, Serum

The bile acid, serum blood test—also known as serum bile acids test or total bile acids test—measures the levels of bile acid in the blood. It is a single analyte that is commonly run when intrahepatic cholestasis of pregnancy (ICP) is suspected.

Bile acids are produced by the liver and play a crucial role in the digestion and absorption of fats.

Specialized liver cells known as hepatocytes initiate the process by synthesizing bile salts from cholesterol. These bile salts are then conjugated with amino acids, such as glycine or taurine, forming bile acid. The hepatocytes release this synthesized bile acid, along with bilirubin and phospholipids, into the gallbladder for storage. The gallbladder contracts to release concentrated bile into the small intestine during digestion. Bile is either reabsorbed and transferred back to the liver for recycling or expelled with the feces.

This test is particularly useful for assessing conditions such as intrahepatic cholestasis of pregnancy (ICP) and liver diseases that affect bile acid synthesis and secretion.

Pregnancy

Serum bile acid increases slightly beginning in the first trimester, and it peaks in the third trimester close to term.[1] This rise is primarily driven by elevated estrogen levels. Estrogens increase the activity of bile acid synthase and inhibit their metabolic enzymes, as well as promote the increase of bile acid content in hepatocytes. This causes an overproduction of bile acid.[2] Progesterone slows gallbladder function.[3] These normal hormonal increases cause an increase in serum bile acid in pregnancy. Due to the normal increase in serum bile acid associated with pregnancy, researchers now suggest that even higher-reference range intervals should be used to diagnose ICP.[4]

Postpartum

In the days and weeks following childbirth, serum bile acid levels typically decrease gradually, returning to baseline levels.

> The serum bile acid test is heavily influenced by fasting, and postprandial levels may be several μmol/L higher than fasting values. Therefore, this test should always be run fasting for accuracy.

STANDARD LAB RANGE: 0 – 10 µmol/L

Trimester	Standard Pregnancy Ranges	**Functional Pregnancy Ranges**
Preconception	0 – 10	**0 – 10**
First Trimester	0 – 4.9	**0 – 4.9**
Second Trimester	0 – 9.1	**0 – 9.1**
Third Trimester	0 – 11	**0 – 11**
Postpartum	0 – 10	**0 – 10**

Causes of Elevated Bile Acid, Serum

Levels up to 11 µmol/L are accepted as normal in late gestation.[5]

Levels exceeding 40 µmol/L have been associated with higher rates of fetal demise.[6]

Selenium Deficiency: Selenium deficiency has been associated with disruptions in bile acid metabolism, which can contribute to elevated serum bile acid. Selenium is a cofactor for the enzyme glutathione peroxidase, which is involved in the recycling of glutathione—a key antioxidant in the liver. Glutathione peroxidase helps protect liver cells from oxidative damage and participates in the breakdown of hydrogen peroxide and lipid hydroperoxides. Some studies show a connection between low selenium and ICP.[7]

Vitamin D Deficiency: While the exact mechanisms are not fully understood, there is evidence suggesting that vitamin D may play a role in cholestatic liver diseases.[8] The liver expresses vitamin D receptors (VDRs), indicating that vitamin D may have direct effects on liver function. VDRs are found in various liver cells, including hepatocytes and biliary epithelial cells. Vitamin D is known for its immunomodulatory effects, and it may influence the immune responses in the liver. Dysregulation of the immune system can contribute to liver inflammation and cholestasis. Research also suggests that vitamin D may influence bile acid metabolism.[9]

Hypothyroidism: Hypothyroidism is associated with cholestasis and an increase in serum bile acid. A decreased biliary output of unconjugated bilirubin further characterizes cholestasis induced by hypothyroidism.

Gut Dysbiosis: Recent studies have connected gut dysbiosis characterized by elevated bacteroides with an increase in ICP.[10]

Other Possible Causes: genetics, gallbladder obstruction, autoimmune disease, toxin exposure

Treatment Strategies for Elevated Bile Acid, Serum

Diet

Rich in pectin and other soluble fibers, apples are thought to stimulate bile production and help with its flow. Additionally, the malic acid found in apples may assist in the prevention of gallstones. Apple cider vinegar may help stimulate bile flow.

Artichokes contain compounds known as cynarin and sesquiterpene lactones, which are believed to stimulate bile production and promote bile flow. Beets are rich in betaine, which supports liver health and bile production. Beet kvass can easily be made and incorporated daily into the diet. Lemon and other citrus fruits contain citric acid, which may stimulate bile production. Dandelion greens have traditionally been used to support liver health and promote bile flow. Radishes contain compounds that may help stimulate bile production and improve digestion.

Supplements

A few studies have shown a positive effect from the use of injectable glutathione in the treatment of ICP.[11] [12] Currently, there is not enough evidence to fully support the use of injectable glutathione in the treatment of ICP, but this limited amount of research is promising for future use.

CoQ10 has been shown to be effective in reducing bile acid in animal models.[13] Milk thistle contains silymarin, a flavonoid with antioxidant and anti-inflammatory properties that may support liver health and bile flow. A typical recommended dosage for milk thistle extract containing between 70% and 80% silymarin is between 200 and 400 milligrams taken two to three times daily.

While research on probiotics' specific effects on gallbladder function and bile flow is still in its early stages, some evidence suggests that certain probiotic strains may have beneficial effects on bile metabolism and gallbladder health. *Lactobacillus (L.) acidophilus* is one of the most widely studied probiotic strains and has been associated with various health benefits, including digestive health. Some research suggests that *L. acidophilus* may help modulate bile acid metabolism and improve bile flow, potentially supporting gallbladder function.

L. rhamnosus GG has been shown to prevent progesterone metabolite-induced hepatic bile acid accumulation. Elevated progesterone levels have been indicated in the pathogenesis of ICP in pregnancy.[14]

Additional Testing

complete blood count (CBC); comprehensive metabolic panel (CMP); vitamin D, 25-hydroxy (25-hydroxycalciferol, 25OH-D); comprehensive thyroid profile II; thyroid peroxidase antibodies (TPOAb); thyroglobulin antibody (TgAb); gamma-glutamyl transpeptidase (GGT); lactate dehydrogenase (LDH); antinuclear antibodies (ANA); comprehensive stool testing

Causes of Low Bile Acid, Serum

Not considered pathogenic

Treatment Strategies for Low Bile Acid, Serum

Not considered pathogenic

References

1. Gagnon M, Trottier J, Weisnagel SJ, et al. Bile acids during pregnancy: Trimester variations and associations with glucose homeostasis. Health Sci Rep. 2021;4(1):e243. Published 2021 Feb 10. doi:10.1002/hsr2.243

2. Zu Y, Yang J, Zhang C, Liu D. The Pathological Mechanisms of Estrogen-Induced Cholestasis: Current Perspectives. Front Pharmacol. 2021;12:761255. Published 2021 Nov 8. doi:10.3389/fphar.2021.761255

3. Tierney S, Nakeeb A, Wong O, et al. Progesterone alters biliary flow dynamics. Ann Surg. 1999;229(2):205–209. doi:10.1097/00000658–199902000-00007

4. Huri M, Seravalli V, Lippi C, et al. Intrahepatic cholestasis of pregnancy—Time to redefine the reference range of total serum bile acids: A cross-sectional study. BJOG. 2022;129(11):1887–1896. doi:10.1111/1471–0528.17174

5. Ambros-Rudolph CM, Glatz M, Trauner M, Kerl H, Müllegger RR. The importance of serum bile acid level analysis and treatment with ursodeoxycholic acid in intrahepatic cholestasis of pregnancy: a case series from central Europe. Arch Dermatol. 2007;143(6):757–762. doi:10.1001/archderm.143.6.757

6. Glantz A, Marschall HU, Mattsson LA. Intrahepatic cholestasis of pregnancy: Relationships between bile acid levels and fetal complication rates. Hepatology. 2004;40(2):467–474. doi:10.1002/hep.20336

7. Wang Z, Liu S, Wang J. Zhonghua Fu Chan Ke Za Zhi. 2000;35(8):476–478

8. Gençosmanoğlu Türkmen G, Vural Yilmaz Z, Dağlar K, et al. Low serum vitamin D level is associated with intrahepatic cholestasis of pregnancy. J Obstet Gynaecol Res. 2018;44(9):1712–1718. doi:10.1111/jog.13693

9. Schmidt DR, Holmstrom SR, Fon Tacer K, Bookout AL, Kliewer SA, Mangelsdorf DJ. Regulation of bile acid synthesis by fat-soluble vitamins A and D. J Biol Chem. 2010;285(19):14486–14494. doi:10.1074/jbc.M110.116004

10. Tang, B., Tang, L., Li, S. et al. Gut microbiota alters host bile acid metabolism to contribute to intrahepatic cholestasis of pregnancy. Nat Commun 14, 1305 (2023). doi.org/10.1038/s41467–023-36981–4

11. Ping, X., Ying, W., and Yanping, Y. (2017). Clinical effect of reduced glutathione combined with S-adenosylmethionine in the treatment of intrahepatic cholesstasis of pregnancy. J. Int. Obstetrics Gynecol. (Chin) 2017, 44

12. Chundong, W., and Bin, W. (2022). Effect of reduced glutathione combined with ademetionine in the treatment of intrahepatic cholestasis of pregnancy and its influences on liver function, oxidative stress indexes, expression of miR-3614–5p, miR-21 and IGFBP-3. Clin. Res. Pract. (Chin) 7, 97–100. doi:10.5114/ceji.2016.65894

13. Shan D, Dai S, Chen Q, Xie Y, Hu Y. Hepatoprotective agents in the management of intrahepatic cholestasis of pregnancy: current knowledge and prospects. Front Pharmacol. 2023;14:1218432. Published 2023 Aug 31. doi:10.3389/fphar.2023.1218432

14. Ren L, Song Q, Liu Y, Zhang L, Hao Z, Feng W. Probiotic Lactobacillus rhamnosus GG prevents progesterone metabolite epiallaopregnanolone sulfate-induced hepatic bile acid accumulation and liver injury. Biochem Biophys Res Commun. 2019;520(1):67–72. doi:10.1016/j.bbrc.2019.09.103

Thyroid-Stimulating Hormone (TSH)

Thyroid-stimulating hormone (TSH), also known as thyrotropin, is found as a single analyte as well as an indice on several different panels that include the Thyroid-Stimulating Hormone (TSH) and Free T4, Thyroid Cascade Profile, thyroid profile with TSH, and the comprehensive thyroid profile II.

It is produced and released by the pituitary gland and plays a fundamental role in regulating the function of the thyroid gland.

TSH secretion is controlled by a feedback system known as the hypothalamic-pituitary-thyroid (HPT) axis. When the levels of thyroid hormones in the bloodstream drop below a certain threshold, the hypothalamus in the brain releases thyrotropin-releasing hormone (TRH), which signals the anterior pituitary gland to produce and release TSH. TSH then travels through the bloodstream to the thyroid gland, where it binds to specific receptors on the surface of thyroid cells, stimulating the production and release of T3 and T4. The release of TSH is tightly regulated by a negative feedback loop, meaning that as the levels of T3 and T4 in the bloodstream increase, they inhibit the production of TSH. On the other hand, when T3 and T4 levels are low, TSH production increases to stimulate the thyroid gland to produce more of these hormones.

The synthesis of T4 and T3 thyroid hormones involves several steps, and the abbreviation ATEICE can be a helpful mnemonic to remember them.

Active Transport: The initial step in thyroid hormone production is the active transport of iodine into the thyroid gland, facilitated by the sodium-iodide symporter (NIS). This symporter actively transports both sodium ions (Na^+) and iodide ions (I^-) from the bloodstream into the thyroid follicular cells against their respective concentration gradients. The sodium-potassium pump maintains the sodium gradient. This process is integral to the accumulation of iodine within the thyroid gland.

Thyroglobulin: Thyroglobulin is a large glycoprotein produced by the thyroid follicular cells. These cells synthesize thyroglobulin by linking together multiple tyrosine molecules through a process known as polymerization. It is then placed into secretory vesicles.

Exocytosis of Thyroglobulin: After the synthesis of thyroglobulin within the thyroid follicular cells and its subsequent iodination, thyroglobulin is transported to the apical membrane of the follicular cells, facing the follicle lumen. Here, exocytosis comes into play. The thyroglobulin-containing vesicles fuse with the apical membrane of the thyroid follicular cells, allowing the release of thyroglobulin into the follicle lumen.

Iodination: Iodination is also known as organification. Iodide is enzymatically activated by thyroid peroxidase (TPO). TPO catalyzes the oxidation of iodide to form reactive iodine. The reactive iodine generated by TPO is then incorporated into the tyrosine residues within the thyroglobulin molecule. The iodination process results in the formation of iodinated tyrosine residues within the thyroglobulin molecule. Depending on the number of iodine molecules attached, these residues can be either monoiodotyrosine (MIT) or diiodotyrosine (DIT).

Coupling: Two iodinated tyrosine residues, one containing MIT and the other containing DIT, are then coupled together by TPO. This coupling forms either triiodothyronine (T3), when one MIT and one DIT combine, or thyroxine (T4), when two DIT molecules combine.

Endocytosis: This process results in the release of free T3 or T4, and the thyroglobulin undergoes recycling.

Abnormal TSH levels, either too high (hypothyroidism) or too low (hyperthyroidism), can indicate underlying thyroid disorders.

Thyroid Patterns of Dysfunction

TSH (Normal) + T4 (Low) + T3 (Normal) = Hypothyroxinemia

TSH (Normal/High) + T4 (Low) + T3 (Low or Normal) = Subclinical Hypothyroid

TSH (High) + T4 (Normal) + T3 (Normal) = Subclinical Hypothyroid

TSH (High) + T4 (Low) + T3 (Low) = Clinical Hypothyroid

TSH (Low) + T4 (Low) + T3 (Low) = Pituitary Hypothyroid

TSH (Normal) + T4 (Normal) + T3 (Low) = T3 Syndrome

TSH (Normal) + T4 (High) + T3 (High or Normal) = Subclinical Hyperthyroid

TSH (Low) + T4 (High) + T3 (High) = Clinical Hyperthyroid

Pregnancy

Changes in thyroid function are primarily regulated by hormones, such as hCG and progesterone. In the early weeks of the first trimester, hCG binds to TSH receptors on the thyroid, increasing stimulation and production of thyroid hormones. This increase in thyroid hormone production, up to 25% in the first trimester, causes a decrease in TSH production. In the second trimester, TSH levels stabilize and slightly increase from first-trimester levels. In the late stages of the third trimester, TSH levels may decrease again as the need for the thyroid hormones increases in preparation for labor and delivery.

Postpartum

In the first 24 to 48 hours after giving birth, TSH levels typically drop significantly. This drop is primarily due to the sudden reduction in the high levels of hCG. Levels usually start to return to their pre-pregnancy baseline within the first week postpartum. The process of returning to normal can take a significant amount of time. For most women, thyroid recovery may take a full year.

STANDARD LAB RANGE: 0.45 – 4.5 mIU/L

Trimester	Standard Pregnancy Ranges	**Functional Pregnancy Ranges**
Preconception	0.45 – 4.5	**0.5 – 3**
First Trimester	0.6 – 3.4	**0.1 – 2.5**
Second Trimester	0.37 – 3.6	**0.2 – 3**
Third Trimester	0.38 – 4.04	**0.3 – 2.5**
Postpartum	0.45 – 4.5	**0.5 – 3**

Causes of Elevated Thyroid-Stimulating Hormone (TSH)

A 2019 case-controlled study found that TSH ranges between 2.5 and 4.87 mIU/L increased the risk of miscarriage. After controlling for the confounding factors, thyroid peroxidase antibodies (TPOAb) positivity status, and FT4, the results were similar.[1]

A 2021 cohort study found that compared to euthyroid pregnancies, those

Autoimmune Disease: Autoimmune disease is the number one cause of hypothyroidism in developed countries, and the number two cause in underdeveloped countries. Autoimmune diseases such as Hashimoto's thyroiditis can lead to an increase in TSH by causing the destruction of the enzymes and proteins needed for thyroid hormone production. In these conditions, the immune system mistakenly identifies the body's own thyroid tissue as a threat and launches an attack. One common target of this autoimmune assault is the thyroid peroxidase (TPO) enzyme.

When TPO is attacked, it impairs the thyroid's ability to synthesize T4 and T3, resulting in reduced thyroid hormone production. This shortage of thyroid hormones is sensed by the pituitary gland, which responds by releasing more TSH to stimulate the thyroid to produce more hormones, thus trying to compensate for the deficiency.

with hypothyroxinemia (<2.5% of the reference range) from the first trimester through the second had an increased risk of preeclampsia.[2]

A 2019 study on hypothyroidism and birth outcomes found postpartum hemorrhage as the most frequent maternal outcome (38.8%). Emergency cesarean section occurred in 23.4% of cases. Risk was increased with a TSH >2.5 mIU/L.[3]

Subclinical hypothyroidism throughout pregnancy is associated with a risk of increased rates of induction, longer first stage of labor, premature rupture of membranes (PROM), "failure to progress," increased chance of hemorrhage, and increased ICU (intensive care unit) stay.[4]

Subclinical hypothyroidism in the third trimester exhibits a significant positive association with the length of the first stage of labor. With each unit increment of TSH (mIU/L) increase, the length of the first stage of labor is 2.44 hours longer after adjusting for potential confounders.[5]

Additionally, in some cases, autoimmune processes can also target thyroglobulin proteins, further exacerbating the thyroid's dysfunction and contributing to higher TSH levels.

Iodine Deficiency: Iodine deficiency is the number one cause of hypothyroidism in underdeveloped countries and the number two cause in developed countries. Iodine deficiency is a well-established cause of hypothyroidism.[6] When iodine intake is insufficient, the thyroid gland is unable to produce an adequate number of thyroid hormones, leading to a decrease in their circulating levels. As a response to the negative feedback mechanisms, the pituitary gland releases more TSH to stimulate the thyroid to produce additional hormones. However, if iodine deficiency persists, this becomes insufficient, resulting in hypothyroidism. In cases of iodine deficiency, T3 production is often prioritized over T4 production. In early presentations, this may cause hypothyroxinemia.

Iron Deficiency: Iron deficiency can be found in up to 40% of hypothyroidism cases. It can have a significant impact on thyroid function, resulting in an increase in TSH levels. This occurs because iron is a structural component of TPO. When the body lacks sufficient iron, the production and activity of TPO becomes compromised, leading to a reduction in thyroid hormone production. Additionally, low iron levels can contribute to hypoxia within the thyroid gland, causing a decrease in its metabolic activity.

Iron Overload/Hemochromatosis: Excess iron can accumulate in various tissues, including the thyroid gland, promoting the generation of reactive oxygen species (ROS) and triggering oxidative stress. This oxidative stress can damage thyroid cells and contribute to inflammation in the thyroid tissue. Furthermore, iron overload has been associated with an increased presence of autoantibodies, suggesting a potential link between elevated iron levels and autoimmune thyroid disorders.[7] (See Iron Section.)

TSH-Secreting Pituitary Adenomas: TSH-secreting pituitary adenomas, also known as thyrotropin-secreting adenomas, are rare tumors that develop in the pituitary gland. These tumors are characterized by their ability to produce excessive amounts of TSH. As a result, the elevated TSH levels signal the thyroid gland to produce and release more thyroid hormones. Consequently, the increased TSH stimulates the thyroid to overproduce these hormones, causing elevated T4 and T3 levels in the bloodstream.

This condition leads to hyperthyroidism, with associated symptoms such as weight loss, nervousness, rapid heart rate, and other signs of an overactive thyroid. The management of TSH-secreting pituitary adenomas often involves treatment strategies such as surgery, medication, or radiation therapy to control excessive hormone production and restore thyroid function to normal levels. The pattern of elevated TSH with elevated T4 and T3 would signal a need for additional specialized assessment and treatment by an endocrinologist/oncologist.

Bromide Exposure: Bromide exposure has been demonstrated to influence TSH values,[8] potentially contributing to thyroid dysfunction. Bromide, a halogen like iodine, can competitively inhibit iodine absorption and utilization by the thyroid gland. Bromide exposure can come from certain flame retardants, pesticides, agricultural practices, or brominated vegetable oils. With reduced iodine availability, the thyroid may produce inadequate amounts of thyroid hormones, prompting an increase in TSH release as the pituitary gland attempts to stimulate the thyroid to compensate.

Glyphosate Exposure: Studies have suggested a link between glyphosate exposure and disruptions in thyroid hormone production and metabolism.[9] Glyphosate may interfere with the enzymatic pathways involved in the synthesis and conversion of thyroid hormones. While research on the direct impact of glyphosate on thyroid health is ongoing, the evidence suggests a complex interplay of factors, including inflammation and disruption of biochemical pathways, which may contribute to hypothyroidism.

Other Possible Causes: other halogen exposures, heavy metals, vitamin A deficiency, magnesium deficiency, low-protein diet, progesterone deficiency, zinc deficiency, selenium deficiency

Treatment Strategies for Elevated Thyroid-Stimulating Hormone (TSH)

See the following sections: Thyroid Peroxidase Antibodies (TPOAb), Thyroglobulin Antibody (TgAb), and Iodine, Serum or Plasma.

Diet

Dietary strategies for managing elevated TSH often focus on supporting thyroid health and reducing inflammation. An anti-inflammatory diet rich in nutrients like iodine, zinc, selenium, iron, and magnesium can be beneficial. Foods high in iodine such as seaweed, fish, and dairy products can help support the production of thyroid hormones. Zinc and selenium-rich foods, including nuts, seeds, and organ meats, play a role in thyroid function and reducing inflammation. Iron from sources like quality meats, beans, and leafy greens is needed for TPO enzyme activity. Magnesium-rich foods like nuts, leafy greens, and whole grains support iodine transport via NIS.

Some studies have found that in a large percentage of women with autoimmune thyroid disease, adhering to a gluten-free diet can help to reduce autoantibodies. Going on a gluten-free diet has been related to improved thyroid function for many without gluten allergies or intolerances. Some theories as to why include modern wheat agriculture practices in the United States (US).

Methyl bromide, a common form of bromide, is used as a soil treatment to eliminate a variety of soil-borne pathogens, nematodes, and weeds. Another factor may be glyphosate exposure. Glyphosate is a widely used herbicide, particularly in the context of wheat agriculture in the US. Reducing exposure to the chemicals by reducing gluten/wheat in the diet may improve thyroid function in a non-gluten-related mechanism.

Lifestyle

The connection between halogens like chlorine, bromine, and fluorine and hypothyroidism lies in their ability to interfere with thyroid function. Exposure to other halogens can displace iodine in the thyroid gland, disrupting hormone production. Chlorine and fluorine are often found in tap water and dental products, while bromine can be present in certain flame retardants and baked goods.

Avoiding these halogens can be challenging, but there are strategies to minimize exposure, such as using a water filter that removes chlorine and fluoride, and opting for natural cleaning and personal care products with reduced halogen content.

Supplements

Supplement strategies depend on the underlying cause. Some supplements such as vitamin D and selenium work better in autoimmune cases, while iodine and magnesium work better for others. Identifying the cause is key to treatment. Proper supplementation will depend on the underlying cause of elevated TSH.

Additional Testing
complete blood count (CBC); thyroid peroxidase antibodies (TPOAb); thyroglobulin antibody (TgAb); comprehensive metabolic panel (CMP); iron and TIBC; ferritin; urinary iodine clearance (UIC); iodine, serum or plasma; oral zinc tolerance test; progesterone

Causes of Low Thyroid-Stimulating Hormone (TSH)

Gestational Transient Thyrotoxicosis (GTT): Human chorionic gonadotrophin (hCG) is composed of two subunits, hCGα and hCGβ. hCGβ is the subtype tested in a pregnancy test and is dominant in early pregnancy. Serum hCGβ is a glycoprotein produced primarily by the placenta and peaks at the end of the first trimester of pregnancy. It binds to the TSH receptor on the thyroid cell membrane and is a weak stimulator, resulting in increased secretion of T4 and T3 and partial suppression of serum TSH.

GTT is a temporary condition that occurs during pregnancy, primarily in the first trimester. It is characterized by an overactive thyroid, leading to an increase in thyroid hormone levels. While this transient thyrotoxicosis is generally benign and self-limiting, it can cause symptoms such as fatigue, weight loss, hyperemesis, and palpitations. As the mother enters the second trimester, generally around 12 or 13 weeks, there is a shift to hCGα production. This decreases the stimulation of the thyroid gland and reduces the total T4 production.

Many women with GTT will experience another increase in symptoms in the third trimester as hCGβ levels increase again. GTT does not usually require treatment and is considered a natural and self-limiting adaptation to the hormonal changes of pregnancy.

Adrenal Hyperfunction: The hypothalamic-pituitary-thyroid (HPT) axis regulates thyroid hormone production. It involves the hypothalamus, pituitary gland, and thyroid gland. In a healthy system, the hypothalamus releases TRH, which signals the pituitary gland to produce and release TSH. TSH then stimulates the thyroid to produce thyroid hormones (T3 and T4).

Cortisol is involved in a negative feedback loop within the HPT axis. When cortisol levels are high, it can directly suppress the production of TSH and TRH. This is an adaptive response to stress, as high cortisol levels prioritize the body's immediate needs over thyroid function. As a result of the decreased TSH stimulation, the thyroid gland produces and releases fewer thyroid hormones. This leads to a decrease in the levels of circulating T3 and T4, causing a state of hypothyroidism. This pattern would be a lower TSH level with lower T4 and T3 levels.

Postpartum Thyroiditis: This is an inflammatory condition that is caused by a buildup of toxicity in the thyroid gland during pregnancy. It is mostly seen in women with preexisting thyroid disease, particularly autoimmune disease, but can occur without preexisting disease. It is defined as the presence of an immune response, typically with thyroid antibodies, that causes an infiltration of immune cells and cytokines. This results in the destruction of the thyroid follicles and a significant release of T4 and T3 into the bloodstream, causing a transient hyperthyroid state that lasts until the thyroid gland is deficient in thyroglobulin and stored T4 and T3.

During this phase of hyperthyroidism, the thyroid gland shuts down thyroid hormone production and there is a decrease in TSH production. This can often turn into hypothyroidism as the thyroid gland is damaged and production is decreased. This negative pattern continues until the inflammation is reduced.

Vitamin A Deficiency: Vitamin A is needed for TSH synthesis. A deficiency in vitamin A can cause a decrease in pituitary synthesis of TSH. This pattern may mimic adrenal hyperfunction with low-normal TSH and low T4 and T3 indices.

Other Possible Causes: Graves' disease, thyroid nodules, medication overdose, pituitary disease, cancer

Treatment Strategies for Low Thyroid-Stimulating Hormone (TSH)

Diet

Dietary treatment for hyperthyroidism, particularly in cases of autoimmune thyroid disease, focuses on supporting thyroid function and addressing autoimmune factors. In these conditions, the immune system mistakenly targets healthy thyroid tissue, leading to increased autoimmune antibodies. Identifying potential triggers, both in foods and the environment, is crucial. Common triggers include gluten, dairy, eggs, soy, and nuts as well as preservatives, food additives, and pesticides. To counter inflammation and cellular damage, incorporating antioxidant-rich foods like berries and green tea is beneficial. Increasing the consumption of omega-3-rich fish can help reduce inflammation.

The role of iodine in Graves' disease treatment is controversial, and it's advisable to avoid iodine-fortified foods like iodized salts, processed grains, and seaweed-based products. Yet some women with hyperthyroidism are iodine deficient and need additional iodine for other functions in the body. It is best to monitor iodine levels with additional blood work. Cruciferous vegetables such as broccoli, cabbage, kale, Brussels sprouts, and kohlrabi contain compounds that reduce iodine absorption and help regulate thyroid hormone production in those with elevated iodine. Additionally, certain culinary herbs like turmeric and green chilies have shown promise in reducing hyperthyroid symptoms in research studies.[10]

Supplements

L-carnitine may be a useful supplement in the management of hyperthyroid patterns. Because hyperthyroidism depletes the body deposits of carnitine—and since carnitine has no toxicity, teratogenicity, contraindications, and/or interactions with drugs—carnitine can be of clinical use in those with hyperthyroid patterns.[11] Studies have used doses between 2 and 4 grams per day. Selenium is another supplement that has been shown to be beneficial in autoimmune hyperthyroid cases.[12] Lemon balm (*Melissa officinalis*), an herb, has also been shown in limited studies to reduce hyperthyroid symptoms and to block TSH receptors, which reduces T4 and T3 production.[13] In cases of vitamin D deficiency, additional vitamin D supplementation may be beneficial in reducing autoimmune antibodies.[14] Hyperthyroid presentation should always be referred to maternal-fetal medicine specialists.

Additional Testing

vitamin D, 25-hydroxy (25-hydroxycalciferol, 25OH-D); thyroid peroxidase antibodies (TPOAb); thyroglobulin antibody (TgAb); thyroid receptor antibodies (TRAb); reverse T3 (rT3); complete blood count (CBC); comprehensive metabolic panel (CMP)

References

1. Li J, Liu A, Liu H, et al. Maternal TSH levels at first trimester and subsequent spontaneous miscarriage: a nested case-control study. Endocr Connect. 2019;8(9):1288–1293. doi:10.1530/EC-19–0316

2. Su X, Liu Y, Li G, et al. Associations of Hypothyroxinemia With Risk of Preeclampsia-Eclampsia and Gestational Hypertension. Front Endocrinol (Lausanne). 2021;12:777152. Published 2021 Nov 4. doi:10.3389/fendo.2021.777152

3. Kiran Z, Sheikh A, Malik S, et al. Maternal characteristics and outcomes affected by hypothyroidism during pregnancy (maternal hypothyroidism on pregnancy outcomes, MHPO-1). BMC Pregnancy Childbirth. 2019;19(1):476. Published 2019 Dec 5. doi:10.1186/s12884–019-2596–9

4. Männistö T, Mendola P, Grewal J, Xie Y, Chen Z, Laughon SK. Thyroid diseases and adverse pregnancy outcomes in a contemporary US cohort. J Clin Endocrinol Metab. 2013;98(7):2725–2733. doi:10.1210/jc.2012–4233

5. Wei H, Guan Q, Yu Q, Chen T, Wang X, Xia Y. Assessing maternal thyroid function and its relationship to duration of the first stage of labor. Eur Thyroid J. 2022;11(2):e210071. Published 2022 Mar 17. doi:10.1530/ETJ-21–0071

6. Zimmermann MB, Boelaert K. Iodine deficiency and thyroid disorders. Lancet Diabetes Endocrinol. 2015;3(4):286–295. doi:10.1016/S2213–8587(14)70225–6

7. Tamagno G, De Carlo E, Murialdo G, Scandellari C. A possible link between genetic hemochromatosis and autoimmune thyroiditis. Minerva Med. 2007;98(6):769–772

8. Allain P, Berre S, Krari N, et al. Bromine and thyroid hormone activity. J Clin Pathol. 1993;46(5):456–458. doi:10.1136/jcp.46.5.456

9. Sirikul, W., Sapbamrer, R. Exposure to pesticides and the risk of hypothyroidism: a systematic review and meta-analysis. BMC Public Health 23, 1867 (2023). doi.org/10.1186/s12889–023-16721–5

10. Jawa, Ali; Jawad, Ali; Riaz, Syed Hunain; Assir, Muhammad Zaman Khan; Chaudhary, Abdul Wahid; Zakria, Muhammad1; Akram, Javed. Turmeric use is associated with reduced goitrogenesis: Thyroid disorder prevalence in Pakistan (THYPAK) study. Indian Journal of Endocrinology and Metabolism 19(3):p 347–350, May–Jun 2015. | DOI: 10.4103/2230–8210.152768

11. Benvenga S, Ruggeri RM, Russo A, Lapa D, Campenni A, Trimarchi F. Usefulness of L-carnitine, a naturally occurring peripheral antagonist of thyroid hormone action, in iatrogenic hyperthyroidism: a randomized, double-blind, placebo-controlled clinical trial. J Clin Endocrinol Metab. 2001;86(8):3579–3594. doi:10.1210/jcem.86.8.7747

12. Duntas LH. The evolving role of selenium in the treatment of Graves' disease and ophthalmopathy. J Thyroid Res. 2012;2012:736161. doi:10.1155/2012/736161

13. Auf'mkolk M, Ingbar JC, Kubota K, Amir SM, Ingbar SH. Extracts and auto-oxidized constituents of certain plants inhibit the receptor-binding and the biological activity of Graves' immunoglobulins. Endocrinology. 1985;116(5):1687–1693. doi:10.1210/endo-116–5-1687

14. Wang S, Wu Y, Zuo Z, Zhao Y, Wang K. The effect of vitamin D supplementation on thyroid autoantibody levels in the treatment of autoimmune thyroiditis: a systematic review and a meta-analysis. Endocrine. 2018;59(3):499–505. doi:10.1007/s12020–018-1532–5

Thyroxine (T4), Total

The thyroxine (T4), total test measures the total amount of T4 in the bloodstream. It is found as a single indice and is associated with thyroid panels such as the comprehensive thyroid profile II, thyroid profile with TSH, thyroxine (T4), and thyroid-stimulating hormone (TSH).

Total T4 = Protein-Bound T4 + Free T4

T4 is the primary thyroid hormone secreted by the thyroid gland. It accounts for between 80% and 90% of thyroid hormone production.

Measuring total T4 levels is essential for assessing thyroid function, as it provides a more accurate reflection of the total hormone output by the thyroid gland.

Thyroxine-binding globulin (TBG) has high-affinity binding sites for T4. When T4 is released by the thyroid gland into the bloodstream, a significant portion of it binds to TBG. The T4-TBG complex is stable, meaning T4 remains bound to TBG during circulation. This binding prevents the rapid clearance of T4 from the bloodstream and extends its half-life. T4 needs to be free from TBG to become biologically active. This unbinding occurs as the T4-TBG complex encounters target tissues or cells, allowing T4 to be released and interact with thyroid hormone receptors within cells.

Pregnancy

There is an increase in total TBG by about 50% in the first half of pregnancy, and subsequently, there should be an increase in total T4 by about 50% during this period.[1] This shift in higher total T4 and lower free T4 plateaus around 20 weeks. TBG production increases again through the second trimester with a total production of two or three times pre-pregnancy ranges.[2]

In the first trimester, maternal thyroid hormones are transferred to the fetal yolk sac. At six weeks gestation, plasma proteins that allow for the transfer of thyroid hormones are detectable. By 12 weeks, the thyroid hormones are transferred directly into fetal circulation.[3]

Maternal T4 is converted by the placenta to T3 by deiodinase enzymes (D2 and D3), and transfer of T3 to the fetus for development occurs as early as six weeks gestation. The passage of thyroid hormones from the placenta to the fetus is reliant on transthyretin, a transport protein with a high affinity for the neurological tissues. Trophoblast cells secrete transthyretin to bind to T4. Transthyretin bypasses D3 enzymes and transports thyroid hormones directly to the fetus. The fetal thyroid begins to accumulate iodine and make small amounts of thyroid hormones by 12 weeks but cannot make enough without maternal supply until around 20 weeks gestation.

Postpartum

As estrogen levels decrease, so does the production of TBG. This reduction in TBG levels can lead to a decrease in the total T4 levels. The decline in TBG may be more pronounced in the immediate postpartum period and will gradually normalize in the weeks that follow. While total T4 levels may fluctuate postpartum, the levels of free T4 are typically maintained within a more stable range.

According to the Endocrine Society, European Thyroid Association, and American Thyroid Association, the use of total T4 to assess thyroid function is more accurate than free T4 in pregnancy.[4] An article published by the *American Journal of Obstetrics & Gynecology* in 2014 concluded that total T4 and free T4 were equally as accurate in diagnosing thyroid disease in pregnancy.[5]

STANDARD LAB RANGE: 5 – 12 μg/dL

Trimester	Standard Pregnancy Ranges	**Functional Pregnancy Ranges**
Preconception	5 – 12	**6 – 12.5**
First Trimester	6.5 – 10.1	**7.5 – 18**
Second Trimester	7.5 – 10.3	**7.5 – 18**
Third Trimester	6.3 – 9.7	**7.5 – 18**
Postpartum	5 – 12	**6 – 12.5**

Causes of Elevated Thyroxine (T4), Total

See the following sections: Thyroid Peroxidase Antibodies (TPOAb), Thyroglobulin Antibody (TgAb), and Thyroid Receptor Antibodies (TRAb).

Other Possible Causes: gestational transient thyrotoxicosis, oxidative stress, hyperthyroidism, Graves' disease, overdose on medications, thyroid nodules, pituitary disease, cancer

Treatment Strategies for Elevated Thyroxine (T4), Total

See the following sections: Thyroid-Stimulating Hormone (TSH), Thyroid Peroxidase Antibodies (TPOAb), Thyroglobulin Antibody (TgAb), and Iodine, Serum or Plasma.

Additional Testing

thyroid peroxidase antibodies (TPOAb); thyroglobulin antibody (TgAb); thyroid receptor antibodies (TRAb); reverse T3 (rT3); complete blood count (CBC); comprehensive metabolic panel (CMP); vitamin D, 25-hydroxy (25-hydroxycalciferol, 25OH-D)

Causes of Low Thyroxine (T4), Total

See the following sections: Thyroid-Stimulating Hormone (TSH), Thyroid Peroxidase Antibodies (TPOAb), Thyroglobulin Antibody (TgAb), and Iodine, Serum or Plasma.

Autoimmune Disease: In Hashimoto's thyroiditis, antibodies primarily target the thyroid peroxidase (TPO) enzyme, which is essential to producing thyroid hormones by catalyzing the iodination of thyroglobulin. By attacking TPO, these antibodies impair the enzyme's activity, leading to decreased thyroid hormone production. Antibodies can also be present against thyroglobulin.

Hypothyroxinemia occurs in around 85% of preterm babies.[6]

Evidence suggests that maternal hypothyroxinemia alone poses an increased risk for fetal neurodevelopmental deficits.[7]

Iodine Deficiency: In cases of iodine deficiency, T3 production is often prioritized over T4 production. In early presentations, this may cause hypothyroxinemia.

Vitamin A Deficiency: Several animal studies have shown that vitamin A deficiency is related to reduced iodine uptake, impaired coupling of iodothyronines, and reduced thyroglobulin synthesis, which can lead to thyroid hypertrophy and goiter and to a decreased intrathyroidal pool of T3 and T4, as well as a decrease in TSH production. This pattern may mimic adrenal hyperfunction with low-normal TSH and low T4 and T3 indices.[8]

Iron Deficiency: TPO contains heme. Iron deficiency can reduce the availability of heme, thereby impairing the activity of TPO. As a result, the process of iodination and coupling of tyrosine residues to form T4 and T3 is compromised. Individuals with iron deficiency may experience decreased production of thyroid hormones, particularly T4. Iron deficiency can exacerbate autoimmune hypothyroidism.

Selenium Deficiency: Glutathione, a major antioxidant produced in cells, relies on selenium for its synthesis. By promoting the production of glutathione, selenium helps to mitigate oxidative stress and inflammation in the thyroid gland, supporting optimal thyroid hormone production and regulation. Inadequate selenium intake has been associated with increased susceptibility to thyroid disorders, including autoimmune thyroid diseases such as Hashimoto's thyroiditis.

Thyroid-Binding Globulin Deficiency: If total T4 is lower in ratio to free T4, this may indicate an issue in the production of TBGs. Estrogen stimulates the synthesis of TBGs by the liver. During pregnancy, estrogen levels increase, leading to elevated TBG production. This contributes to the increased total thyroid hormone levels observed during pregnancy. Vitamin B6 is involved in protein metabolism and synthesis, including the synthesis of TBGs. This may be shown as lower globulins in the comprehensive metabolic panel (CMP).

T3 Syndrome: Triiodothyronine (T3) can upregulate TBG production. Increased thyroid hormone levels signal the liver to produce more TBGs to bind and transport thyroid hormones in the bloodstream. T3 syndrome can create a vicious cycle of functional hypothyroidism and thyroid dysfunction.

Environmental Toxins: Certain environmental toxins such as polychlorinated biphenyls (PCBs), dioxins, or polybrominated diphenyl ethers (PBDEs) can interfere with the synthesis of thyroid hormones in the thyroid gland. These toxins may disrupt iodine uptake, impair thyroid hormone production, or inhibit the activity of TPO.

Other Possible Causes: low-protein diet, vitamin D deficiency, zinc deficiency, magnesium deficiency, adrenal hypofunction

Treatment Strategies for Low Thyroxine (T4), Total

See the following sections: Thyroid-Stimulating Hormone (TSH), Thyroid Peroxidase Antibodies (TPOAb), Thyroglobulin Antibody (TgAb), and Iodine, Serum or Plasma.

Additional Testing

thyroid peroxidase antibodies (TPOAb); thyroglobulin antibody (TgAb); complete blood count (CBC); iron and TIBC; ferritin; comprehensive metabolic panel (CMP); vitamin D, 25-hydroxy (25-hydroxycalciferol, 25OH-D); urinary iodine clearance (UIC); iodine, serum or plasma; oral zinc tolerance test

References

1. Yap YW, Onyekwelu E, Alam U. Thyroid disease in pregnancy. Clin Med (Lond). 2023;23(2):125–128. doi:10.7861/clinmed.2023–0018

2. Alemu A, Terefe B, Abebe M, Biadgo B. Thyroid hormone dysfunction during pregnancy: A review. Int J Reprod Biomed. 2016;14(11):677–686

3. Zuñiga LFF, Muñoz YS, Pustovrh MC. Thyroid hormones: Metabolism and transportation in the fetoplacental unit. Mol Reprod Dev. 2022;89(11):526–539. doi:10.1002/mrd.23647

4. De Groot L, Abalovich M, Alexander EK, et al. Management of thyroid dysfunction during pregnancy and postpartum: an Endocrine Society clinical practice guideline [published correction appears in J Clin Endocrinol Metab. 2021 May 13;106(6):e2461]. J Clin Endocrinol Metab. 2012;97(8):2543–2565. doi:10.1210/jc.2011–2803

5. Wilson KL, Casey BM, McIntire DD, Cunningham FG. Is total thyroxine better than free thyroxine during pregnancy? Am J Obstet Gynecol. 2014;211(2):132.e1–132.e1326. doi:10.1016/j.ajog.2014.02.029

6. Bernal J., 5.08—Thyroid Hormones and Brain Development. In: Bernal J. Hormones, Brain and Behavior, 3rd ed. Academic Press, 2017: 159–184, ISBN 9780128036082. doi.org/10.1016/B978–0-12–803592-4.00100–0

7. Negro R, Soldin OP, Obregon MJ, Stagnaro-Green A. Hypothyroxinemia and pregnancy. Endocr Pract. 2011;17(3):422–429. doi:10.4158/EP10309.RA

8. Capriello S, Stramazzo I, Bagaglini MF, Brusca N, Virili C, Centanni M. The relationship between thyroid disorders and vitamin A: A narrative minireview. Front Endocrinol (Lausanne). 2022;13:968215. Published 2022 Oct 11. doi:10.3389/fendo.2022.968215

Thyroxine (T4), Free

Thyroxine (T4), free is a test that measures only the free T4 (FT4) in the blood sample. It is a single analyte or found with other thyroid panels such as thyroid-stimulating hormone (TSH) and free T4 and the Thyroid Cascade Profile.

In serum, 99.98% of T4 is bound to binding proteins, and 0.02% of T4 is free or unbound. Free T4 is the active form of the hormone. Only free T4 can enter the cells.

Measuring free T4 levels is essential for assessing thyroid function, as it provides a more accurate reflection of the active thyroid hormone available to tissues.

Pregnancy

In the first trimester, there is a slight increase in FT4 levels, with a decrease after this initial phase of between 10% and 15%.[1]

Postpartum

While total T4 levels may fluctuate postpartum, free T4 levels are typically maintained within a more stable range. As the thyroid enters a small hypothyroidism period of recovery, there may be a relatively small drop in free T4 in conjunction with decreased progesterone levels.

STANDARD LAB RANGE: 0.82 – 1.77 ng/dL*

Trimester	Standard Pregnancy Ranges	**Functional Pregnancy Ranges**
Preconception	0.82 – 1.77	**1 – 1.9**
First Trimester	0.8 – 1.2	**0.8 – 1.2**
Second Trimester	0.6 – 1	**0.6 – 1**
Third Trimester	0.5 – 0.8	**0.5 – 0.8**
Postpartum	0.82 – 1.77	**1 – 1.9**

*Studies have shown that automated free T4 is often overestimated in pregnancy. They may underdiagnose those with subclinical hypothyroidism. According to a 2002 ACOG bulletin on thyroid disease, TSH and FT4 or FTI testing should be performed in pregnant women with suspected hyperthyroidism or hypothyroidism.[2 3]

Causes of Elevated Thyroxine (T4), Free

See the following sections: Thyroid-Stimulating Hormone (TSH), Thyroxine (T4), Total, Thyroid Peroxidase Antibodies (TPOAb), Thyroglobulin Antibody (TgAb), and Iodine, Serum or Plasma.

Hyperthyroidism is defined as a suppressed TSH with elevated FT4. If left untreated in pregnancy, there is an increased risk of miscarriage, stillbirth, low birth weight, and preterm delivery. Maternal complications include thyroid storm and a fivefold increase in the risk of preeclampsia and congestive heart failure.[4]

Other Possible Causes: gestational transient thyrotoxicosis, oxidative stress, hyperthyroidism, Graves' disease, overdose on medications

Treatment Strategies for Elevated Thyroxine (T4), Free

See the following sections: Thyroid-Stimulating Hormone (TSH), Thyroxine (T4), Total, Thyroid Peroxidase Antibodies (TPOAb), Thyroglobulin Antibody (TgAb), and Thyroid Receptor Antibodies (TRAb).

Additional Testing

thyroid peroxidase antibodies (TPOAb); thyroglobulin antibody (TgAb); thyroid receptor antibodies (TRAb); reverse T3 (rT3); complete blood count (CBC); comprehensive metabolic panel (CMP); vitamin D, 25-hydroxy (25-hydroxycalciferol, 25OH-D)

Causes of Low Thyroxine (T4), Free

See the following sections: Thyroid-Stimulating Hormone (TSH), Thyroxine (T4), Total, Thyroid Peroxidase Antibodies (TPOAb), Thyroglobulin Antibody (TgAb), and Iodine, Serum or Plasma.

Women with hypothyroidism have an increased risk of infertility, miscarriage, spontaneous

Progesterone Deficiency: A deficiency in progesterone could potentially influence the binding of thyroxine T4 to TBG. Progesterone competes with T4 for binding sites on TBG. In the absence of sufficient progesterone, there may be less competition for these binding sites. With reduced competition, more T4 molecules may

abortion, stillbirth, placental abruption, hypertension, anemia, and postpartum hemorrhage.[5]

Hypothyroxinemia is defined as FT4 <2.5th percentile of the gestational reference range with a normal TSH. Hypothyroxinemia in the first trimester is associated with potential neurological damage in the child.[6]

bind to TBG. This can lead to an increase in the total T4 levels in the bloodstream, as a larger proportion of T4 is bound to TBG. In cases of progesterone deficiency, total T4 levels may appear higher due to increased binding to TBG, but free T4 levels may be lower because of reduced displacement from TBG. Because of the reduction in free T4, TSH levels may remain normal or be elevated.

Other Possible Causes: low-protein diet, iodine deficiency, autoimmune disease, selenium deficiency, vitamin D deficiency, zinc deficiency, iron deficiency, vitamin A deficiency, vitamin B6 (pyridoxine) deficiency, magnesium deficiency, estrogen deficiency

Treatment Strategies for Low Thyroxine (T4), Free

See the following sections: Thyroid-Stimulating Hormone (TSH), Thyroxine (T4), Total, Thyroid Peroxidase Antibodies (TPOAb), Thyroglobulin Antibody (TgAb), and Iodine, Serum or Plasma.

Additional Testing

thyroid peroxidase antibodies (TPOAb); thyroglobulin antibody (TgAb); complete blood count (CBC); iron and TIBC; ferritin; comprehensive metabolic panel (CMP); vitamin D, 25-hydroxy (25-hydroxycalciferol, 25OH-D); urinary iodine clearance (UIC); iodine, serum or plasma; progesterone; oral zinc tolerance test

References

1. Moleti M, Trimarchi F, Vermiglio F. Thyroid physiology in pregnancy. Endocr Pract. 2014;20(6):589–596. doi:10.4158/EP13341.RA

2. Jansen, H. I., van Herwaarden, A. E., Huijgen, H. J., Painter, R. C., Hillebrand, J. J., Boelen, A., & Heijboer, A. C. (2022). Pregnancy disrupts the accuracy of automated FT4 immunoassays. European Thyroid Journal, 11(6), e220145. Retrieved Feb 11, 2024, from doi.org/10.1530/ETJ-22–0145

3. Schroeder BM; American College of Obstetricians and Gynecologists. ACOG practice bulletin on thyroid disease in pregnancy. Am Fam Physician. 2002;65(10):2158–2162

4. Moore LE. Thyroid disease in pregnancy: A review of diagnosis, complications and management. World J Obstet Gynecol 2016; 5(1): 66–72 [DOI: 10.5317/wjog.v5.i1.66]

5. Sahay RK, Nagesh VS. Hypothyroidism in pregnancy. Indian J Endocrinol Metab. 2012;16(3):364–370. doi:10.4103/2230–8210.95667

6. De Escobar GM, Obregón MJ, del Rey FE. Maternal thyroid hormones early in pregnancy and fetal brain development. Best Pract Res Clin Endocrinol Metab. 2004;18(2):225–248. doi:10.1016/j.beem.2004.03.012

Triiodothyronine (T3), Total

The triiodothyronine (T3), total test measures the total amount of T3 in the bloodstream. It is found as a single indice as the comprehensive thyroid profile II.

Total T3 = Protein-Bound T3 + Free T3

Approximately 10% of total thyroid hormone production is triiodothyronine (T3).

T3 is considered the active form of thyroid hormones. It affects every physiological process in the body. Around 80% of circulating T3 isn't produced by the thyroid but by the liver and other tissues by deiodinase enzymes.

TBG has a low affinity for T3, while albumin has a high affinity for T3; therefore, more T3 is bound to albumin for transport than TBG.

Deiodinase enzymes catalyze the removal of an iodine atom from T4, converting it to an inactive form called reverse triiodothyronine (rT3) and the active form, T3.

There are three types of deiodinase enzymes involved in this process.

Deiodinase Type	Location	Function
Type 1 (D1)	Liver, kidneys, thyroid, and pituitary, but notably absent in the central nervous system	Converting T4 to T3 circulation in some tissues
Type 2 (D2)	Central nervous system, pituitary, brown adipose tissue, thyroid, placenta, skeletal muscle, and heart	Converting T4 to T3 in tissues
Type 3 (D3)	Central nervous system, skin, hemangiomas, fetal liver, placenta, and fetal tissues	Converting T4 to reverse T3

Measuring free T3 levels is essential for assessing thyroid function, as it provides a more accurate reflection of total thyroid hormone output, as well as conversion of T4 to T3.

Pregnancy

Total T3 increases gradually and steadily throughout pregnancy, peaking in the third trimester.

Postpartum

During the postpartum phase, there is a period of minor hypothyroidism that should correct itself in the first few weeks of postpartum. Total T3 levels should return to normal between four and six weeks postpartum.[1]

STANDARD LAB RANGE: 71 – 180 ng/dL

Trimester	Standard Pregnancy Ranges	**Functional Pregnancy Ranges**
Preconception	71 – 180	**80 – 190**
First Trimester	97 – 149	**92 – 218**
Second Trimester	117 – 169	**112 – 278**
Third Trimester	123 – 162	**111 – 265**
Postpartum	71 – 180	**80 – 190**

Causes of Elevated Triiodothyronine (T3), Total

See the following sections: Thyroid-Stimulating Hormone (TSH) and Reverse T3 (rT3).

Other Possible Causes: gestational transient thyrotoxicosis, oxidative stress, hyperthyroidism, Graves' disease, overdose on medications, thyroid storm, pituitary disease

Treatment Strategies for Elevated Triiodothyronine (T3), Total

See the following sections: Thyroid-Stimulating Hormone (TSH) and Reverse T3 (rT3).

Additional Testing

thyroid peroxidase antibodies (TPOAb); thyroglobulin antibody (TgAb); thyroid receptor antibodies (TRAb); reverse T3 (rT3); complete blood count (CBC); comprehensive metabolic panel (CMP); c-reactive protein

Causes of Low Triiodothyronine (T3), Total

See Thyroid-Stimulating Hormone (TSH) Section.

Low T3 levels have been shown to have negative effects on fetal brain development, particularly the hippocampus.[23]

Selenium Deficiency: Selenium is an essential trace element required for the proper structure and function of deiodinase enzymes, especially types D1 and D2. Selenium is incorporated into the catalytic center of these enzymes, supporting their activity. A deficiency in selenium would cause a decrease in the synthesis of deiodinase enzymes and decrease in T4 to T3 conversion.

Magnesium Deficiency: Magnesium serves as a cofactor for various enzymes, including the deiodinase enzymes involved in the conversion of T4 to T3. Magnesium also supports the sodium-iodide symptoms (NIS) needed for iodine cellular absorption.

T3 Syndrome: T3 syndrome is a condition in which T3 levels are decreased with no present thyroid disease and with normal T4 levels. This is primarily seen in a condition known as euthyroid sick syndrome (ESS) or non-thyroidal illness syndrome (NTIS). Euthyroid sick syndrome is a complex alteration in thyroid hormone levels that occurs in the setting of acute or chronic systemic illness. It can also be seen in those with chronic inflammatory stress reactions not related to systemic illness.

Total and free triiodothyronine (T3) levels may be decreased, while thyroxine (T4) levels are typically normal or low-normal. This reflects a decrease in the conversion of T4 to the biologically active T3 form, which may be due to decreased peripheral conversion of T4 to T3 or increased conversion of T4 to reverse T3 (rT3), an inactive form of T3. This same pattern can be seen in both zinc and selenium deficiency, as they are both needed for deiodinase enzyme function.

Vitamin A Deficiency: Vitamin A deficiency reduces T3 binding and uptake by tissues and decreases hepatic conversion of T4 to T3. This can present with lower total T3 with normal or elevated free T3, as well as elevated reverse T3.

High Reverse T3: RT3 is known to destroy deiodinase enzymes, reducing the conversion of T4 to T3.

Other Possible Causes: low-protein diet, iodine deficiency, autoimmune disease, vitamin D deficiency, vitamin B6 (pyridoxine) deficiency, iron deficiency

Treatment Strategies for Low Triiodothyronine (T3), Total

See Thyroid-Stimulating Hormone (TSH) Section.

Additional Testing

thyroid peroxidase antibodies (TPOAb); thyroglobulin antibody (TgAb); reverse T3 (rT3); complete blood count (CBC); iron and TIBC; ferritin; comprehensive metabolic panel (CMP); vitamin D, 25-hydroxy (25-hydroxycalciferol, 25OH-D); urinary iodine clearance (UIC); iodine, serum or plasma; oral zinc tolerance test

References

1. Soldin OP, Hilakivi-Clarke L, Weiderpass E, Soldin SJ. Trimester-specific reference intervals for thyroxine and triiodothyronine in pregnancy in iodine-sufficient women using isotope dilution tandem mass spectrometry and immunoassays. Clin Chim Acta. 2004;349(1–2):181–189. doi:10.1016/j.cccn.2004.06.021

2. Gould E, Woolley CS, McEwen BS. The hippocampal formation: morphological changes induced by thyroid, gonadal and adrenal hormones. Psychoneuroendocrinology. 1991;16(1–3):67–84. doi:10.1016/0306–4530(91)90071-z

3. Hellstrom, I. C., Dhir, S. K., Diorio, J. C., & Meaney, M. J. (2012). Maternal licking regulates hippocampal glucocorticoid receptor transcription through a thyroid hormone–serotonin–NGFI-A signalling cascade. Philosophical Transactions of the Royal Society of London. Series B, Biological Sciences, 367, 2495–2510. doi.org/10.1098/rstb.2012.0223

Triiodothyronine (T3), Free

The triiodothyronine (T3), free test measures only the free T3 in the blood sample. It is a single analyte or found with other thyroid panels, such as the Thyroid Cascade Profile.

Only 0.3% of T3 is free, yet free T3 is not influenced by variations in protein binding (e.g., TBG and albumin levels), and measuring free T3 provides a more accurate representation of the biologically available and active thyroid hormone levels.

Measuring free T3 levels is essential for assessing thyroid function, as it provides a more accurate reflection of bound versus unbound thyroid hormone and the conversion of T4 to T3.

Pregnancy

Free T3 increases in the first trimester and then decreases through the second and third trimesters.

Postpartum

Free T3 can decrease in the first few weeks postpartum, as the thyroid recovers from pregnancy.

STANDARD LAB RANGE: 2 – 4.4 pg/mL

Trimester	Standard Pregnancy Ranges	**Functional Pregnancy Ranges**
Preconception	2 – 4.4	**2 – 4.4**
First Trimester	4.1 – 4.4	**4.1 – 4.4**
Second Trimester	4 – 4.2	**4 – 4.2**
Third Trimester	4 – 4.2	**4 – 4.2**
Postpartum	2 – 4.4	**2 – 4.4**

Causes of Elevated Triiodothyronine (T3), Free

See the following sections: Thyroid-Stimulating Hormone (TSH) and Triiodothyronine (T3), Total.

Low Albumin: Free T3 represents the unbound, biologically active fraction of T3. A decrease in albumin levels may result in an increase in free T3 as a higher proportion of T3 becomes unbound. This would be seen with a low-normal total T3 and a higher free T3, as well as low serum albumin levels.

Thyroid Hormone Resistance: Thyroid hormone resistance syndrome is characterized by reduced tissue responsiveness to thyroid hormones despite normal or elevated circulating levels. In these cases, FT3 levels may be disproportionately elevated compared to TT3 levels due to impaired tissue uptake or utilization of thyroid hormones.

Other Possible Causes: gestational transient thyrotoxicosis, low-protein diet, oxidative stress, hyperthyroidism, Graves' disease, overdose on medications, insulin resistance

Treatment Strategies for Elevated Triiodothyronine (T3), Free

See the following sections: Thyroid-Stimulating Hormone (TSH) and Triiodothyronine (T3), Total.

Additional Testing

thyroid peroxidase antibodies (TPOAb); thyroglobulin antibody (TgAb); thyroid receptor antibodies (TRAb); reverse T3 (rT3); complete blood count (CBC); comprehensive metabolic panel (CMP); vitamin D, 25-hydroxy (25-hydroxycalciferol, 25OH-D)

Causes of Low Triiodothyronine (T3), Free

See the following sections: Thyroid-Stimulating Hormone (TSH) and Triiodothyronine (T3), Total.

T3 Syndrome: Low T3 syndrome is characterized by low T3 indices with normal T4 indices. This can be found in cases of euthyroid sick syndrome (ESS), associated with elevated rT3, or it can be an issue with the conversion of T4 to T3. In some cases, it is a prioritization in the thyroid production to T4 over T3. This may be associated with other things, such as vitamin A deficiency. Generally, the prioritization for T4 over T3 is found in cases of chronic inflammation and stress.

Low T3 syndrome is commonly seen in individuals experiencing acute or chronic illnesses, such as severe infections, trauma, major surgery, or critical illnesses. It may also be observed in conditions like heart failure, chronic kidney disease, and other systemic diseases. The decrease in T3 levels is considered an adaptive response to stress or illness. The body redirects its resources to prioritize vital functions.[1]

Other Possible Causes: low-protein diet, magnesium deficiency, selenium deficiency, vitamin B6 (pyridoxine) deficiency, zinc deficiency, progesterone deficiency, oxidative stress

Treatment Strategies for Low Triiodothyronine (T3), Free

See the following sections: Thyroid-Stimulating Hormone (TSH) and Triiodothyronine (T3), Total.

Additional Testing

thyroid peroxidase antibodies (TPOAb); thyroglobulin antibody (TgAb); comprehensive thyroid profile II; reverse T3 (rT3); complete blood count (CBC); iron and TIBC; ferritin; comprehensive metabolic panel (CMP); progesterone; c-reactive protein (CRP); oral zinc tolerance test

References

1. Moura Neto A, Zantut-Wittmann DE. Abnormalities of Thyroid Hormone Metabolism during Systemic Illness: The Low T3 Syndrome in Different Clinical Settings. Int J Endocrinol. 2016;2016:2157583. doi:10.1155/2016/2157583

Reverse T3 (rT3)

Reverse T3 (rT3) measures the amount of rT3 in the bloodstream and is found as a single analyte.

Reverse T3 is considered an "inactive" thyroid hormone. But it works as a regulation of thyroid function at a cellular level. The conversion of T4 to rT3 is considered an adaptive mechanism in response to certain conditions such as stress, illness, or changes in thyroid hormone levels. Measuring rT3 can help assess cellular function and utilization of thyroid hormones.

RT3 is produced from T4 and T3 by the type 3 deiodinase enzymes (D3). D3 converts T4 to rT3 by removing an iodine atom from the outer ring of T4, creating rT3. D3 can also convert T3 to an inactive metabolite called 3,3'-diiodothyronine (T2).

Although both T3 and rT3 contain three iodine atoms, the difference lies in the arrangement of these atoms. T3 is composed of a tyrosine molecule with three iodine atoms attached to its aromatic rings. The iodine atoms are typically attached at positions 3, 5, and 3'. The structure of T3 allows it to be an active thyroid hormone, binding to thyroid hormone receptors and influencing cellular metabolism. On the other hand, rT3 is also composed of a tyrosine molecule, but the iodine atoms are arranged at positions 3, 3', and 5' on the two aromatic rings. This altered arrangement makes rT3 biologically inactive compared to T3, as it cannot effectively bind to thyroid hormone receptors and exert metabolic effects.

Pregnancy

Increasing cortisol levels reduce serum levels of free T4 and T3 while increasing rT3. In the first trimester, rT3 increases significantly, decreasing slightly and plateauing in the second trimester, then increasing again in the third trimester. This is partially driven by the increase in thyroid hormone production and cellular saturation that is stimulated by hCG.

Postpartum

Reverse T3 levels may initially remain elevated in the immediate postpartum period due to the catabolic state associated with labor and delivery stress. However, they typically return to baseline or lower levels as the body resolves the stress response.

STANDARD LAB RANGE: 9.2 - 24.1 ng/dL

Trimester	Standard Pregnancy Ranges	**Functional Pregnancy Ranges**
Preconception	9.2-24.1	**9.2 - 24.1**
First Trimester	Not Established	**34.8 - 83.4**
Second Trimester	Not Established	**18.2 - 74.7**
Third Trimester	Not Established	**20.1 - 84.5**
Postpartum	9.2-24.1	**9.2 - 24.1**

Causes of Elevated Reverse T3 (rT3)

The primary mechanism leading to elevated rT3 levels is the increased production of rT3 from T4 rather than its conversion to the active form of triiodothyronine T3. This is a mechanism to protect the mother from hyperthyroidism associated with increasing thyroid hormone production in pregnancy.

Inflammation/Illness: During acute illness or periods of critical illness, the body may prioritize the conversion of T4 to rT3 over the active T3 as a protective mechanism. This phenomenon is known as euthyroid sick syndrome (ESS) or non-thyroidal illness syndrome (NTIS). This may follow a period of illness, such as a viral infection during pregnancy. In this pattern, there will be low FT3 and elevated rT3. Normal increases of rT3 during pregnancy can make it difficult to diagnose inflammation with rT3, but it can still be a helpful tool.

Chronic Stress: Prolonged exposure to chronic stress can lead to elevated cortisol levels. High cortisol levels may affect the conversion of T4 to T3 and favor the production of rT3. Chronic stress can include physical, emotional, or psychological stressors. The elevation of rT3 during chronic stress is thought to be an adaptive response aimed at conserving energy. By reducing the production of active T3, the body may prioritize resources for coping with the stressor.

Environmental Toxins: Exposure to certain environmental toxins and pollutants has been associated with disruptions in hormone metabolism, including thyroid hormone metabolism. Specifically, polychlorinated biphenyls, polybrominated diphenyl ethers, polyfluoroalkyl substances (PFASs), bisphenol A (BPA), and phthalates.[1] [2] Other chemicals, such as glyphosates, have also been shown to affect thyroid function and increase rT3.[3]

Vitamin A Deficiency: Vitamin A regulates thyroid hormone receptor (THR) expression and function in target tissues. THR activation by thyroid hormones is essential for mediating thyroid hormone actions on metabolism, growth, and development. Vitamin A deficiency may disrupt THR signaling pathways, leading to alterations in thyroid hormone responsiveness and metabolism and elevated rT3 production.

Other Possible Causes: overmedication, hyperthyroidism, gestational transient thyrotoxicosis, autoimmune disease, zinc deficiency, selenium deficiency, fibromyalgia, chronic inflammatory diseases, adrenal hyperfunction, genetics

Treatment Strategies for Elevated Reverse T3 (rT3)

Diet

The primary goal with elevated rT3 is to heal cellular damage and reduce oxidative stress, improving the conversion of T4 to T3 at a cellular level. Berries such as strawberries, blueberries, raspberries, and blackberries are rich in antioxidants like vitamin C, flavonoids, and anthocyanins, which help neutralize free radicals and reduce oxidative stress. Vitamin C acts as an antioxidant and regulates thyroid receptor expression.

Liver, particularly beef liver, is one of the most concentrated sources of vitamin A. Additionally, colorful fruits and vegetables are excellent sources of beta-carotene. Sweet potatoes, carrots, and dark leafy greens like spinach and kale are packed with this antioxidant precursor.

Lifestyle

Because the primary cause of elevated rT3 is cellular stress and inflammation, lifestyle improvements can help. Poor sleep quality or inadequate sleep duration should be addressed. Increase mild exercise such as walking or hiking. Activities that also help to reduce stress can be important.

Additional Testing

comprehensive thyroid profile II; thyroid peroxidase antibodies (TPOAb); thyroglobulin antibody (TgAb); thyroid receptor antibodies (TRAb); complete blood count (CBC); comprehensive metabolic panel (CMP); vitamin D, 25-hydroxy (25-hydroxycalciferol, 25OH-D); c-reactive protein (CRP); antinuclear antibodies (ANA); oral zinc tolerance test

Causes of Low Reverse T3 (rT3)

Fasting/Malnutrition: Severe caloric restriction or prolonged fasting can lead to a decrease in rT3 levels. This is considered an adaptive response, as the body conserves energy during times of reduced food intake.

Other Possible Causes: hypothyroidism, genetics

Treatment Strategies for Low Reverse T3 (rT3)

Diet

If reverse T3 is low, assess other thyroid parameters and assess for caloric and nutritional deficiencies.

Additional Testing

comprehensive thyroid profile II; thyroid peroxidase antibodies (TPOAb); thyroglobulin antibody (TgAb); complete blood count (CBC); comprehensive metabolic panel (CMP); vitamin D, 25-hydroxy (25-hydroxycalciferol, 25OH-D); urinary iodine clearance (UIC); iodine, serum or plasma; iron and TIBC; ferritin

References

1. Calsolaro V, Pasqualetti G, Niccolai F, Caraccio N, Monzani F. Thyroid Disrupting Chemicals. Int J Mol Sci. 2017;18(12):2583. Published 2017 Dec 1. doi:10.3390/ijms18122583

2. Lee JE, Choi K. Perfluoroalkyl substances exposure and thyroid hormones in humans: epidemiological observations and implications. Ann Pediatr Endocrinol Metab. 2017;22(1):6–14. doi:10.6065/apem.2017.22.1.6

3. Llop S, Murcia M, Alvarez-Pedrerol M, et al. Association between exposure to organochlorine compounds and maternal thyroid status: Role of the iodothyronine deiodinase 1 gene. Environ Int. 2017;104:83–90. doi:10.1016/j.envint.2016.12.013

T3 Resin Uptake (T3 Uptake)

Despite its name, T3 uptake does not directly measure the amount of T3 in the blood but rather evaluates the capacity of TBG to bind thyroid hormones. It is found as a single indice or in panels such as the thyroid profile and comprehensive thyroid profile II.

This can give a measure of the ratio between thyroid hormones and transport proteins. During the T3 uptake test, a radioactive or nonradioactive thyroxine (T4) analog is added to the blood sample. This analog competes with endogenous T4 in the blood for binding sites on thyroid-binding proteins like TBG and albumin. The percentage of T4 analogs bound to these proteins is then measured. A higher percentage of bound T4 analogs indicates a lower binding capacity of the proteins, while a lower percentage suggests a higher binding capacity.

While T3 uptake is less commonly used today to assess the thyroid, it has historically been used to understand the binding capacity of thyroid-binding proteins in the blood.

TBG has a high binding affinity for both T4 and T3 but more readily binds T4 over T3. Changes in the production of TBG or thyroid hormone production can cause changes to other thyroid indices, such as total T4 and total T3. Adding the T3 uptake can be useful to assess the ratio between the thyroid hormones and the transport proteins.

> The T3 uptake is used to help assess the amount of TBG and not the amount of thyroid hormone.

Pregnancy

Estrogen stimulates TBG synthesis. As estrogen levels increase during pregnancy, TBG production also rises, leading to higher circulating levels of TBG-bound thyroid hormones. There is a slight drop in T3 uptake during pregnancy due to this rise. This increase is also the cause of increased total T4/T3 and decreased free T4/T3. The percentage should not decrease below standard ranges.[1]

Postpartum

The T3 uptake is affected in the days and weeks postpartum, as the production of TBG decreases with the drop in estrogen and the transient decrease in thyroid hormone production in thyroid recovery.

STANDARD LAB RANGE: 24% – 39%

Trimester	Standard Pregnancy Ranges	**Functional Pregnancy Ranges**
Preconception	24 – 39%	**27 – 39%**
First Trimester	24 – 39%	**24 – 39%**
Second Trimester	24 – 39%	**24 – 39%**
Third Trimester	24 – 39%	**24 – 39%**
Postpartum	24 – 39%	**27 – 39%**

Causes of Elevated T3 Resin Uptake (T3 Uptake)

See Thyroid-Stimulating Hormone (TSH) Section.

An overproduction of thyroid hormones or a decrease in TBG = more thyroid hormones in ratio to thyroid-binding proteins.

Other Possible Causes: gestational transient thyrotoxicosis, low TBG production, protein deficiency diet, oxidative stress, hyperthyroidism, Graves' disease, overdose on medications, low estrogen, vitamin B6 (pyridoxine) deficiency

Treatment Strategies for Elevated T3 Resin Uptake (T3 Uptake)

See Thyroid-Stimulating Hormone (TSH) Section.

Additional Testing

reverse T3 (rT3); thyroid peroxidase antibodies (TPOAb); thyroglobulin antibody (TgAb); thyroid receptor antibodies (TRAb); complete blood count (CBC); comprehensive metabolic panel (CMP)

Causes of Low T3 Resin Uptake (T3 Uptake)

See Thyroid-Stimulating Hormone (TSH) Section.

Other Possible Causes: hypothyroidism, progesterone deficiency

Fewer thyroid hormones or an overproduction of TBG = fewer thyroid hormones in ratio to thyroid-binding proteins.

Treatment Strategies for Low T3 Resin Uptake (T3 Uptake)

See Thyroid-Stimulating Hormone (TSH) Section.

Additional Testing

thyroid peroxidase antibodies (TPOAb); thyroglobulin antibody (TgAb); comprehensive thyroid profile II; reverse T3 (rT3); complete blood count (CBC); comprehensive metabolic panel (CMP); iron and TIBC; progesterone; c-reactive protein (CRP)

References

1. Souma JA, Green PJ, Coppage AT, Donner RS, Hogg AL. Changes in thyroid function in pregnancy and with oral contraceptive use. South Med J. 1981;74(6):684–687. doi:10.1097/00007611–198106000-00013

Free Thyroxine Index (FTI/FT4I)

The Free Thyroxine Index (FTI) estimates the actual free T4. It is an indice found in the thyroid profile and comprehensive thyroid profile II.

$$FTI = Total\ T4/T3\ Uptake \times 100$$

The direct measurement of FT4 is, conventionally, considered a more accurate assessment of the biologically active form of thyroxine. Based on the hormonal changes in pregnancy that affect the total and free T4 levels, some researchers suggest that FTI is a more accurate measure to assess FT4 in pregnancy.[1]

Pregnancy

FTI increases in conjunction with total and free T4. TT4 and FTI should maintain an inverse relationship to TSH during pregnancy.[2] Studies have found that FT4 values are falsely elevated and that FTI is a better measure of accurate T4 levels.[3]

Postpartum

In the postpartum period, as estrogen levels decrease, there is a subsequent reduction in thyroxine-binding globulin (TBG) production, as well as a decrease in thyroid hormone production. Depending on birth experience and breastfeeding status, thyroid hormone production may vary. FTI should remain fairly stable through pregnancy and postpartum.

According to a 2002 American College of Obstetricians and Gynecologists bulletin on thyroid disease, TSH and FT4 or FTI testing should be performed in pregnant women with suspected hyperthyroidism or hypothyroidism.[4]

STANDARD LAB RANGE: 4.8 – 12.7 μg/dL OR 1.2 – 4.9 UNITS*

Trimester	Standard Pregnancy Ranges	**Functional Pregnancy Ranges**
Preconception	4.8 – 12.7	**4.8 – 12.7**
First Trimester	5 – 10.5	**5 – 10.5**
Second Trimester	5 – 10.5	**5 – 10.5**
Third Trimester	5 – 10.5	**5 – 10.5**
Postpartum	4.8 – 12.7	**4.8 – 12.7**

*Reference ranges for FTI can vary between laboratories, and the specific range for FTI might depend on the assay method used. It's crucial to interpret FTI results in the context of the laboratory's reference range and the individual's clinical situation. Currently, only a few studies have identified trimester-specific reference ranges. These also vary. Currently ACOG and other organizations have stated that FTI is a better assessment of true availability of FT4, yet do not offer a trimester-specific reference range for guidance.

Causes of Elevated Free Thyroxine Index (FTI/FT4I)

See the following sections: Thyroxine (T4), Total and Thyroxine (T4), Free.

Hyperthyroidism: This could be due to either gestational transient thyrotoxicosis or Graves' disease. Diagnosis is generally based on an elevated FT4 or FTI, with suppression of TSH in the absence of thyroid mass or nodular goiter. It is important in these cases to test for thyroid antibodies. This is a very common finding in the first trimester, especially in those with severe nausea and vomiting.

Other Possible Causes: stress, inflammation, acute illness, medication overdose

Treatment Strategies for Elevated Free Thyroxine Index (FTI/FT4I)

See the following sections: Thyroxine (T4), Total and Thyroxine (T4), Free.

Additional Testing

thyroid peroxidase antibodies (TPOAb); thyroglobulin antibody (TgAb); thyroid receptor antibodies (TRAb); complete blood count (CBC); comprehensive metabolic panel (CMP); comprehensive thyroid profile II; reverse T3 (rT3)

Causes of Low Free Thyroxine Index (FTI/FT4I)

See the following sections: Thyroxine (T4), Total and Thyroxine (T4), Free.

Other Possible Causes: hypothyroidism, progesterone deficiency

Treatment Strategies for Low Free Thyroxine Index (FTI/FT4I)

See the following sections: Thyroxine (T4), Total and Thyroxine (T4), Free.

Additional Testing

thyroid peroxidase antibodies (TPOAb); thyroglobulin antibody (TgAb); comprehensive thyroid profile II; reverse T3 (rT3); complete blood count (CBC); comprehensive metabolic panel (CMP); iron and TIBC; progesterone; c-reactive protein (CRP)

References

1. Azizi F, Mehran L, Amouzegar A, et al. Establishment of the trimester-specific reference range for free thyroxine index [published correction appears in Thyroid]. 2013 Jul;23(7):915. Fereidoun, Azizi [corrected to Azizi, Fereidoun]; Ladan, Mehran [corrected to Mehran, Ladan]; Atieh, Amouzegar [corrected to Amouzegar, Atieh]; Hossein, Delshad [corrected to Delshad, Hossein]; Maryam, Tohidi [corrected to Tohidi, Maryam]; Sahar, Askari [c]. Thyroid. 2013;23(3):354–359. doi:10.1089/thy.2012.0407

2. Lee RH, Spencer CA, Mestman JH, et al. Free T4 immunoassays are flawed during pregnancy. Am J Obstet Gynecol. 2009;200(3):260.e1–260.e2606. doi:10.1016/j.ajog.2008.10.042

3. Liberman, C. S., Pino, S. C., Fang, S. L., Braverman, L. E., & Emerson, C. H. (1998). Circulating iodide concentrations during and after pregnancy. The Journal of clinical endocrinology and metabolism, 83(10), 3545–3549. doi.org/10.1210/jcem.83.10.5163

4. Schroeder BM; American College of Obstetricians and Gynecologists. ACOG practice bulletin on thyroid disease in pregnancy. Am Fam Physician. 2002;65(10):2158–21

Thyroid Peroxidase Antibodies (TPOAb)

The thyroid peroxidase antibodies (TPOAb) test measures the presence of antibodies against the thyroid peroxidase enzyme. This is a single analyte, or it can be found in specific thyroid panels such as thyroid antibodies and the Thyroid Cascade Profile.

Thyroid peroxidase catalyzes the iodination of tyrosine residues within thyroglobulin. This iodination occurs in the colloid of thyroid follicles. Coupling of the iodinated residues leads to the formation of thyroxine (T4) and triiodothyronine (T3). Thyroid peroxidase is a heme-containing enzyme. The iodination process is reliant on the heme group in the TPO enzyme. Selenium is an essential cofactor for TPO activity. It is a component of the enzyme's active site and is required for its proper function.

TPO antibodies are the hallmark of autoimmune thyroid disease, which is characterized by chronic inflammation in the thyroid gland. In Hashimoto's thyroiditis, the immune system mistakenly targets and attacks the thyroid gland. TPO antibodies can also be found in Graves' disease, which is characterized by hyperthyroidism.

TPO antibodies have been associated with an increased risk of thyroid dysfunction during pregnancy and postpartum, regardless of preconception thyroid-stimulating hormone (TSH) levels. They have also been associated with adverse pregnancy outcomes that include miscarriage and preterm labor.

Hashimoto's thyroiditis is a progressive autoimmune disease and is described in five stages.

Stage 1: Genetic Predisposition

Genetics play a role in the progression of all autoimmune diseases. Having a predisposition does not mean disease is inevitable; it just means someone carries the genetics that increase the risk of developing the condition. Diet, lifestyle, or chemical exposure could activate the subsequent stages. Some genetic factors that have been associated with an increased risk of developing TPO antibodies include the HLA genes (HLA-DR3, HLA-DR4, HLA-DQA1, and HLA-DQB1), CTLA-4, PTPN22, FCRL3, and FOXP3, as well as genetic variants in the TPO gene itself.

Stage 2: Immune Infiltration

At this stage, a patient may still have normal thyroid function and lab values, although mild thyroiditis symptoms may exist. During this stage, the genetic predisposition is activated, and the immune system starts to turn toward the thyroid gland. If you were to do a fine-needle aspiration at this point, you would find WBCs in the thyroid tissue. This is also known as the "trigger" stage. This happens when the body is stressed, with an increased immune response and decreased discrimination. For many people, autoimmune thyroid disease is triggered after an event such as pregnancy, viral infection, parasitic infection, high-emotion stress, or trauma.

Stage 3: Subclinical Hypothyroidism

At this stage, we begin to see mild rises in TSH production. T4 and T3 may be normal or slightly decreased, but typically no value will signal hypothyroidism. At this point, we are going to see more and more symptoms and potentially higher thyroid antibodies. These are cases in which patients complain of hypothyroidism symptoms but do not have lab values that diagnose them with hypothyroidism.

Stage 4: Overt Hypothyroidism

In this stage, we begin to see elevations in TSH and decreases in T4 and T3 indices. Stage 4 is when most people are diagnosed with hypothyroidism but not always Hashimoto's. Antibodies can also be significantly elevated at this point.

Stage 5: Progression to Other Autoimmune Diseases

Research shows that once a person is diagnosed with one autoimmune disease, they typically develop more throughout their life. Following strict guidelines will help prevent autoimmune progression and slow the development of future autoimmune diseases.

Pregnancy

Any elevation in TPOAb should be monitored throughout pregnancy. It is not uncommon for TPO antibodies to increase in the first trimester if present preconception. For some, with the change in lymphocyte production and function as well as globulin production changes, there can be a drop in TPO enzymes late first trimester through the remainder of pregnancy.[1] Pregnancy increases the demand on the thyroid gland. Making thyroid hormones is an oxidative process, and it creates high amounts of reactive oxygen species (ROS). This increase in demand, increase in ROS, and overall state of mild inflammation coupled with immunoglobulin and white blood cell changes can lead to an increased risk of developing autoantibodies toward the end of pregnancy and into the postpartum phase.

Postpartum

A woman's TPO antibody levels may increase significantly after giving birth. Postpartum thyroiditis affects between 5% and 10% of women in the first year after giving birth. Around

60% of Graves' disease patients have onset in the postpartum phase.[2] With birth, the demand for thyroid hormones decreases, and the immune system returns to normal. In cases of heightened oxidative stress in the thyroid gland from inflammation, the immune system responds. This is when antibodies to the TPO enzymes can increase or be triggered. Postpartum thyroid inflammation can continue for one to two years postpartum.

STANDARD LAB RANGE: 0 – 34 IU/mL

Trimester	Standard Pregnancy Ranges	**Functional Pregnancy Ranges**
Preconception	0–34	**0–34**
First Trimester	0–34	**0–34**
Second Trimester	0–34	**0–34**
Third Trimester	0–34	**0–34**
Postpartum	0–34	**0–34**

Causes of Elevated Thyroid Peroxidase Antibodies (TPOAb)

See Thyroid-Stimulating Hormone (TSH) Section.

The presence of TPO antibodies in women with euthyroid function lead to a higher prevalence of infertility, anemia, preterm delivery, subclinical hypothyroidism, and birth complications.

Studies have shown that thyroid autoantibodies, especially TPOAb, can lead to adverse obstetric outcomes such as miscarriage and preterm delivery, even when thyroid function is normal.[3]

TPO antibodies >35 IU/mL are associated

Environmental Chemical Exposure: Various environmental factors have been implicated in the development of autoimmune disease, including thyroid peroxidase antibodies. This includes perchlorate,[6] bisphenol A (BPA),[7] and polybrominated diphenyl esters (PBDEs).[8]

BPA is found in plastics, epoxy resins, and other commonly used products. Studies in animals have suggested that BPA may be associated with autoimmune thyroid disease.

Perchlorate is a chemical used in fireworks and industrial processes. It can be a water or food contaminant. Perchlorate competes with iodide uptake by the thyroid. Exposure to perchlorate has been associated with thyroid dysfunction and autoantibody production, including TPO antibodies. Perchlorate contains chlorine, a halogen compound.

Other halogens include bromine and fluorine. Bromine is found in PBDEs as well as in brominated flour, brominated vegetable oil, and pesticides. Bromide competes with iodine in the thyroid. High exposure has been associated with thyroid dysfunction, goiter, and hypothyroidism. It is hypothesized that bromide-induced thyroid

with an increased risk of pregnancy complications. The risk increases with increasing antibody levels.[4]

A systematic review published in 2011 of over 12,000 women showed that the presence of thyroid autoantibodies leads to significantly increased odds of miscarriage for women from all populations compared to women without autoantibodies.[5]

dysfunction may contribute to immune dysregulation and the development of autoimmune thyroid disease.

Fluoride is commonly found in drinking water and in oral hygiene products. While fluoride is generally considered safe at low doses, excess exposure has been associated with thyroid dysfunction.

Overall, halogen replacement of iodine in the T4/T3 structure has been shown to trigger autoimmune reactions.[9]

Latent Viral Infections: Latent viruses are those that "hibernate" in the host cells until they are reactivated after initial infection. A primary example of this is the herpesvirus family of viruses (herpes simplex, varicella zoster, Epstein-Barr, cytomegalovirus). Others include HIV (human immunodeficiency virus), hepatitis B, hepatitis C, HPV (human papillomavirus), and polyomaviruses. Often these viruses are found in thyroid tissues, thus triggering autoimmune reactions in various ways.[10] The exact mechanisms are not fully understood but may include molecular mimicry. This is where viral antigens share a similar structure to self-antigens such as TPO.

During a viral infection, the immune system may misidentify the TPO enzyme as the viral antigen, and generate antibodies and T cells in response to both. This would result in TPO antibodies. Another potential mechanism would be where the viral load damages the thyroid tissue and increases the immune-system response to the thyroid tissues. The heightened immune system reacting to the damage activates autoimmune responses against the thyroid gland to facilitate apoptosis of the damaged cells.

Persistent viral infections can dysregulate the immune system and reduce immune tolerance, leading to reduced self-tolerance. Since latent viruses persist in host cells, with periodic reactivation, this may trigger immune responses to the host cells and surrounding tissues. If the virus is dormant in the thyroid cells, this would elicit a response to the thyroid cells.

Iron Deficiency: Iron deficiency can affect the thyroid in various ways. It can exacerbate TPO antibody presentations by limiting the production of TPO enzymes. In addition, studies find that low iron levels are associated with higher antibody levels.[11]

Magnesium Deficiency: Studies have shown a significant association between serum magnesium levels and thyroid antibodies. Magnesium may play a role in immune regulation. Hypomagnesemia has been shown to increase pro-inflammatory cytokines. Lower serum magnesium levels are associated with incremental positivity of thyroiditis antibodies.[12]

Iodine Overdose: In cases of autoimmune thyroid disease, there is a bell curve with iodine use; both low iodine and elevated iodine have been associated with higher antibody levels.

Vitamin D Deficiency: Patients with vitamin D deficiency have significantly higher TPOAb levels.[13]

Other Possible Causes: heavy metal exposure, thyroid injury, iodine overdose, chronic stress, gut dysbiosis, chronic bacterial infections, parasitic infections, high-dose vitamin B7 (biotin), certain medications (Accutane, interferon), selenium deficiency

Treatment Strategies for Elevated Thyroid Peroxidase Antibodies (TPOAb)

See Thyroid-Stimulating Hormone (TSH) Section.

Diet

A gluten-free diet trial is advised for those with TPOAb presentations. Generally, this is done over three months, and antibodies are retested to assess for reductions. A 2023 meta-analysis concluded that a gluten-free diet was associated with a reduction in TPO antibodies in those without celiac disease diagnosis or symptoms.[14] One study on Hashimoto's patients found that 88% of those who adopted a gluten-free diet had a reduction of symptoms and improved lab values, even though only 3.5% of them were diagnosed with celiac disease. Patients should avoid iodized salts. Several different gut conditions have been associated with the increased progression of Hashimoto's. There is a connection between gut inflammation and an overactive immune response. Probiotics and probiotic-rich foods can help balance gut bacteria and prevent gut inflammation.

Supplements

Several studies have shown a relationship between selenium supplementation and thyroid antibodies, specifically TPOAb. Supplementing with selenium reduces TPOAb and the severity of symptoms. The standard dosage is 200 µg/day.[15] When vitamin D is low, supplementation may help lower TPOAb but will not change thyroid indices.[16] In cases of autoimmune hyperthyroidism, L-carnitine supplements may be beneficial.

Note that hyperthyroidism due to autoimmune disease should be monitored and treated by a maternal-fetal medicine physician and endocrinologist. L-carnitine at 2 to 4 grams per day has been shown to reverse hyperthyroid symptoms. L-carnitine inhibits thyroid hormone action, reducing thyroid hormone entry into the cells.[17] This should also be cautioned in those with hypothyroidism.

Additional Testing

thyroglobulin antibody (TgAb); comprehensive thyroid profile II; reverse T3 (rT3); thyroid receptor antibodies (TRAb); thyroid imaging; complete blood count (CBC); iron and TIBC; ferritin; comprehensive metabolic panel (CMP); vitamin D, 25-hydroxy (25-hydroxycalciferol, 25OH-D); heavy metal testing; antinuclear antibodies (ANA); urinary iodine clearance (UIC); iodine, serum or plasma

Causes of Low Thyroid Peroxidase Antibodies (TPOAb)

Not considered pathogenic

Treatment Strategies for Low Thyroid Peroxidase Antibodies (TPOAb)

Not considered pathogenic

References

1. Meena M, Chopra S, Jain V, Aggarwal N. The Effect of Anti-Thyroid Peroxidase Antibodies on Pregnancy Outcomes in Euthyroid Women. J Clin Diagn Res. 2016;10(9):QC04-QC07. doi:10.7860/JCDR/2016/19009.8403

2. Di Bari F, Granese R, Le Donne M, Vita R, Benvenga S. Autoimmune Abnormalities of Postpartum Thyroid Diseases. Front Endocrinol (Lausanne). 2017;8:166. Published 2017 Jul 13. doi:10.3389/fendo.2017.00166

3. Liu M, Wang D, Zhu L, et al. Association of thyroid peroxidase antibodies with the rate of first-trimester miscarriage in euthyroid women with unexplained recurrent spontaneous abortion. Front Endocrinol (Lausanne). 2022;13:966565. Published 2022 Aug 31. doi:10.3389/fendo.2022.966565

4. Fernández Martínez P, Aguado García R, Barajas Galindo DE, et al. Influence of thyroid peroxidase antibodies on TSH levels of pregnant women and maternal-fetal complications. Influencia de los anticuerpos antiperoxidasa tiroidea en los valores de TSH de gestantes y en las complicaciones materno-fetales. Endocrinol Diabetes Nutr (Engl Ed). 2018;65(8):444–450. doi:10.1016/j.endinu.2018.05.004

5. Thangaratinam S, Tan A, Knox E, Kilby MD, Franklyn J, Coomarasamy A. Association between thyroid autoantibodies and miscarriage and preterm birth: meta-analysis of evidence. BMJ. 2011;342:d2616. Published 2011 May 9. doi:10.1136/bmj.d2616

6. Knight BA, Shields BM, He X, et al. Effect of perchlorate and thiocyanate exposure on thyroid function of pregnant women from South-West England: a cohort study. Thyroid Res. 2018;11:9. Published 2018 Jul 6. doi:10.1186/s13044–018-0053-x

7. Chailurkit LO, Aekplakorn W, Ongphiphadhanakul B. The Association of Serum Bisphenol A with Thyroid Autoimmunity. Int J Environ Res Public Health. 2016;13(11):1153. Published 2016 Nov 17. doi:10.3390/ijerph13111153

8. Makey CM, McClean MD, Braverman LE, et al. Polybrominated Diphenyl Ether Exposure and Thyroid Function Tests in North American Adults. Environ Health Perspect. 2016;124(4):420–425. doi:10.1289/ehp.1509755

9. Andrade LJdO, de Oliveira LM, Bittencourt AMV, de Oliveira LCM, de Oliveira GCM. Halogens as Potential Thyroid Disruptors – In Sílico Simulation and Mathematical Model for Triggering Autoimmune Thyroiditis. Research Square; 2023. DOI: 10.21203/rs.3.rs-2614009/v1

10. Weider T, Genoni A, Broccolo F, et al. High Prevalence of Common Human Viruses in Thyroid Tissue. Front Endocrinol (Lausanne). 2022;13:938633. Published 2022 Jul 14. doi:10.3389/fendo.2022.938633

11. Gupta N, Narayan A, Tonk RS, Gupta SK, Narayan A. Study of Relationship Between Iron Deficiency and Thyroid Function in Pregnant Females. Cureus. 2022;14(12):e32411. Published 2022 Dec 11. doi:10.7759/cureus.32411

12. Luo Y, Zeng H, Ye Y, et al. Associations of metal profiles in blood with thyroiditis: a cross-sectional study. Environ Sci Pollut Res Int. 2023;30(8):21072–21080. doi:10.1007/s11356–022-23625–1

13. Czarnywojtek A, Florek E, Pietrończyk K, et al. The Role of Vitamin D in Autoimmune Thyroid Diseases: A Narrative Review. J Clin Med. 2023;12(4):1452. Published 2023 Feb 11. doi:10.3390/jcm12041452

14. Piticchio T, Frasca F, Malandrino P, et al. Effect of gluten-free diet on autoimmune thyroiditis progression in patients with no symptoms or histology of celiac disease: a meta-analysis. Front Endocrinol (Lausanne). 2023;14:1200372. Published 2023 Jul 24. doi:10.3389/fendo.2023.1200372

15. Hu Y, Feng W, Chen H, et al. Effect of selenium on thyroid autoimmunity and regulatory T cells in patients with Hashimoto's thyroiditis: A prospective randomized-controlled trial. Clin Transl Sci. 2021;14(4):1390–1402. doi:10.1111/cts.12993

16. Jiang H, Chen X, Qian X, Shao S. Effects of vitamin D treatment on thyroid function and autoimmunity markers in patients with Hashimoto's thyroiditis-A meta-analysis of randomized controlled trials. J Clin Pharm Ther. 2022;47(6):767–775. doi:10.1111/jcpt.13605

17. Benvenga S, Amato A, Calvani M, Trimarchi F. Effects of carnitine on thyroid hormone action. Ann N Y Acad Sci. 2004;1033:158–167. doi:10.1196/annals.1320.015

Thyroglobulin Antibody (TgAb)

The thyroglobulin antibody (TGAb) test measures the presence of antibodies against thyroglobulin. This is a single analyte, or it can be found in specific thyroid panels such as thyroid antibodies.

Thyroglobulin is a large glycoprotein complex. It consists of 140 tyrosine residues. Its genetic transcription requires vitamin A. Thyroglobulin serves as the storage form of thyroid hormones within the colloid space of thyroid follicles. Ionization of the thyroglobulin with iodine is facilitated by the thyroid peroxidase enzyme.

Thyroglobulin antibodies are those that target thyroglobulin. These antibodies can be present in both hypothyroidism and hyperthyroidism.

Pregnancy

It is not uncommon for thyroglobulin antibodies to increase in the first trimester if present preconception. TgAb levels tend to mimic the increase and decrease seen with thyroid peroxidase antibodies (TPOAb), with a potential increase in the early first trimester and a subsequent decrease throughout the remainder of pregnancy.

Postpartum

Elevated thyroid antibodies are found in 60% to 85% of women presenting with postpartum thyroiditis.[1]

STANDARD LAB RANGE: 0.0 – 0.9 IU/mL

Trimester	Standard Pregnancy Ranges	**Functional Pregnancy Ranges**
Preconception	0.0 – 0.9	**0.0 – 0.9**
First Trimester	0.0 – 0.9	**0.0 – 0.9**
Second Trimester	0.0 – 0.9	**0.0 – 0.9**
Third Trimester	0.0 – 0.9	**0.0 – 0.9**
Postpartum	0.0 – 0.9	**0.0 – 0.9**

Causes of Elevated Thyroglobulin Antibody (TgAb)

See Thyroid Peroxidase Antibodies (TPOAb) Section.

Most studies have focused on the presence of TPOAb and less on the presence of TgAb, therefore there is limited research on the effects of these antibodies on pregnancy outcomes. A 2023 systemic review and meta-analysis did find a correlation between TgAb and recurrent pregnancy loss.[2]

Genetics: In all cases of autoimmune thyroid disease, there is an element of genetics that predisposes someone to an increased risk of developing thyroid self-antibodies. In the case of thyroglobulin antibodies, genetic mutations in the HLA (HLA-DR3 and HLA-DR4), TG, CTLA-4, FOXP3, PTPN22, CD40, and CD20 (MS4A1) have been correlated with thyroglobulin antibodies.

Other Possible Causes: environmental chemical exposure, latent viral infection, heavy metal exposure, thyroid injury, iodine overdose, chronic stress, gut dysbiosis, chronic bacterial infections, parasitic infections, high-dose vitamin B7 (biotin), certain medications (Accutane, interferon), selenium deficiency, vitamin D deficiency

Treatment Strategies for Elevated Thyroglobulin Antibody (TgAb)

See Thyroid Peroxidase Antibodies (TPOAb) Section.

Diet

Excess iodine seems to affect the TgAb antibodies more severely than TPOAb. Avoiding excess iodine supplementation when TgAb is present may be important for maintaining levels. This does not mean avoiding iodine-rich foods, but possibly avoiding or limiting excess iodine in the form of iodized salts and in supplemental form in those with hyperthyroidism or severe antibody presentations. Iodine is crucial for fetal brain development and IQ, so complete avoidance is not advised.[3] Overall, diets high in vegetables, fruit, nuts, and seeds are associated with lower levels of thyroglobulin antibodies.

Supplements

Interestingly, studies on smoking and thyroid have shown a protective effect with tobacco use against thyroglobulin antibodies. Tobacco contains an alkaloid called anatabine. In studies, anatabine at a dosage of 0.17 to 0.25 mg/kg was shown to reduce the thyroid antibodies. Currently, there are no studies on the use of anatabine in pregnancy, and smoking in pregnancy is not advised. Vegetables that contain anatabine include tomatoes, peppers, eggplants, and other members of the nightshade family.

Additional Testing
thyroid peroxidase antibodies (TPOAb); comprehensive thyroid profile II; reverse T3 (rT3); thyroid receptor antibodies (TRAb); thyroid imaging; complete blood count (CBC); iron and TIBC; ferritin; comprehensive metabolic panel (CMP); vitamin D, 25-hydroxy (25-hydroxy-calciferol, 25OH-D); heavy metal testing; antinuclear antibodies (ANA); urinary iodine clearance (UIC); iodine, serum or plasma

Causes of Low Thyroglobulin Antibody (TgAb)

Not considered pathogenic

Treatment Strategies for Low Thyroglobulin Antibody (TgAb)

Not considered pathogenic

References

1. Naji Rad S, Deluxe L. Postpartum Thyroiditis. [Updated 2023 Jun 12]. In: StatPearls [Internet]. Treasure Island (FL): StatPearls Publishing; 2024 Jan-. www.ncbi.nlm.nih.gov/books/NBK557646

2. Huisman P, Krogh J, Nielsen CH, Nielsen HS, Feldt-Rasmussen U, Bliddal S. Thyroglobulin Antibodies in Women with Recurrent Pregnancy Loss: A Systematic Review and Meta-Analysis. Thyroid. 2023;33(11):1287–1301. doi:10.1089/thy.2023.0292

3. Francesco Latrofa, Emilio Fiore, Teresa Rago, Lucia Antonangeli, Lucia Montanelli, Debora Ricci, Maria Annateresa Provenzale, Maria Scutari, Monica Frigeri, Massimo Tonacchera, Paolo Vitti, Iodine Contributes to Thyroid Autoimmunity in Humans by Unmasking a Cryptic Epitope on Thyroglobulin, The Journal of Clinical Endocrinology & Metabolism, Volume 98, Issue 11, 1 November 2013, Pages E1768–E1774. doi.org/10.1210/jc.2013-2912

Thyroid Receptor Antibodies (TRAb)

The thyroid receptor antibodies (TRAb) test measures the levels of antibodies that target the thyroid-stimulating hormone (TSH) receptor, also known as the thyrotropin receptor, on the surface of thyroid cells.

This test detects two main types of thyroid receptor antibodies.

Thyroid-Stimulating Immunoglobulin (TSI)

TSI antibodies mimic the actions of TSH by binding to and stimulating that TSH receptor. The continuous stimulation causes a decrease in TSH and an increase in T4 and T3 indices, generally with an increased reverse T3.

Thyroid-Binding Inhibitory Immunoglobulins (TBIIs)

TBIIs completely bind to TSH receptors but do not stimulate the thyroid. Instead, they lead to a decrease in the production of thyroid hormones. In rare cases, they have been associated with hyperstimulation, but this is typically in association with TSI.

TSI can be measured on its own. It is a separate and specified analyte.

TRAb is typically used to rule out Graves' disease or autoimmune hyperthyroidism.

Pregnancy

It is not uncommon for all thyroid antibodies to increase in the first trimester if present pre-conception. Levels may then increase or decrease based on individual presentations. With changes in immune-system function and globulin production, in normal pregnancy, antibodies generally decrease slightly in the second trimester and increase again toward the end of the third trimester through postpartum.

Postpartum

Postpartum thyroiditis typically occurs in the first 1 to 4 months postpartum, but Graves' disease may develop between 4 and 12 months postpartum.[1]

STANDARD LAB RANGE: 0.0 – 1.75 IU/L

Trimester	Standard Pregnancy Ranges	**Functional Pregnancy Ranges**
Preconception	0.0 – 1.75	**0.0 – 1.75**
First Trimester	0.0 – 1.75	**0.0 – 1.75**
Second Trimester	0.0 – 1.75	**0.0 – 1.75**
Third Trimester	0.0 – 1.75	**0.0 – 1.75**
Postpartum	0.0 – 1.75	**0.0 – 1.75**

Causes of Elevated Thyroid Receptor Antibodies (TRAb)

See Thyroid Peroxidase Antibodies (TPOAb) Section.

All Graves' disease patients should be medically managed by physician specialists.

During pregnancy, TRAb crosses the placenta and may induce fetal hyperthyroidism. TRAb levels over three times the normal limit are associated with hyperthyroidism in the fetus and newborn.[2]

Gut Parasites: Several parasitic infections have been associated with an increased rate of Graves' disease diagnosis. The exact mechanism is unknown, but a few associations include helminths and *Toxoplasma gondii.*

Other Possible Causes: environmental chemical exposure, latent viral infection, heavy metal exposure, thyroid injury, iodine overdose, chronic stress, gut dysbiosis, chronic bacterial infections, parasitic infections, high-dose vitamin B7 (biotin), certain medications (Accutane, interferon), selenium deficiency, vitamin D deficiency

Treatment Strategies for Elevated Thyroid Receptor Antibodies (TRAb)

See Thyroid Peroxidase Antibodies (TPOAb) Section.

Diet

Currently, there are no studies linking a gluten-free diet with a decrease of TRAb, yet based on the connection to the HLA gene and the benefits seen in the reduction of other thyroid autoantibodies, a gluten-free diet trial may be beneficial. The role of iodine is controversial. On one hand, iodine may further increase thyroid hormone production; on the other hand, hyperthyroidism may further deplete the body of iodine. Graves' disease patients have a higher risk of cancer, particularly thyroid and breast. The breast tissue and the reproductive organs need iodine, and it is theorized that the antimicrobial effects of iodine help to reduce the risk of cancer in these tissues.

Patients should eat more cruciferous vegetables. These veggies contain compounds that may reduce iodine absorption into the thyroid. Some culinary spices, such as green chilies and turmeric, have been shown to reduce the frequency of hyperthyroid episodes in those with diagnosed Graves' disease.

Supplements

Low selenium is associated with increased risk of Graves' disease. Selenium supplementation has been shown to have short-term benefits in improving symptoms, but long-term use has not been found to be beneficial. Maximum benefit and TRAb reduction is seen at six months of use.[3] Vitamin D supplementation may benefit those with low vitamin D. Studies have shown an inverse relationship between vitamin D levels and TRAb.[4]

Additional Testing

thyroid peroxidase antibodies (TPOAb); thyroglobulin antibody (TgAb); comprehensive thyroid profile II; reverse T3 (rT3); thyroid imaging; complete blood count (CBC); iron and TIBC; ferritin; comprehensive metabolic panel (CMP); vitamin D, 25-hydroxy (25-hydroxy-calciferol, 25OH-D); heavy metal testing; antinuclear antibodies (ANA); urinary iodine clearance (UIC); iodine, serum or plasma

Causes of Low Thyroid Receptor Antibodies (TRAb)

Not considered pathogenic

Treatment Strategies for Low Thyroid Receptor Antibodies (TRAb)

Not considered pathogenic

References

1. Amino N, Arata N. Thyroid dysfunction following pregnancy and implications for breastfeeding. Best Pract Res Clin Endocrinol Metab. 2020;34(4):101438. doi:10.1016/j.beem.2020.101438

2. Nguyen CT, Sasso EB, Barton L, Mestman JH. Graves' hyperthyroidism in pregnancy: a clinical review. Clin Diabetes Endocrinol. 2018;4:4. Published 2018 Mar 1. doi:10.1186/s40842–018-0054–7

3. Zheng H, Wei J, Wang L, et al. Effects of Selenium Supplementation on Graves' Disease: A Systematic Review and Meta-Analysis. Evid Based Complement Alternat Med. 2018;2018:3763565. Published 2018 Sep 26. doi:10.1155/2018/3763565

4. Zhang H, Liang L, Xie Z. Low Vitamin D Status is Associated with Increased Thyrotropin-Receptor Antibody Titer in Graves' Disease. Endocr Pract. 2015;21(3):258–263. doi:10.4158/EP14191.OR

Iodine, Serum or Plasma

The iodine, serum or plasma test, also known as the serum iodine concentration (SIC) test, is used to analyze the amount of iodine present in a blood sample. It is an individual analyte.

Iodine, serum or plasma testing is less commonly used in research to assess iodine deficiency. The more common measure is urinary iodine clearance (UIC). Studies show that the iodine, serum or plasma test accurately correlates with the UIC/creatinine ratio. It measures the iodine pool. Research is being done to determine the effective reference ranges for SIC in pregnancy, as it is an easier test to perform.[1]

Iodine is a mineral and a chemical element with the symbol "I" that belongs to the halogen family. The halogen family is a group of nonmetallic elements of the periodic table. It includes fluorine (F), chlorine (Cl), bromine (Br), iodine (I), and astatine (At). These elements readily bond to other compounds such as minerals.

Iodine content in the soil is fairly low, but it is found in higher amounts in oceans. It is found naturally as iodide. Iodide is iodine bound to other minerals to create a salt, such as sodium or potassium.

Iodide is absorbed through the stomach and small intestines, with between 70% and 90% of dietary iodide being absorbed. Iodine absorption is lower and may vary depending on other factors, as it is not naturally found in the diet as iodine.

The sodium-iodide symporter (NIS) is a transport protein responsible for the active transport of iodide ions across cell membranes. They are found in the gastric mucosa, salivary glands, liver, mammary tissues, eyes, thyroid gland, endometrium, ovaries, brain, and cervix. The function of NIS is reliant on magnesium. The symporter exchanges the potassium found commonly in iodide for sodium and transports the sodium iodide through the membrane. The expression of NIS is tightly regulated by thyroid hormones, which upregulate NIS expression when iodine levels are low.

Once absorbed, iodide enters the bloodstream and becomes part of the iodide pool, which is the serum-accumulated iodide that the body can pull from. This can be recycled iodide from the deiodination of thyroxine as well as recent intake. A significant portion is taken up by the thyroid gland. The rest of the iodide is either taken up by other organs with NIS proteins or excreted through the urine. About 90% of iodide is excreted through the urine within 24 to 48 hours.

In the US, between 2011 and 2021, 38% of the population was classified as iodine deficient. A 2021 sampling of pregnant women in Michigan found that 23% had inadequate iodine intake.[2]

It is estimated that an average of 44% of Europeans are iodine deficient, and more than 50% of those in central and western Europe are deficient.[3]

A 2011 study from Spain found that only 14.4% of pregnant women in the first trimester and 26.8% in the second trimester had adequate iodine levels.[4]

In Southeast Asia and the Eastern Mediterranean, iodine deficiency is estimated to be present in 36% to 43% of the general population.[5]

Up to 80% of children in South American countries are estimated to be iodine deficient.

Pregnancy

During pregnancy, there is a 50% increase in the dietary need for iodine.[6] Much of the iodine is used for the increase in maternal thyroid hormone production. Another portion of iodine is transferred to the fetus for storage starting around 10 to 12 weeks gestation, until they begin producing their own thyroid hormones around 16 to 20 weeks gestation. Iodine is also essential for the development of the fetal brain and nervous system.[7] There are limited studies on serum iodine levels throughout pregnancy. There is a mild increase in serum iodine levels between the first and second trimester and a decrease in the third trimester.[8]

Postpartum

Serum iodine levels should be stable postpartum. If breastfeeding, the need for iodine increases slightly.

STANDARD LAB RANGE: 40 – 92 µg/L

Trimester	Standard Pregnancy Ranges	**Functional Pregnancy Ranges**
Preconception	40 – 92	**70 – 110**
First Trimester	Not Established	**70 – 110**
Second Trimester	Not Established	**70 – 110**
Third Trimester	Not Established	**70 – 110**
Postpartum	40 – 92	**70 – 110**

Causes of Elevated Iodine, Serum or Plasma

Elevated serum iodine levels, particularly in the first trimester, may be associated with a slight negative impact on motor and physical development and infant intellect, according to a 2024 study.[9]

It has been suggested that excess iodine in the first trimester may be a cause of nausea as a means of preventing excess consumption. Pregnancy nausea is closely linked to iodine intake and thyroid function.[10]

Overconsumption of Supplemental Iodine: It is difficult to overdose on iodine in the diet, even when consuming large amounts of foods like seaweed. Those consuming potassium iodide supplements are susceptible to iodine overdose.

Magnesium Deficiency: Magnesium is required for the function of NIS proteins. When magnesium is deficient, there are hypothyroidism patterns with elevated serum iodine. This shows a decrease in the uptake of iodine into the thyroid cells.[11] In this case, you may see a higher TSH, lower thyroid hormone profile, and elevated serum iodine with no excess iodine consumption or supplementation.

Kidney Disease: There is a rapid turnover rate of serum iodine with nearly 90% being excreted within 24 to 48 hours after consumption through the urine. When the kidneys are unable to function properly, there can be an increase in serum iodine due to a reduction of excretion.[12] (See Estimated Glomerular Filtration Rate (eGFR) Section.)

Goitrogen Exposure: Goitrogens are substances that affect thyroid function in various ways. Thiocyanate is the most researched in its effects on the thyroid and has been shown to compete with iodine for thyroid uptake. Glucosinolates also compete for iodine uptake into the thyroid. These two are found in foods and may result in higher serum iodine levels and decreased thyroid function if consumed in excessive amounts. Thiocyanate is found in cassava, lima beans, linseed, sorghum, and sweet potatoes.

Studies show a decrease in iodine uptake when goitrin ingestion is ≥194 μmol, and there was no difference if consumption was ≤77 μmol. Vegetables with the highest goitrogen content, >100 μmol/100 grams of *fresh* vegetable matter, include collards, kale, and certain types of Brussels sprouts. Those with moderate levels, between 10 and 100 μmol/100 grams of fresh vegetable matter, include Chinese cabbage, some varieties of collard greens, and some varieties of Brussels sprouts. Those with lower levels, <10 μmol/100 grams of fresh vegetable matter, include turnip greens, broccoli rabe, broccoli, and kale.

Thiocyanate and other goitrogens belong to a family of compounds called indoles. Many are protective against cancer and estrogen dominance, and not all of them have iodine block capacity.[13] Blanching foods before consumption reduces these compounds. In order to elicit negative iodine uptake effects, a person would have to consume one kilogram of raw broccoli per day. More likely exposure would come from smoking, perchlorate, nitrates, polychlorinated (PCB) and polybrominated (PBB) biphenyls, 2,4-dinitrophenol, disulfides, and lithium use. Smoking increases serum thiocyanate. Perchlorate and nitrates inhibit iodine uptake. Nitrates are found in processed and cured meats and other preserved foods. PCB and biphenyls alter thyroid hormone metabolism. Disulfides reduce thyroid iodine uptake. Lithium inhibits thyroid hormone synthesis.[14]

Other Possible Causes: water contamination from industrial sources, oxidative stress, progesterone deficiency

Treatment Strategies for Elevated Iodine, Serum or Plasma

Diet

First, assess the diet and supplements for iodine excess. If iodine excess has been ruled out, assess for magnesium deficiency. Increasing magnesium intake through the diet may have a positive impact on the ability of symporters to use serum iodine effectively. Foods rich in magnesium include leafy green vegetables (chard, kale, spinach) as well as nuts and seeds (almonds, pumpkin seeds, sunflower seeds). Legumes (lentils, chickpeas) are also an excellent source. Additionally, quinoa and oats can provide a good amount of magnesium. Many magnesium food sources are high in antinutrients that hold magnesium and other minerals in the plants, limiting absorption and bioavailability.

Certain preparation and cooking methods can help increase bioavailability. For example, soaking and sprouting nuts, seeds, and grains can help reduce phytic acid, which inhibits magnesium absorption. Similarly, steaming or blanching green leafy vegetables can reduce oxalates, increasing bioavailability. If levels are elevated, hydrating and eating foods with diuretic effects may help clear excess iodine quickly. Avoid processed foods that may be high in nitrite and nitrates.

Lifestyle

Reduce environmental chemical exposure. Perchlorate can be found in drinking water, particularly in areas near industrial runoff or in produce grown in contaminated soil. Nitrates are commonly used as fertilizers in agricultural practices and can also be found in contaminated groundwater. It is a common preservative in processed foods such as bacon, hot dogs, and other preserving salts.

PCBs are commonly found in hydraulic fluids and industrial processes. Depending on animal exposure, fish and dairy products can contain high amounts of PCBs. PBBs are flame retardants commonly found in home appliances and furniture. Due to water contamination, they can also accumulate in the meat and dairy of exposed animals. The organic compound 2,4-dinitrophenol was historically used as a pesticide and a weight-loss medication. It is now illegal. Exposure is limited to contaminated groundwater.

Additional Testing

thyroid peroxidase antibodies (TPOAb); thyroglobulin antibody (TgAb); comprehensive thyroid profile II; reverse T3 (rT3); thyroid receptor antibodies (TRAb); thyroid imaging; comprehensive metabolic panel (CMP); water quality testing; urinary iodine clearance (UIC)

Causes of Low Iodine, Serum or Plasma

Low Iodine Intake: Decreased iodine intake is the most common cause of low serum iodine. Assess the diet for decreased intake.

Vitamin A Deficiency: Vitamin A, in the form of retinoic acid, is required for the genetic expression of NIS proteins. When vitamin A is deficient, there is an overall decrease in NIS production. NIS is required for gastric absorption of iodine, and thus when there is a decrease in vitamin A, there is a decrease in overall iodine absorption.[16]

Other Possible Causes: inflammatory bowel diseases (celiac disease), certain medications (lithium, diuretics), environmental chemical exposure

Maternal iodine deficiency in pregnancy is associated with childhood cognitive delays, lower IQ, and increased learning disabilities in children.

Serum iodine levels are associated with urinary iodine clearance (UIC) and thyroid function in pregnancy. Low serum iodine is associated with an increased risk for iodine deficiency and hypothyroxinemia.[15]

Treatment Strategies for Low Iodine, Serum or Plasma

Diet

The World Health Organization recommends a dietary intake of 250 µg of iodine per day during pregnancy and 290 µg daily while breastfeeding. Iodine deficiency is more common in certain dietary philosophies, including the Paleo diet, Autoimmune Protocol (AIP) diet, and vegan diets. These diets often exclude iodine-rich foods such as legumes and dairy. There has also been a movement to switch from iodized salts to sea salts that do not have naturally occurring iodine. Removing dairy from the diet is a big cause of a decrease in iodine intake, causing a 44% drop in iodine consumption.[17]

Supplements

The best supplement form is potassium iodide. It is highly absorbable through the gastrointestinal tract and readily taken up by NIS. Seaweed and kelp supplements can also provide iodine in its natural form. Because the amount of iodine present in these forms can vary, they are not commonly used. Dietary intake of iodine has an absorption rate between 70% and 90%, while potassium iodide supplements have nearly a 100% absorption rate. This does increase the risk of overdose. Some studies have shown that potassium iodide is absorbed more quickly but is also excreted at a faster rate than naturally occurring iodine in seaweed supplements.[18]

Additional Testing

comprehensive thyroid profile II; urinary iodine clearance (UIC); comprehensive stool testing; toxin testing

References

1. Li X, Tu P, Gu S, et al. Serum Iodine as a Potential Individual Iodine Status Biomarker: A Cohort Study of Mild Iodine-Deficient Pregnant Women in China. Nutrients. 2023;15(16):3555. Published 2023 Aug 11. doi:10.3390/nu15163555

2. Hatch-McChesney A, Lieberman HR. Iodine and Iodine Deficiency: A Comprehensive Review of a Re-Emerging Issue. Nutrients. 2022;14(17):3474. Published 2022 Aug 24. doi:10.3390/nu14173474

3. Ittermann T, Albrecht D, Arohonka P, et al. Standardized Map of Iodine Status in Europe [published correction appears in Thyroid. 2022 May;32(5):603]. Thyroid. 2020;30(9):1346–1354. doi:10.1089/thy.2019.0353

4. Vila L, Serra-Prat M, de Castro A, et al. Iodine nutritional status in pregnant women of two historically different iodine-deficient areas of Catalonia, Spain. Nutrition. 2011;27(10):1029–1033. doi:10.1016/j.nut.2010.11.012

5. Vitti P., Rago T., Aghini-Lombardi F., Pinchera A. Iodine deficiency disorders in Europe. Public Health Nutr. 2001;4:529–535. doi: 10.1079/PHN2001138

6. Zimmermann MB. The Importance of Adequate Iodine during Pregnancy and Infancy. World Rev Nutr Diet. 2016;115:118–124. doi:10.1159/000442078

7. Leung AM. Thyroid function in pregnancy. J Trace Elem Med Biol. 2012;26(2–3):137–140. doi:10.1016/j.jtemb.2012.03.004

8. Ji S, Wu X, Wu J, Chen D, Chen Z. Serum iodine concentration and its associations with thyroid function and dietary iodine in pregnant women in the southeast coast of China: a cross-sectional study. Front Endocrinol (Lausanne). 2023;14:1289572. Published 2023 Nov 9. doi:10.3389/fendo.2023.1289572

9. Wang S, Bu Y, Shao Q, Cai Y, Sun D, Fan L. A Cohort Study on the Effects of Maternal High Serum Iodine Status During Pregnancy on Infants in Terms of Iodine Status and Intellectual, Motor, and Physical Development. Biol Trace Elem Res. 2024;202(1):133–144. doi:10.1007/s12011–023-03677–1

10. Forbes S. Embryo quality: the missing link between pregnancy sickness and pregnancy outcome. Evol. Hum. Behav. 2017;38(2):265–278. dio:10.1016/j.evolhumbehav.2016.10.003

11. Wang K, Wei H, Zhang W, et al. Severely low serum magnesium is associated with increased risks of positive anti-thyroglobulin antibody and hypothyroidism: A cross-sectional study. Sci Rep. 2018;8(1):9904. Published 2018 Jul 2. doi:10.1038/s41598–018-28362–5

12. Al Fahdi I, Al Salmi I, Al Rahbi F, Shaheen F, Hannawi S. Thyroid Dysfunction and Kidney Dysfunction. Oman Med J. 2022;37(3):e377. Published 2022 May 31. doi:10.5001/omj.2022.55

13. Felker P, Bunch R, Leung AM. Concentrations of thiocyanate and goitrin in human plasma, their precursor concentrations in brassica vegetables, and associated potential risk for hypothyroidism. Nutr Rev. 2016;74(4):248–258. doi:10.1093/nutrit/nuv110

14. Bertinato J. Iodine nutrition: Disorders, monitoring and policies. Adv Food Nutr Res. 2021;96:365–415. doi:10.1016/bs.afnr.2021.01.004

15. Pan Z, Cui T, Chen W, et al. Serum iodine concentration in pregnant women and its association with urinary iodine concentration and thyroid function. Clin Endocrinol (Oxf). 2019;90(5):711–718. doi:10.1111/cen.13945

16. Capriello S, Stramazzo I, Bagaglini MF, Brusca N, Virili C, Centanni M. The relationship between thyroid disorders and vitamin A: A narrative minireview. Front Endocrinol (Lausanne). 2022;13:968215. Published 2022 Oct 11. doi:10.3389/fendo.2022.968215

17. Mansilla R, Long G, Welham S, et al. Identifying and understanding dietary transitions and nutrient deficiency from loyalty card digital footprints. Int J Popul Data Sci. 2023;8(3):2266. Published 2023 Sep 11. doi:10.23889/ijpds.v8i3.2266

18. Combet E, Ma ZF, Cousins F, Thompson B, Lean MEJ. Low-level seaweed supplementation improves iodine status in iodine-insufficient women. British Journal of Nutrition. 2014;112(5):753–761. doi:10.1017/S0007114514001573

Iodine, Urinary Clearance

The urinary iodine clearance (UIC) test measures the amount of iodine present in a urine sample. It can be done using a random sample, a 24-hour sample, or an iodine/creatinine ratio.

The random UIC is the most common assessment for iodine deficiency used in research.

The 24-hour UIC is considered slightly more accurate than the random UIC, but it is rarely assessed in research and can be variable based on consumption and methodological errors. There are no established pregnancy ranges.

The iodine/creatinine ratio corrects for urinary output and kidney function, adding accuracy to the UIC spot test.

Iodine is a small molecule that is capable of passing through the sieve of the glomeruli, making it easy to filter from the bloodstream. Some iodine is reabsorbed through the proximal tubules. NIS proteins are located on the apical membrane of the proximal tubules and actively transport iodine from the tubular fluid to the tubular cells for cellular function. The thyroid hormones control the reabsorption of iodine. Thyroid hormones regulate the expression of NIS proteins in the proximal tubules (as well as the gastrointestinal mucosa).

In cases of iodine deficiency, more iodine is reabsorbed and less is excreted. When iodine levels are sufficient, more iodine is excreted through the urine.

Approximately 38% of Americans are classified as iodine deficient, with a UIC <100 µg/L.[1]

RANDOM URINARY IODINE TEST (SPOT TEST)

<150 µg/L indicates mild iodine deficiency.

<100 µg/L indicates moderate iodine deficiency.

<50 µg/L indicates severe iodine deficiency.

>250 µg/L indicates iodine excess in nonpregnant individuals.

Pregnancy

Urinary iodine clearance increases during pregnancy, with the highest clearance seen during the first trimester.[2]

Postpartum

Iodine needs increase while breastfeeding, and there may be a slight decrease in UIC with increased demand.

Iodine, Random Urine

STANDARD LAB RANGE: 28 – 544 µg/L

Trimester	Standard Pregnancy Ranges	**Functional Pregnancy Ranges**
Preconception	100 – 200	**150 – 250**
First Trimester	100 – 250	**150 – 250**
Second Trimester	100 – 250	**150 – 250**
Third Trimester	100 – 250	**150 – 250**
Postpartum	100 – 200	**150 – 250**

Iodine, 24-Hour Urine

STANDARD LAB RANGE: 100 – 460 µg/24 HOURS

Trimester	Standard Pregnancy Ranges	**Functional Pregnancy Ranges**
Preconception	100 – 460	**150 – 460**
First Trimester	100 – 460	**150 – 460**
Second Trimester	100 – 460	**150 – 460**
Third Trimester	100 – 460	**150 – 460**
Postpartum	100 – 460	**150 – 460**

Iodine: Creatinine Ratio

STANDARD LAB RANGE: 29 – 536 µg/g

Trimester	Standard Pregnancy Ranges	**Functional Pregnancy Ranges**
Preconception	100 – 200	**150 – 250**
First Trimester	100 – 200	**150 – 250**
Second Trimester	100 – 200	**150 – 250**
Third Trimester	100 – 200	**150 – 250**
Postpartum	100 – 200	**150 – 250**

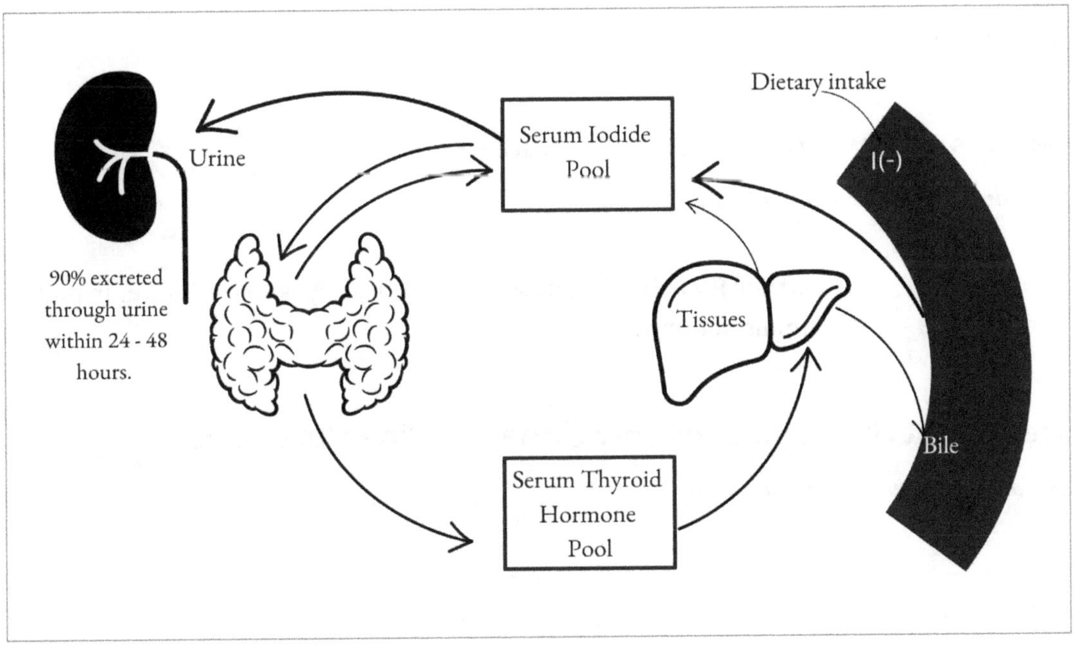

Figure 10: Iodine Cycle

Causes of Elevated Urinary Iodine Clearance

See Iodine, Serum or Plasma Section.

Levels <250 μg/L are protective against hyperthyroidism. There is a bell curve in iodine and thyroid function. Excess iodine limits iodine uptake to the thyroid.[3]

Other Possible Causes: excess iodine intake or supplementation, certain medications (diuretics, progesterone), vitamin A deficiency, hyperthyroidism, dehydration

Treatment Strategies for Elevated Urinary Iodine Clearance

See Iodine, Serum or Plasma Section.

Causes of Low Urinary Iodine Clearance

See Iodine, Serum or Plasma Section.

Other Possible Causes: iodine deficiency, kidney disease, hypothyroidism, overhydration

Treatment Strategies for Low Urinary Iodine Clearance

See Iodine, Serum or Plasma Section.

References

1. Hatch-McChesney A, Lieberman HR. Iodine and Iodine Deficiency: A Comprehensive Review of a Re-Emerging Issue. Nutrients. 2022;14(17):3474. Published 2022 Aug 24. doi:10.3390/nu14173474

2. Bu Y, Cai Y, Ji C, et al. Evaluation of iodine nutritional status during pregnancy by estimated 24-h urinary iodine excretion: population variation range and individual accuracy. Public Health Nutr. 2022;25(2):237–247. doi:10.1017/S1368980021003335

3. Pearce EN, Lazarus JH, Moreno-Reyes R, Zimmermann MB. Consequences of iodine deficiency and excess in pregnant women: an overview of current knowns and unknowns. Am J Clin Nutr. 2016;104 Suppl 3(Suppl 3):918S-23S. doi:10.3945/ajcn.115.110429

Progesterone

The serum progesterone test is used to measure the levels of the hormone progesterone in the blood. It is an individual analyte.

Progesterone synthesis is a complex biochemical process called steroidogenesis. It occurs in the adrenal glands, corpus luteum of the ovaries, and the placenta. First, cholesterol is transported into the mitochondria of steroid-producing cells, where it is converted to pregnenolone. The enzyme responsible for this conversion is the cholesterol side-chain cleavage enzyme (CYP11A1). CYP11A1 is modulated by vitamin D. The enzyme 3β-hydroxysteroid dehydrogenase (3β-HSD) catalyzes the conversion of pregnenolone to progesterone. NAD^+ (nicotinamide adenine dinucleotide) is a cofactor for 3β-HSD. Other nutrients that have been shown to affect progesterone production via enzymatic action include vitamin A, vitamin K, vitamin B2 (riboflavin), and iron.

Pregnancy

During pregnancy, progesterone levels increase, starting at conception.

Progesterone in early pregnancy helps prime the endometrial tissues for implantation. While estrogen grows tissue, progesterone gives it life. After ovulation, the endometrial cells produce a thick and nutrient-dense liquid. This uterine "milk" nourishes the trophoblast cells until the placenta and uterine arteries are connected. Progesterone also stimulates the endometrial cells to produce activin A. Activin A is a glycoprotein that helps stimulate the differentiation and remodeling of the endometrial cells.

During pregnancy, the immune system undergoes significant adaptations to support and protect the developing fetus, including a shift toward a more tolerant and anti-inflammatory state to prevent rejection of the baby by the mother's body. Progesterone is a driver of immune system changes that help facilitate this action.

Beginning in early pregnancy, there is an increased production of neutrophils. Neutrophils are the first line of defense for the immune system. Their job is to neutralize pathogens. To do this, they produce neutrophil extracellular traps (NETs). NETs are weblike structures that ensnare and immobilize pathogens, preventing their spread. This process is called NETosis. Progesterone prevents NETosis.

Progesterone-induced blocking factor (PIBF) is a chemical produced by lymphocytes when stimulated by progesterone. PIBF is produced in response to progesterone; it increases the synthesis of progesterone receptors on lymphocytes. Progesterone helps to decrease lymphocyte activity to prevent reactions to the placenta.

Vascular development is crucial for placental implantation and growth during the initial and middle stages of pregnancy. Progesterone actively encourages angiogenesis, the formation of new blood vessels, and facilitates vasodilation. Furthermore, progesterone aids in preserving the structural integrity and proper functioning of the uterine arteries.

Progesterone stimulates the kidneys to aid in electrolyte balance via filtration, clearance, and reabsorption. Progesterone receptors are found on the glomeruli and tubules. Stimulation by progesterone increases glomerular filtration rate (GFR) and diuresis. There is also an increase in the production of aldosterone without stimulating the rest of the renin-angiotensin-aldosterone system (RAAS). Regardless of pregnancy, progesterone stimulates bone-building osteoclasts and increases the production of parathyroid hormones. Parathyroid hormones release stored calcium into the bloodstream and activate calcitriol production from the kidneys to increase calcium absorption through the gut.

The production of progesterone steadily increases throughout pregnancy as the placenta increases in size and health. Levels peak around 34 weeks and decrease toward the onset of labor.

Postpartum

Within hours after delivery, following the birth of the placenta, maternal progesterone levels decrease abruptly. These levels reach their lowest point within the first 24 to 48 hours. This drop in progesterone helps to signal the initiation of lactation and uterine involution. Over the next several weeks and months, progesterone levels remain low. In women who are breastfeeding, the progesterone levels will remain low until the return of menstrual cycles.

STANDARD LAB RANGE: 0.1 – 12 ng/mL

Trimester	Standard Pregnancy Ranges	**Functional Pregnancy Ranges**
Preconception	0.1 – 12	**0.3 – 15**
First Trimester	11 – 44.3	**15 – 35***
Second Trimester	25.4 – 83.3	**30 – 95***
Third Trimester	58.7 – 214	**90 – 175***
Postpartum	0.1 – 0.9	**0.1 – 0.9**

*Progesterone levels vary greatly in the preconception phase based on menstrual patterns.
Levels taken from National Hormone Laboratory, Pope Paul VI Institute.

Causes of Elevated Progesterone

Other Possible Causes: overdose on medication, molar pregnancy, multiples, ovarian cysts, adrenal disorders, pituitary disease

Treatment Strategies for Elevated Progesterone

Additional Testing

imaging studies

Causes of Low Progesterone

Vitamin D Deficiency: Vitamin D has been shown to modulate several enzymes in the steroidogenesis pathways.[1] A deficiency in vitamin D has also been shown to cause lower progesterone and estrogen levels. The placenta has vitamin D receptors, and studies have shown that vitamin D is essential for placental function. There is a cyclical relationship between progesterone and vitamin D. Progesterone is important for the synthesis of the vitamin D receptors within the cells, and vitamin D is needed for progesterone synthesis.[2 3]

T3 Syndrome: T3 syndrome is a condition in which subclinical hypothyroidism presents with normal T4 and low T3 levels. T3 is specifically needed for the synthesis of progesterone from the corpus luteum and the placenta. Hypothyroidism, specifically low T3, can be a cause of low progesterone production.[4] Interestingly, a 2022 study pointed to a cross talk between thyroid hormones and progesterone during pregnancy. The administration of progesterone in the first trimester has been shown to increase T4 levels. In addition, the administration of thyroid hormones in the first trimester has been shown to increase progesterone levels.[5]

Stress: Survival is more important than reproduction. Studies have linked first-trimester maternal stress, cortisol, and pregnancy loss.[6] During times of stress, whether physical or emotional, the body initiates a complex response known as the stress response or the "fight or flight" reaction. This response involves the release of stress hormones, primarily cortisol and cortisone. Cortisol is often associated with the "fight or flight" response, while cortisone is often associated with our inflammatory responses.

In this context, the body prioritizes survival over reproductive functions, and one way it achieves this is by modulating hormone levels. Progesterone may be diverted to produce cortisol to cope with the stressor. This shift in hormone production reflects the body's adaptive strategy, prioritizing immediate survival needs over long-term reproductive functions during stressful situations. This can be seen in inflammation as well. If the body is prioritizing reducing inflammation, it will steal progesterone to convert to cortisone so it can reduce inflammation for maternal survival.

Small Placenta: The size of the placenta can have a direct impact on the amount of progesterone that can be produced.

Other Possible Causes: genetics, malnutrition, iron deficiency with or without anemia, vitamin B2 (riboflavin) deficiency

Treatment Strategies for Low Progesterone

Diet

Vitamin C and vitamin E levels are often decreased in cases of miscarriage and certain pregnancy complications that are also associated with progesterone deficiency. Increasing dietary intake of these antioxidants may help support the antioxidant functions of the body. Full-fat dairy contains natural progesterone in the fat of the milk. It also contains cholesterol, which is important for hormone synthesis. Other cholesterol foods include eggs and skin-on meats. Cholesterol needs increase during pregnancy. The role of cholesterol in the diet is controversial, but it is essential for several biological functions that include brain and neurological health, steroid hormone synthesis, cell membrane function and strength, as well as tissue healing, making it an important aspect of the maternal diet. Reducing caffeine can also help, because it raises cortisol levels.

Lifestyle

Binge eating has been shown to lower progesterone levels. Stretching of the stomach with large meals elicits a stress response and an increase in steroid hormones. This stress response causes a decrease in progesterone levels for acute need. When progesterone levels are decreased, smaller more frequent meals are important.

Supplements

Animal studies have shown that selenium supplementation of 200 μg/day increases progesterone levels in the second and third trimesters. Alpha-lipoic acid in combination with progesterone was shown to reduce subchorionic hemorrhage bleeding and symptoms by >70% within one week and by 100% within three weeks.[7] If progesterone levels are below reference ranges, it is advised to consult a NaPro (natural procreative) physician for assessment and progesterone prescriptions. If vitamin D deficiency is discovered, vitamin D supplementation should be recommended.

Additional Testing

comprehensive thyroid profile II; iron and TIBC; vitamin D, 25-hydroxy (25-hydroxycalciferol, 25OH-D); complete blood count (CBC); comprehensive metabolic panel (CMP); c-reactive protein (CRP)

References

1. Lundqvist J. Vitamin D as a regulator of steroidogenic enzymes [version 1; peer review: 1 approved, 1 approved with reservations]. F1000Research 2014, 3:155. doi.org/10.12688/f1000research.4714.1

2. Kim CH. A functional relay from progesterone to vitamin D in the immune system. DNA Cell Biol. 2015;34(6):379–382. doi:10.1089/dna.2015.2857

3. Shin JS, Choi MY, Longtine MS, Nelson DM. Vitamin D effects on pregnancy and the placenta. Placenta. 2010;31(12):1027–1034. doi:10.1016/j.placenta.2010.08.015

4. Datta M, Roy P, Banerjee J, Bhattacharya S. Thyroid hormone stimulates progesterone release from human luteal cells by generating a proteinaceous factor. J Endocrinol. 1998;158(3):319–325. doi:10.1677/joe.0.1580319

5. Ren B, Zhu Y. A New Perspective on Thyroid Hormones: Crosstalk with Reproductive Hormones in Females. Int J Mol Sci. 2022;23(5):2708. Published 2022 Feb 28. doi:10.3390/ijms23052708

6. Nepomnaschy PA, Welch KB, McConnell DS, Low BS, Strassmann BI, England BG. Cortisol levels and very early pregnancy loss in humans. Proc Natl Acad Sci U S A. 2006;103(10):3938–3942. doi:10.1073/pnas.0511183103

7. Petca A, Bot M, Maru N, et al. Benefits of α-lipoic acid in high-risk pregnancies (Review). Exp Ther Med. 2021;22(5):1232. doi:10.3892/etm.2021.10666

Vitamin D, 25-Hydroxy (25-Hydroxycalciferol, 25OH-D)

The 25OH vitamin D (25OH-D) is considered the most accurate test to assess vitamin D status. It is a single analyte.

When the skin is exposed to UVB radiation from sunlight, 7-dehydrocholesterol, a compound present in the skin, absorbs the UVB rays. UVB radiation converts 7-dehydrocholesterol into previtamin D3. Previtamin D3 undergoes thermal isomerization (a change in structure induced by heat) in the skin, converting it into vitamin D3 (cholecalciferol). Vitamin D3 is then transported into the bloodstream, bound to a carrier protein.

Dietary vitamin D is found primarily in the form of vitamin D2 (ergocalciferol) or vitamin D3 (cholecalciferol). In the small intestine, dietary vitamin D is incorporated into mixed micelles with bile salts and is exposed to pancreatic enzymes. The micelles facilitate the absorption of vitamin D through the intestinal lining into the enterocytes. Once absorbed, vitamin D is incorporated into chylomicrons, which are lipoprotein particles that transport dietary fats through the lymphatic and blood circulation. Chylomicrons transport vitamin D to the liver and other tissues.

In the liver, vitamin D3 undergoes hydroxylation (addition of a hydroxyl group) by the enzyme 25-hydroxylase, converting it into 25-hydroxyvitamin D3 (25(OH)D3), also known as calcidiol. Calcidiol is then bound to vitamin D-binding protein (DBP) in the blood for transport to various tissues. (This is what is tested in the 25OH-D serum blood test.)

In the kidneys, calcidiol undergoes another hydroxylation step, catalyzed by the enzyme 1-alpha-hydroxylase, forming the biologically active form of vitamin D, known as calcitriol or 1,25-dihydroxyvitamin D3 (1,25(OH)2D3).

Elevated levels of calcitriol inhibit further synthesis by suppressing the activity of 1-alpha-hydroxylase. This negative feedback loop helps maintain optimal vitamin D levels.

Some tissues, such as the placenta, have the capacity to locally convert calcidiol into calcitriol.

Vitamin D, being fat-soluble, can be stored in adipose tissue for future use. When needed, vitamin D can be released from storage and converted to its active form based on the body's requirements.

Pregnancy

During pregnancy, serum calcitriol rises from the first trimester, doubling by the end of the third trimester.[1] This increase is due to a true increase in production and not a reduction in renal clearance. This rise is driven by both maternal kidney production and placental production, with most of the conversion from maternal sources.[2] While serum calcitriol levels rise, serum 25OH-D levels decrease due to increased demands.[3]

Postpartum

Maternal need for dietary vitamin D increases in the breastfeeding period. A study found that a maternal intake of 6,400 IU of vitamin D was equivalent to supplementing 400 IU in the infant. This means that the higher consumption of vitamin D delivered the required 400 IU of vitamin D needed in breast milk to supply infant needs.[4]

The Institute of Medicine recommendations suggest a normal level of 20 ng/ml in pregnancy, while the Endocrine Society recommends 30 ng/ml or more.

VITAMIN D CONVERSION TABLE

Serum Levels nmol/L	Seum Levels ng/mL
<30 nmol/L	<12 ng/mL
between 30 and 50 nmol/L	between 12 and 20 ng/ml
50 nmol/L	20 ng/mL
75 nmol/L	30 ng/ml
100 nmol/L	40 ng/mL
125 nmol/L	50 ng/mL
150 nmol/L	60 ng/mL
175 nmol/L	70 ng/mL
200 nmol/L	80 ng/mL
225 nmol/L	90 ng/mL
250 nmol/L	100 ng/mL

*Research studies used varied measurements of nmol/L and ng/mL.

STANDARD LAB RANGE: 30 – 100 ng/mL

Trimester	Standard Pregnancy Ranges	**Functional Pregnancy Ranges**
Preconception	30 – 100	**40 – 100**
First Trimester	20 – 100	**40 – 80**
Second Trimester	20 – 100	**40 – 80**
Third Trimester	20 – 100	**40 – 80**
Postpartum	30 – 100	**40 – 100**

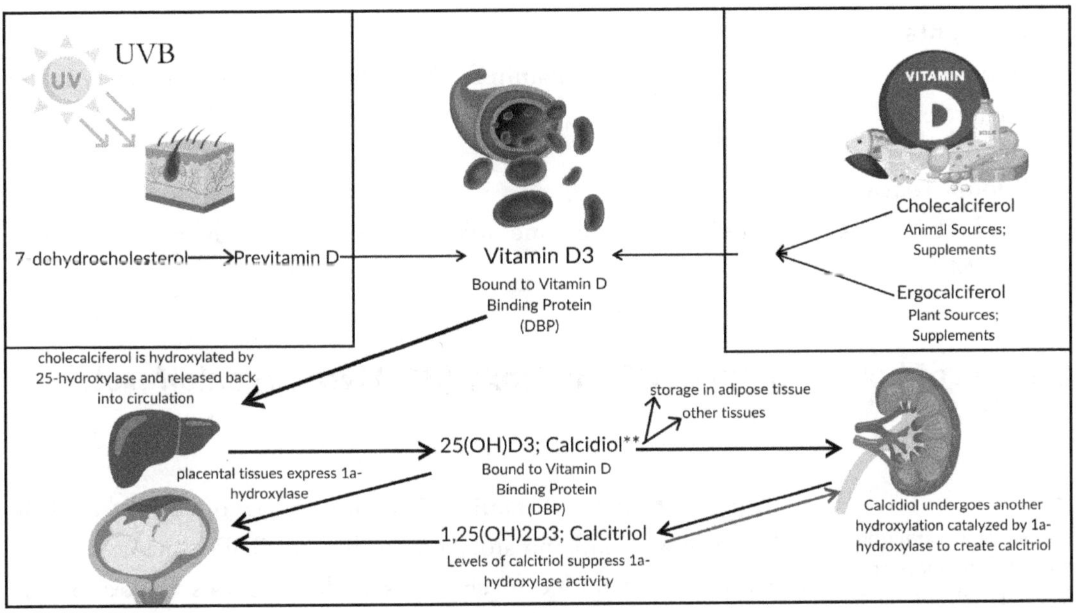

Figure 11: Vitamin D

Causes of Elevated Vitamin D, 25-Hydroxy (25-Hydroxycalciferol, 25OH-D)

—

Studies have shown no negative effects in pregnancy with serum levels <80 ng/mL.[5] Greater than 100 ng/mL is associated with hyperkalemia risk.[6] That being said, no studies have found

Magnesium Deficiency: Magnesium is involved in the activation of vitamin D in the body. Magnesium-dependent enzymes convert vitamin D into its active form (calcitriol) as well as inactive vitamin D when levels are elevated. It is possible for magnesium deficiency to impair the utilization of vitamin D and cause serum excess.

Zinc Deficiency: Zinc is required for the synthesis of vitamin D-binding protein (DBP), which transports vitamin D in the blood-

supplementation in pregnancy to cause severe elevations or risk.

stream. Zinc deficiency can impair vitamin D binding and cause a buildup of vitamin D in the bloodstream. High-dose zinc supplementation may falsely elevate serum vitamin D levels, causing inaccuracy in test results.

Other Possible Causes: overdose, poor conversion by the kidneys or placenta, genetics, cancer

Treatment Strategies for Elevated Vitamin D, 25-Hydroxy (25-Hydroxycalciferol, 25OH-D)

Supplements

When this is elevated, have the patient stop vitamin D, zinc, and magnesium supplementation and then retest.

Additional Testing

calcitriol (1,25 di-OH vitamin D); oral zinc tolerance test; comprehensive metabolic panel (CMP)

Causes of Low Vitamin D, 25-Hydroxy (25-Hydroxycalciferol, 25OH-D)

Women living at higher altitudes, or above the 37th parallel, are more likely to have vitamin D deficiency.[7 8] These individuals need to focus on increasing vitamin D-rich foods as well as supplements. Those with higher melanin levels living at higher altitudes and latitudes are at an even higher risk of vitamin D deficiency.

Studies have found that vitamin D deficiency increases the risk of preeclampsia,

Gut Inflammation: Vitamin D deficiency is often observed in individuals with inflammatory bowel diseases (IBD) such as Crohn's and celiac disease. The mechanisms underlying this association are multifaceted. In the context of IBD, chronic inflammation within the gastrointestinal tract can lead to impaired absorption of nutrients, including vitamin D. The inflammation and structural changes in the intestine can compromise the functionality of the mucosal surface, where nutrient absorption primarily occurs.

Additionally, the liver and kidneys, which play key roles in converting vitamin D into its active form, may be affected by inflammation or dysfunction in individuals with IBD.[14]

Other Possible Causes: low dietary intake, low-fat diet, low sun exposure, advanced maternal age, magnesium deficiency gestational diabetes, low birth weight, and preterm birth. Maternal vitamin D deficiency in pregnancy is also associated with long-term health risks for babies.[9]

Vitamin D levels higher than 30 ng/mL are associated with reduced preeclampsia risk when compared with vitamin D levels <30 ng/mL or <20 ng/mL, suggesting that women may benefit from the supplementation of vitamin D to a level of ≥30 ng/mL in early and middle pregnancy. The risk of preeclampsia was higher if the serum vitamin D was at lower levels mid-pregnancy.[10]

A 2023 study from Sweden found that serum vitamin D levels ≤30.1 nmol/L were associated with an increased risk of preeclampsia.[11] Vitamin D status prior to 20 weeks is associated with gestational diabetes risk, with >30 ng/mL being protective.[12]

Studies have also found that a serum concentration of 40 ng/mL is needed to maintain calcitriol balance in pregnancy.[13] To maintain these levels, a supplemental dosage of 4,000 IU per day was required.

Treatment Strategies for Low Vitamin D, 25-Hydroxy (25-Hydroxycalciferol, 25OH-D)

Diet

Fatty fish such as salmon, mackerel, and tuna are excellent sources of vitamin D, with a single serving providing a significant portion of the daily requirement. Additionally, pasture-raised pork fat, particularly from pigs exposed to sunlight, can be a valuable source, offering approximately 1,000 IU of vitamin D per tablespoon. Mushrooms, when exposed to ultraviolet (UV) light during growth or processing, can also provide varying amounts of vitamin D2.

It is intriguing to observe a correlation between the traditional dietary habits of populations in higher latitude and altitude regions and their reliance on vitamin D-rich foods. Nordic countries, situated at high latitudes, have a diet traditionally rich in fatty fish, such as salmon and mackerel, which are abundant sources of vitamin D. Similarly, northern European countries often incorporate pork, particularly fat from pasture-raised pigs, and mushrooms into their diets, both of which provide significant amounts of vitamin D. This dietary adaptation aligns with the need for these populations to supplement the limited sunlight exposure, especially during long, dark winters.

Lifestyle

Sunlight exposure is a crucial and natural means of synthesizing vitamin D in the human body. Exposing large parts of the skin to sunlight daily can help to increase vitamin D production naturally in the body. Even 10 to 15 minutes of sun exposure produces approximately 1,000 IU of vitamin D. This production amount is dependent on other factors as well, such as skin tone and geographical location.

Supplements

In pregnancy, a minimum dosage of 4,000 IU is typically required to maintain levels. In cases of deficiency, higher doses may be used temporarily to achieve functional levels. Caution should be used with high doses, as vitamin D can have an antagonistic effect on vitamin A.

Additional Testing

comprehensive metabolic panel (CMP); calcitriol (1,25 di-OH vitamin D)

References

1. Olmos-Ortiz A, Avila E, Durand-Carbajal M, Díaz L. Regulation of calcitriol biosynthesis and activity: focus on gestational vitamin D deficiency and adverse pregnancy outcomes. Nutrients. 2015;7(1):443–480. Published 2015 Jan 9. doi:10.3390/nu7010443

2. Wagner CL, Hollis BW. The extraordinary metabolism of vitamin D. Elife. 2022;11:e77539. Published 2022 Mar 8. doi:10.7554/eLife.77539

3. Pérez-López FR, Pilz S, Chedraui P. Vitamin D supplementation during pregnancy: an overview. Curr Opin Obstet Gynecol. 2020;32(5):316–321. doi:10.1097/GCO.0000000000000641

4. Hollis BW, Wagner CL, Howard CR, et al. Maternal Versus Infant Vitamin D Supplementation During Lactation: A Randomized Controlled Trial [published correction appears in Pediatrics. 2019 Jul;144(1):]. Pediatrics. 2015;136(4):625–634. doi:10.1542/peds.2015–1669

5. Al Emadi S, Hammoudeh M. Vitamin D study in pregnant women and their babies. Qatar Med J. 2013;2013(1):32–37. Published 2013 Nov 1. doi:10.5339/qmj.2013.7

6. Dias BA, Fraga CAC, de Rezende Goston HSR, Guerra PB, Heringer VCCR, Rodrigues YS, Panconi CR, Coutinho LM, de Souza HD, Batalha SH, Silva CS, Zimmermmann JB. Blood Dosage of Vitamin D in Pregnant Women and Association with Preeclampsia and Fetal Low Weight. Asp Biomed Clin Case Rep. 2020 Feb 21;3(1):51–61

7. Mata-Greenwood E, Westenburg HCA, Zamudio S, Illsley NP, Zhang L. Decreased Vitamin D Levels and Altered Placental Vitamin D Gene Expression at High Altitude: Role of Genetic Ancestry. Int J Mol Sci. 2023;24(4):3389. Published 2023 Feb 8. doi:10.3390/ijms24043389

8. Schwalfenberg G. Not enough vitamin D: health consequences for Canadians. Can Fam Physician. 2007;53(5):841–854

9. Vestergaard, A.L., Christensen, M., Andreasen, M.F. et al. Vitamin D in pregnancy (GRAVITD) – a randomised controlled trial identifying associations and mechanisms linking maternal Vitamin D deficiency to placental dysfunction and adverse pregnancy outcomes – study protocol. BMC Pregnancy Childbirth 23, 177 (2023): doi.org/10.1186/s12884–023-05484-x

10. Hu KL, Zhang CX, Chen P, Zhang D, Hunt S. Vitamin D Levels in Early and Middle Pregnancy and Preeclampsia, a Systematic Review and Meta-Analysis. Nutrients. 2022;14(5):999. Published 2022 Feb 27. doi:10.3390/nu14050999

11. Malm G, Lindh CH, Hansson SR, Källén K, Malm J, Rylander L (2023) Maternal serum vitamin D level in early pregnancy and risk for preeclampsia: A case-control study in Southern Sweden. PLoS ONE 18(2): e0281234. doi.org/10.1371/journal.pone.0281234

12. Yue, CY., Ying, CM. Sufficience serum vitamin D before 20 weeks of pregnancy reduces the risk of gestational diabetes mellitus. Nutr Metab (Lond) 17, 89 (2020). doi.org/10.1186/s12986–020-00509–0

13. Hollis, B., Wagner, C. New insights into the vitamin D requirements during pregnancy. Bone Res 5, 17030 (2017). doi.org/10.1038/boneres.2017.30

14. Del Pinto R, Pietropaoli D, Chandar AK, Ferri C, Cominelli F. Association Between Inflammatory Bowel Disease and Vitamin D Deficiency: A Systematic Review and Meta-analysis. Inflamm Bowel Dis. 2015;21(11):2708–2717. doi:10.1097/MIB.0000000000000546

Vitamin B12 (Cobalamin)

The vitamin B12 (cobalamin) test measures the amount of vitamin B12 in a serum sample. It is a single analyte. It can also be found in the Vitamin B12 Deficiency Cascade.

Vitamin B12 is also known as cobalamin because, structurally, it contains cobalt surrounded by a corrin ring structure.

Vitamin B12 is released from food by the actions of stomach acid and proteolytic enzymes in the mouth and stomach. Transcobalamin I is a haptocorrin protein produced by the salivary glands and stomach mucosa that binds to B12 to help stabilize it and facilitate absorption. It is synthesized via the TCN1 gene. In the stomach, B12 binds to a protein called intrinsic factor, which is produced in conjunction with hydrochloric acid. The complex protects B12 from degradation by stomach acids and facilitates absorption in the small intestines.

In the small intestine, the B12 intrinsic factor complex binds to intrinsic factor receptors and is transported through the digestive lining and into the bloodstream. The absorption rate of B12 varies based on the amount of intrinsic factor produced and the binding capacity of intrinsic factor. Approximately 50% of 1 or 2 μg doses are absorbed, 2% of 500 μg doses, and 1.3% of 1,000 μg doses.[1 2] Once in the bloodstream, transcobalamin I-bound vitamin B12 is transferred to transcobalamin II, and the complex binds to transcobalamin, a transport protein that delivers the vitamin to various tissues. Transcobalamin II is produced by the liver and circulates in the bloodstream. TCN2 codes for the synthesis of transcobalamin II. It has a high affinity for B12 and readily binds to it.

At a cellular level, transcobalamin II binds to transcobalamin receptors and the cells can internalize the B12. Once in the cells, B12 is released from transcobalamin II, where it is further processed into its active coenzyme forms.

The first step is the conversion of cobalamin to hydroxocobalamin. This form serves as a precursor to the coenzyme forms. Hydroxocobalamin contains a hydroxyl group attached to the cobalt ion. Unlike the active coenzymes, hydroxocobalamin does not have a specific coenzyme function. It is considered a storage form of vitamin B12.

The main coenzyme forms are methylcobalamin and adenosylcobalamin.

Methylcobalamin is cobalamin with a methyl group attached to the cobalt ion. This form serves as a cofactor for the enzyme methionine synthase, which is involved in the conversion of homocysteine to methionine. Genes that are associated with these actions include MTR and MTRR. MTR is responsible for the regeneration of methionine form homocysteine through the synthesis of methionine synthase. Methionine synthase creates methionine from homocysteine using 5-MTHF methyl donor and vitamin B12. MTRR is responsible for maintaining methionine synthase function, by removing used B12. MTRR codes for the enzyme 5-methyltetrahydrofolate-homocysteine methyltransferase reductase.

Adenosylcobalamin is a derivative in which a 5'-deoxyadenosyl group is attached to the cobalt ion. This form serves as a cofactor for the enzyme methylmalonyl-CoA mutase, which is involved in the conversion of methylmalonyl-CoA to succinyl-CoA. A deficiency or dysfunction in methylmalonyl-CoA mutase can lead to elevated methylmalonic acid levels.

Vitamin B12 (cobalamin) testing in pregnancy is not accurately reflective of cellular vitamin B12 status.

Pregnancy

Serum vitamin B12 levels drop drastically throughout pregnancy as cellular need increases and there is increased hemodilution. During normal pregnancies, serum B12 levels drop 30% by the third trimester, yet dietary needs have increased twofold.

Postpartum

In the first few days postpartum, there is a sharp rise in serum vitamin B12 levels, as the hemodilution of pregnancy resolves. Levels return to normal pre-pregnancy levels by a few weeks postpartum.

STANDARD LAB RANGE: 232 – 1,245 pg/mL*

Trimester	Standard Pregnancy Ranges	**Functional Pregnancy Ranges**
Preconception	232 – 1,245	**400 – 1,245**
First Trimester	118 – 438	**280 – 800**
Second Trimester	130 – 656	**280 – 800**
Third Trimester	99 – 526	**280 – 800**
Postpartum	232 – 1,245	**400 – 1,245**

*The conversion ratio for vitamin B12 (cobalamin) is 1.35 pg/mL = 1 pmol/L.

Causes of Elevated Vitamin B12 (Cobalamin)

See the following sections: Homocysteine and Methlymalonic Acid.

High maternal vitamin B12 (>600 pmol/L or 810 pg/mL) and vitamin B9 (folate) have been associated with an increased risk for childhood autism.[3] This is an interesting correlation with no known etiology or mechanism of action yet. Other studies are in process regarding genetic variations and analysis of other biomarkers, as well as the link to unmetabolized folates.

TCN2 Genetic Variation: Studies assessing vitamin B12 functionality via methylmalonic acid found that those with TCN2 gene variants had a reduction in the cellular bioavailability of vitamin B12, leading to elevated serum B12 and decreased cellular function.[4] This may be associated with other blood indices that suggest B12 insufficiency and deficiency symptoms while serum B12 levels are elevated. Most cases of hypercobalaminemia are associated with issues in transcobalamin II, especially when presenting with B12 deficiency symptoms.

MTR or MTRR Genetic Variation: Poor utilization of methylcobalamin may cause backing up of B12 into the bloodstream. In this case, there may be elevated homocysteine due to poor recycling and methionine conversion. MTR gene variation would cause a decrease in the formation of methylcobalamin.[5]

Liver Disease: Acute hepatitis is accompanied by elevated serum B12 in between 25% and 45% of cases.[6] In liver disease, particularly cirrhosis, serum vitamin B12 levels can be five times the upper limit.

Other Possible Causes: excess supplementation, recent consumption prior to blood draw, other genetic variants in vitamin B12 (cobalamin) metabolism, kidney disease, hypereosinophilic syndrome, myeloproliferative blood disorders (polycythemia vera), autoimmune disease, smoking, cancer

Treatment Strategies for Elevated Vitamin B12 (Cobalamin)

See the following sections: Homocysteine and Methlymalonic Acid.

Diet

If someone has genetic issues that cause serum vitamin B12 levels to be elevated, there is no need to reduce vitamin B12 (cobalamin) in the diet or in supplementation. Dietary protocols may be centered around supporting liver and kidney function.

Supplements

If the cause of elevated vitamin B12 is an overuse of supplements, decrease or remove supplements and focus on only dietary intake. If it is associated with genetic causes, additional vitamin B12 supplementation may still be warranted, as the risk of overdose is decreased due to reduced cellular utilization. In cases of MTR or MTRR mutations, methylcobalamin supplementation may be a better option. For those with TCN2 mutations, intramuscular injections of hydroxocobalamin have been successful in treating symptoms and correcting functional biomarkers.[7] If genetic variants and vitamin B12 oral supplementation in high doses are ruled out, supplemental protocols may be centered around liver and kidney function. In these cases, the patient should also be referred to medical specialists for assessment.

Additional Testing

complete blood count (CBC); homocysteine; methylmalonic acid; comprehensive metabolic panel (CMP); antinuclear antibodies (ANA); functional genomic analysis

Causes of Low Vitamin B12 (Cobalamin)

See the following sections: Homocysteine and Methlymalonic Acid.

Vegan Diet: Not all women who follow a vegan diet are at risk for vitamin B12 deficiency. Those who are at high risk are those who have maintained a vegan diet long-term, those who avoid fortified foods, those with reduced intake of fermented foods, and those who are pregnant and breastfeeding due to increased dietary needs. The Academy of Nutrition and Dietetics advises the monitoring of iron, zinc, vitamin B12 (cobalamin), and essential fatty acids in pregnant women choosing a vegan diet, due to the increased risk of deficiency.[11]

TCN1 Genetic Variation: Transcobalamin I is needed to transport vitamin B12 from the gut to the bloodstream. Mutations in this gene can disrupt proper synthesis of transcobalamin I, thus decreasing proper absorption.

Hypochlorhydria: Stomach acid is needed to release vitamin B12 from foods, allowing it to bind to intrinsic factor. Those with low stomach acid production or those taking medicine that reduces stomach acid production are at a higher risk of vitamin B12 deficiencies. Hypochlorhydria is more common in women of advanced maternal age, as stomach acid production decreases with age. H. pylori infections cause inflammation in the stomach, can lead to stomach acid production dysfunction, and increase the risk of vitamin B12 deficiency. Chronic stress can also affect the production of stomach acid.

Outside of pregnancy, vitamin B12 (cobalamin) deficiency symptoms have been noted at levels <400 pg/mL. Other studies have shown that the microscopic correction of vitamin B12 deficiency is seen at 400 pg/mL, nearly twice the current lower limit for serum vitamin B12, as well as the reduction of symptoms associated with vitamin B12 deficiency.[8,9]

Vitamin B12 deficiency has been associated with cognitive alterations in fetal brains, causing cognitive impairment that includes poor memory, language, and motor skills as well as preterm birth, anemia, and insulin resistance.[10]

Other medical conditions, such as thyroid disorders and autoimmune diseases, can also cause a decrease in stomach acid production.

Pernicious Anemia: This is a specific form of anemia characterized by vitamin B12 (cobalamin) deficiency. It is caused by the inability to absorb vitamin B12 due to various factors but typically related to a decrease in the production of intrinsic factor. In pernicious anemia, the immune system attacks and destroys parietal cells, which are responsible for producing both stomach acid and intrinsic factor. This is typically treated with vitamin B12 injections.

Dysbiosis: Vitamin B12 is synthesized by specific bacteria such as *Propionibacterium freudenreichii* subsp. *shermanii* or certain strains of lactobacilli such as *Lactobacillus leichmannii.* Other than in certain algae, vitamin B12 is absent from most plant foods, unless they have been fermented. Bacteria produce various forms of B12, of which only a few are bioavailable in human physiology. Pathogenic bacteria can also utilize and even metabolize B12, reducing availability.

Other Possible Causes: low dietary intake, inflammatory bowel diseases (ulcerative colitis, celiac disease, Crohn's), pancreatic insufficiency, antiacid medication use, bariatric surgery, H. pylori infections

Treatment Strategies for Low Vitamin B12 (Cobalamin)

See the following sections: Homocysteine and Methlymalonic Acid.

> There is no gold standard for the diagnosis of vitamin B12 (cobalamin) deficiency. Generally, diagnosis is determined via functional testing as well as serum B12 levels. These can include biomarkers found in the complete blood count (CBC), homocysteine, methylmalonic acid, and serum B12, in conjunction with symptomology.

Diet

A 2010 study found that in people with normal absorption and no genetic variation associated with vitamin B12 (cobalamin) metabolism, a dietary intake between 4 and 7 μg/day was needed to reach and maintain serum levels of >400 pg/ml. This suggests that the current RDA for vitamin B12 of 2.4 μg/day may be inadequate and more may be needed, especially in pregnancy. Incorporating foods such as beef liver, shellfish (clams, oysters, mussels), fish (mackerel, tuna, sardines, salmon), and eggs can help boost vitamin B12 levels.

For vegans, who abstain from animal products, obtaining sufficient vitamin B12 can be a bit challenging, as it is primarily found in animal-based foods. Some seaweed and algae contain small amounts of vitamin B12, although the bioavailability is questionable. Nutritional yeast and certain fermented foods may also help contribute to vitamin B12 levels in vegan patients.

Adequate absorption of vitamin B12 from food depends on adequate chewing and proper levels of stomach acid and proteolytic enzymes. Advise patients to sit and eat with consciousness, taking the time to thoroughly chew each bite of their food.

Supplements

The most common forms of vitamin B12 found in supplements are cyanocobalamin, hydroxocobalamin, adenocobalamin, and methylcobalamin.

Cyanocobalamin is a synthetic form of vitamin B12 that is often used in food fortification and in supplementation. Its name is due to the cyanide residue found in the structure. It is a small amount, but long-term use can cause an increased risk of vitamin B1 (thiamine) deficiency, and it does take extra work for the body to remove this residue before it can be utilized. The production of cyanocobalamin is through bacterial fermentation that produces adenosylcobalamin and methylcobalamin. These are then treated with potassium cyanide to keep them stable in supplements and food fortification.

Hydroxocobalamin is naturally found in animal proteins. It is a bioavailable form. This form used to be only available for those with severe vitamin B12 deficiency, but it has become more readily available in supplements and intramuscular injections. In fact, a *Lancet* review has proposed the discontinuation of cyanocobalamin because hydroxocobalamin has become readily available in supplementation.[12]

All forms have been clinically shown to improve vitamin B12 status. As with other synthetic vitamins, what happens once it is absorbed becomes the question. Animal studies that compare methylcobalamin to cyanocobalamin have shown that both forms are equally absorbed, but urinary excretion of cyanocobalamin was three times higher than methylcobalamin, and methylcobalamin supplementation increases vitamin B12 storage in the liver by 13%.[13] This also makes methylcobalamin sources easier to overdose on, so caution may be needed for high doses. Supplementing with any of the natural bioidentical forms of B12 (methylcobalamin, hydroxocobalamin, and/or adenosylcobalamin) is preferred instead of the use of cyanocobalamin, due to their superior bioavailability and safety.[14]

Because research on polymorphs and preferential vitamin B12 supplementation research is limited, there may be a trial-and-error approach to supplementation to find the form that improves functional biomarkers of vitamin B12. The rate of vitamin B12 absorption is heavily reliant on the dose given. With doses <0.5 μg, about 50% is typically absorbed; with doses of 1 μg, about 20% is absorbed; and for doses of >500 μg, only 1% is absorbed. It is estimated that for doses of 1,000 μg, approximately 10 to 12 μg are absorbed. This seems to be consistent among all forms.

Those with TCN1 variation that limits absorption or intestinal inflammation, or those who are taking antiacid medications, may need intravenous or intramuscular (IM) injections of vitamin B12. Lozenge or sublingual supplementation absorption rate is approximately the same as oral dosing. Some studies have found that sublingual supplementation was superior to IM injections of B12.[15] In the end, supplementation type may vary on the individual's genetic predispositions and needs. Probiotic supplements have also been shown to improve serum vitamin B12 levels.[16]

Additional Testing

homocysteine; methylmalonic acid; complete blood count (CBC); comprehensive stool testing; functional genomic analysis

References

1. Carmel R. How I treat Vitamin B12 (Cobalamin) deficiency. Blood 2008;112:2214–21

2. Paul C, Brady DM. Comparative bioavailability and utilization of particular forms of B(12) Supplements with potential to mitigate B(12)-related genetic polymorphisms. Integr Med 2017;16:42–9

3. Sourander A, Silwal S, Surcel HM, et al. Maternal Serum Vitamin B12 during Pregnancy and Offspring Autism Spectrum Disorder. Nutrients. 2023;15(8):2009. Published 2023 Apr 21. doi:10.3390/nu15082009

4. Matteini AM, Walston JD, Bandeen-Roche K, et al. Transcobalamin-II variants, decreased vitamin B12 availability and increased risk of frailty. J Nutr Health Aging. 2010;14(1):73–77. doi:10.1007/s12603–010-0013–1

5. Froese DS, Gravel RA. Genetic disorders of vitamin B12 metabolism: eight complementation groups—eight genes. Expert Rev Mol Med. 2010;12:e37. Published 2010 Nov 29. doi:10.1017/S1462399410001651

6. E. Andrès, K. Serraj, J. Zhu, A.J.M. Vermorken, The pathophysiology of elevated vitamin B12 in clinical practice, QJM: An International Journal of Medicine, Volume 106, Issue 6, June 2013, Pages 505–515, doi.org/10.1093/qjmed/hct051

7. Martino, F., Magenta, A., Troccoli, M.L. et al. Long-term outcome of a patient with transcobalamin deficiency caused by the homozygous c.1115_1116delCA mutation in TCN2 gene: a case report. Ital J Pediatr 47, 54 (2021): doi.org/10.1186/s13052–021-01007–6

8. Fenech MF, Dresoti IE, Rinaldi JR. Folate, vitamin B12, homocysteine status and chromosome damage rate in lymphocytes of older men, Carcinogenesis, 1997, vol. 18 (pg. 1329–36)

9. Solomon LR. Diabetes as a cause of clinically significant functional cobalamin deficiency, Diabetes Care, 2011, vol. 34 (pg. 1077–80)

10. Lai J.S., Mohamad Ayob M.N., Cai S., Quah P.L., Gluckman P.D., Shek L.P., Yap F., Tan K.H., Chong Y.S., Godfrey K.M., et al. Maternal Plasma Vitamin B12 Concentrations during Pregnancy and Infant Cognitive Outcomes at 2 Years of Age. Br. J. Nutr. 2019;121:1303–1312. doi: 10.1017/S0007114519000746

11. Melina V, Craig W, Levin S. Position of the Academy of Nutrition and Dietetics: Vegetarian Diets. J Acad Nutr Diet. 2016;116(12):1970–1980. doi:10.1016/j.jand.2016.09.025

12. Foulds WS, Freeman AG, Phillips CI, Wilson J. Cyanocobalamin: A case for withdrawal. Lancet. 1970;1(7636):35

13. Okuda K, Yashima K, Kitazaki T, Takara I. Intestinal absorption and concurrent chemical changes of methylcobalamin. J Lab Clin Med. 1973;81(4):557–567

14. Paul C, Brady DM. Comparative Bioavailability and Utilization of Particular Forms of B12 Supplements With Potential to Mitigate B12-related Genetic Polymorphisms. Integr Med (Encinitas). 2017;16(1):42–49

15. Bensky MJ, Ayalon-Dangur I, Ayalon-Dangur R, et al. Comparison of sublingual vs. intramuscular administration of vitamin B12 for the treatment of patients with vitamin B12 deficiency. Drug Deliv Transl Res. 2019;9(3):625–630. doi:10.1007/s13346–018-00613-y

16. Barkhidarian B, Roldos L, Iskandar MM, Saedisomeolia A, Kubow S. Probiotic Supplementation and Micronutrient Status in Healthy Subjects: A Systematic Review of Clinical Trials. Nutrients. 2021;13(9):3001. Published 2021 Aug 28. doi:10.3390/nu13093001

Methylmalonic Acid (MMA)

The methylmalonic acid (MMA) test measures the amount of MMA in a sample. This can be tested via serum/plasma or through a urine test in ratio to creatinine. It is a single analyte or found in the Vitamin B12 Deficiency Cascade, if serum vitamin B12 is between 200 and 400 pg/mL.

MMA is a compound produced through the breakdown of certain amino acids and fats. Propionyl-CoA is derived from the breakdown of amino acids and fatty acids. It undergoes carboxylation by the enzymes propionyl-CoA carboxylase, using vitamin B7 (biotin) as a cofactor to form D-methylmalonyl-CoA. This reaction also requires bicarbonate. D-methylmalonyl-CoA epimerase then converts D-methylmalonyl-CoA to L-methylmalonyl-CoA, while D-methylmalonyl-CoA hydrolase forms methylmalonic acid.

Methylmalonic acid is a derivative of malonic acid in which one of the methylene hydrogens is replaced by a methyl group. L-methylmalonyl-CoA is then isomerized to form succinyl-CoA. This reaction is catalyzed by the enzyme methylmalonyl-CoA mutase, which requires adenocobalamin. This reaction is reversible. Succinyl-CoA enters the Kreb's cycle, where it is converted to succinate, releasing energy. A dysfunction in the isomerization step can cause an increase in methylmalonic acid.

Only 22% of elevated MMA cases can be attributed to overt vitamin B12 (cobalamin) deficiency, yet elevated MMA and homocysteine are found in 98% of vitamin B12 deficiency cases.[1]

> Urinary methylmalonic acid/creatinine is a useful biomarker of vitamin B12 status in cases in which other methods may not be accurate[2] such as in renal disease and pregnancy.

Pregnancy

There is a gradual increase in methylmalonic acid levels throughout pregnancy, with a peak in the third trimester. There is a twofold increase in the need for vitamin B12 (cobalamin) by the third trimester, with much of this being distributed to the fetus. Maternal vitamin B12 stores are depleted, thus causing a normal elevation in methylmalonic acid with a decrease in serum vitamin B12. In addition, there are changes in renal excretion of MMA.

Postpartum

Postpartum research on MMA levels is limited, but some studies suggest a sharp decrease in both serum and urinary methylmalonic acid immediately after delivery.[3]

Serum, Plasma

STANDARD LAB RANGE: 0 – 378 μmol/L*

Trimester	Standard Pregnancy Ranges	**Functional Pregnancy Ranges**
Preconception	0 – 378	**0 – 370**
First Trimester	Not Established	**0.5 – 275****
Second Trimester	Not Established	**0.75 – 275****
Third Trimester	Not Established	**0.75 – 350****
Postpartum	Not Established	**0 – 370**

*The cutoff for MMA in the diagnosis of vitamin B12 (cobalamin) deficiency has not been universally agreed upon. Upper ranges can vary between >250 and >350 as diagnostic of vitamin B12 deficiency.[4]
**Based on limited data

Urine

STANDARD LAB RANGE: 0.3 – 2.8 μmol/mmol CRT
(MICROMOLES PER mmol OF CREATININE)

Trimester	Standard Pregnancy Ranges	**Functional Pregnancy Ranges**
Preconception	0.3 – 2.8	**0.4 – 2.5**
First Trimester	0.3 – 2.8	**0.4 – 2.5***
Second Trimester	0.3 – 2.8	**0.4 – 3.5***
Third Trimester	0.3 – 2.8	**0.4 – 3.5***
Postpartum	0.3 – 2.8	**0.4 – 2.5**

*Based on limited data

Causes of Elevated Methylmalonic Acid

See the following sections: Vitamin B12 (Cobalamin) and Homocysteine.

Amniotic fluid and maternal urine MMA concentrations in the middle term of neural-tube defect (NTD)-affected pregnancies (22.1 +/-12.6 nmol/mmol creatinine) are significantly higher than that of normal pregnancies (2.5 +/-1.1 nmol/mmol creatinine).[5]

One study from Turkey found that 36% of the women tested had urinary MMA levels >6 µmol/mmol crt. Of those, 50% had serum vitamin B12 levels <180 pg/mL.[6]

Vitamin B12 (Cobalamin) Deficiency: MMA is a strong biomarker of vitamin B12 (cobalamin) deficiency. In cases of vitamin B12 deficiency, there may also be elevated homocysteine levels. Adenosylcobalamin is a cofactor for methylmalonyl-CoA mutase. Anything that causes a decrease in absorption or cellular availability of cobalamin can cause elevated MMA.

Kidney Dysfunction: Methylmalonic acid is primarily excreted by the kidneys. Impaired renal function can result in elevated levels in the bloodstream. Higher levels may be seen in cases of renal damage due to preeclampsia.

Advanced Maternal Age: As we age, we absorb vitamin B12 less effectively and have a decrease in its metabolism. MMA levels increase slightly with age.

Gene Variation: Those with genetic variants in the HIBCH gene may have MMA levels that are almost 50% higher, regardless of B12 levels.[7] The most common gene variant associated with elevated MMA is methylmalonyl-CoA mutase (MUT) deficiency. CblA (cobalamin A factor) and CblB (cobalamin B factor) mutations impair the synthesis of adenosylcobalamin and cause elevated methylmalonic acid.

Vitamin B7 (Biotin) Deficiency: Defects in biotin metabolism due to biotinidase deficiency can also cause elevated MMA levels. Biotin is a cofactor for the synthesis of adenosylcobalamin. A decrease in biotin can thus impair adenocobalamin synthesis. A decrease in adenocobalamin will cause elevated MMA levels.

Other Possible Causes: insulin resistance, bicarbonate deficiency, glutathione deficiency, methylmalonic acidemia, other genetics

Treatment Strategies for Elevated Methylmalonic Acid

See Vitamin B12 (Cobalamin) Section.

Additional Testing

vitamin B12 (cobalamin); homocysteine; complete blood count (CBC); comprehensive metabolic panel (CMP); functional genomic analysis

Causes of Low Methylmalonic Acid

Not considered pathogenic

Treatment Strategies for Low Methylmalonic Acid

Not considered pathogenic

References

1. Stabler S.P. Clinical practice. Vitamin B12 deficiency. N. Engl. J. Med. 2013;368:149–160. doi: 10.1056/NEJMcp1113996

2. Supakul S, Chabrun F, Genebrier S, et al. Diagnostic Performances of Urinary Methylmalonic Acid/Creatinine Ratio in Vitamin B12 Deficiency. J Clin Med. 2020;9(8):2335. Published 2020 Jul 22. doi:10.3390/jcm9082335

3. Soda, H., Ohura, T., Yoshida, I. et al. Prenatal diagnosis and therapy for a patient with vitamin B12-responsive methylmalonic acidaemia. J Inherit Metab Dis 18, 295–298 (1995). doi.org/10.1007/BF00710418

4. Choi R, Choi S, Lim Y, et al. A Prospective Study on Serum Methylmalonic Acid and Homocysteine in Pregnant Women. Nutrients. 2016;8(12):797. Published 2016 Dec 8. doi:10.3390/nu8120797

5. Luo X, Zhang L, Wei H, Liu W, Wang M, Ning Q. Methylmalonic acid in amniotic fluid and maternal urine as a marker for neural tube defects. J Huazhong Univ Sci Technolog Med Sci. 2004;24(2):166–169. doi:10.1007/BF02885420

6. GÜLTEPE, Mustafa & Özcan, Ömer. (2007). Cobalamin Deficiency During Pregnancy Expressed as Elevated Urine Methylmalonic Acid Levels Determined by a Photometric Assay. Turkish Journal of Medical Sciences. 37

7. Molloy AM, Pangilinan F, Mills JL, et al. A Common Polymorphism in HIBCH Influences Methylmalonic Acid Concentrations in Blood Independently of Cobalamin. Am J Hum Genet. 2016;98(5):869–882. doi:10.1016/j.ajhg.2016.03.005

Homocysteine

The homocysteine test measures the amount of homocysteine in the bloodstream. It is a single analyte.

Homocysteine is a metabolic intermediate produced by the demethylation of methionine. It is commonly found in the blood in three forms: free, bound to albumin, and in a complex with other homocysteine thiols.

Homocysteine is then further metabolized in the body through two main pathways: remethylation, which converts homocysteine back to methionine, and transsulfuration, which converts homocysteine to cysteine.

There are two pathways of remethylation and one pathway of transsulfuration.

The remethylation of homocysteine to methionine on the vitamin B9 (folate) side involves a series of enzymatic reactions that require the presence of folate (specifically, 5-methyltetrahydrofolate) and the cofactors vitamin B2 (riboflavin) and vitamin B12 (cobalamin). Folate is first converted to 5,10-methylenetetrahydrofolate through a reaction catalyzed by the enzyme dihydrofolate reductase (DHFR). Then 5,10-methylenetetrahydrofolate is converted to 5-methyltetrahydrofolate (5-methyl-THF) by the enzyme methylenetetrahydrofolate reductase (MTHFR), which requires riboflavin. This step involves the transfer of a methyl group. The methyl group carried by 5-methyl-THF is transferred to homocysteine in a reaction catalyzed by the enzyme methionine synthase (also known as cobalamin-dependent methionine synthase). This transfer is facilitated by vitamin B12, which serves as a cofactor for methionine synthase. Vitamin B12 is converted to its active form (methylcobalamin) during this process. After donating its methyl group to homocysteine, 5-methyl-THF is converted back to tetrahydrofolate (THF) through a series of reactions, making it available for further cycles of the remethylation process.

> Homocysteine + Methyl Group from 5-methyl-THF → (Methionine Synthase) →
> Methionine + Tetrahydrofolate (THF)

The choline betaine pathway, also known as the alternative or non-folate remethylation pathway, is another mechanism for remethylating homocysteine. In the liver, choline is oxidized to betaine in a reaction catalyzed by the enzyme choline oxidase. This step occurs in the mitochondria. Betaine donates a methyl group to homocysteine in a reaction catalyzed by the enzyme betaine-homocysteine methyltransferase (BHMT). This methyl transfer from betaine to homocysteine results in the formation of dimethylglycine (DMG) and methionine. Dimethylglycine, produced in the previous step, can be further metabolized to form sarcosine and then converted back to betaine in subsequent reactions.

Homocysteine + Methyl Group from Betaine → (BHMT) → Methionine + Dimethylglycine (DMG)

The transsulfuration pathway involves the conversion of homocysteine to glutathione. The transsulfuration pathway begins with the conversion of homocysteine to cystathionine. This reaction is catalyzed by the enzyme cystathionine beta-synthase (CBS), which requires vitamin B6 (in the form of pyridoxal phosphate) as a cofactor. The reaction involves the condensation of homocysteine with serine to form cystathionine. Cystathionine is then converted to cysteine in a reaction catalyzed by the enzyme cystathionine gamma-lyase. This step involves the cleavage of cystathionine into cysteine, alpha-ketobutyrate, and ammonia. Cysteine is a key precursor for the synthesis of glutathione. Glutathione synthesis involves the condensation of cysteine with glycine, followed by the addition of another cysteine molecule to form glutathione. The reaction is catalyzed by the enzymes gamma-glutamylcysteine synthetase and glutathione synthetase.

Homocysteine + Serine → (CBS with B6) > Cystathionine

Cystathionine → (Cystathionine Gamma-Lyase) → Cysteine + Alpha-Ketobutyrate + Ammonia

Cysteine + Glycine → (Gamma-Glutamylcysteine Synthetase) → Gamma-Glutamylcysteine

Gamma-Glutamylcysteine + Cysteine → (Glutathione Synthetase) → Glutathione

Pregnancy

Homocysteine levels decrease in normal pregnancies. This drop is attributed to both hemodilution and increased use during pregnancy. Homocysteine levels decrease during early pregnancy, reaching the lowest point during the second trimester, and steadily increase during the later third trimester reaching early pregnancy levels.[1]

Postpartum

There is limited data on the normalization of homocysteine in the postpartum period.

> Hypohomocysteinemia is medically defined as a homocysteine <6 µmol/L, while hyperhomocysteinemia is medically defined as a homocysteine >15 µmol/L in nonpregnant adults.[2]

STANDARD LAB RANGE: 0 – 14.5 µmol/L

Trimester	Standard Pregnancy Ranges	**Functional Pregnancy Ranges**
Preconception	0 – 14.5	**5 – 12**
First Trimester	3.34 – 11	**4 – 7.3**
Second Trimester	2 – 26.9	**3.5 – 5.3**
Third Trimester	3.2 – 21.4	**4 – 7.3**
Postpartum	Not Established	**5 – 12**

Causes of Elevated Homocysteine

See Vitamin B12 (Cobalamin) Section.

Nutritional Deficiency: Any nutritional deficiency that affects proper methylation status can cause an increase in homocysteine. Vitamin B9 (folate), vitamin B12 (cobalamin), vitamin B2 (riboflavin), vitamin B6 (pyridoxine), and choline/betaine are the vitamin deficiencies most commonly associated with elevated homocysteine.

Hypothyroidism: Overt hypothyroidism has been associated with hyperhomocysteinemia with correction of homocysteine levels with levothyroxine use.[8] The exact mechanism is unknown. It is possible

Although studies find increased complication risk with higher homocysteine levels, the ranges used in these studies are not consistent, and developing a range based on these studies is not accurate. Generally, studies find that levels >10 μmol/L are associated with increased risks of varying severity.

There is an association between elevated homocysteine levels and pregnancy complications such as early miscarriage, preeclampsia, IUGR, and placental abruption, as well as in certain cases of maternal and fetal mortality.[3]

Preconception homocysteine levels >12.4 μmol/L increase the prevalence of preterm labor by four times.[4]

A 5 μmol/L increase in homocysteine concentration was associated with 63% increased odds of placental mediated complications.[5 6]

Studies have found that higher homocysteine levels within six weeks postpartum are associated with postpartum depression, regardless of vitamin B9 (folate) and vitamin B12 (cobalamin) levels.[7]

that a decrease in GFR causes a buildup of homocysteine in the bloodstream. There may also be an effect on the production of enzymes needed in homocysteine metabolism by the liver.

Genetic Variants: There has been a large focus on the MTFHR genetic variants in connection to elevated homocysteine levels in previous years. MTHFR mutation is generally present with elevated homocysteine and decreased or normal methionine levels. MTHFR is just one of several genes and enzymes needed for proper recycling and metabolism of homocysteine. A dysfunction in any enzyme synthesis may impair the function of the chemical cycle. CBS genetic variants are associated with elevated homocysteine but with elevated methionine levels. Another condition called CblC (cobalamin C factor) deficiency can cause an elevation in homocysteine as well as methylmalonic acid, with normal to low decreased methionine.[9] This has been associated with various genetic variations in vitamin B12 (cobalamin) metabolism.

Other Possible Causes: kidney disease, certain medications, genetics, age, oxidative stress, smoking history, heavy metal exposure, certain medications (antacids)

Treatment Strategies for Elevated Homocysteine

See Vitamin B12 (Cobalamin) Section.

Diet

Although vitamin B9 (folate) has traditionally been used to reduce elevated homocysteine levels, not everybody needs a methyl folate supplement. Proper genetic and nutritional diagnostics may be needed to determine whether folate, vitamin B12 (cobalamin), vitamin B6 (pyridoxine), or choline pathways are responsible for the elevated homocysteine levels. Generally, without understanding what genetics and nutritional components may be at play, other dietary guidelines can be used to help support proper methylation status. The Mediterranean-style diet has shown the most benefit in reducing homocysteine levels. Betaine-rich foods such as beets can also be a good addition for those with elevated homocysteine. A fermented drink called beet kvass can be made and drunk as a tonic daily.

Lifestyle

Short sleep duration has been associated with higher homocysteine levels. Sleeping seven hours or more was shown to be protective, while sleeping less than five was shown to increase homocysteine levels.[10] Heavy metal exposure has also been shown to increase homocysteine levels. Assessing the diet for exposure to heavy metals such as lead and mercury may also be needed, especially when other more common causes are ruled out.[11]

Supplements

Research supports that folic acid is more absorbable than natural folate, or even methylfolate, raising serum folate levels quicker and to higher levels. A 2014 study found that up to 86% of folic acid remains unmetabolized in the liver, while 100% of natural folate was metabolized correctly.[12] [13] Unmetabolized folic acid can be found in the bloodstream with dosages as small as 200 μg.

The question isn't "Does folic acid supplementation result in high levels of unmetabolized folic acid?" but "What does unmetabolized folic acid do in the body? Is it neutral or pathogenic?" Concern is starting to rise about the effects of these unmetabolized folic acid compounds in both maternal and fetal health. Unmetabolized folic acid compounds can be found in cord blood, and some studies suggest it may affect epigenetics.[14] [15] In addition, researchers are beginning to do comparative studies between methylfolate and folic acid supplementation. However, no studies have been done directly on neural-tube defect prevention. A study in the *Journal of Perinatal Medicine* concluded that methylfolate was superior to folic acid in improving folate biomarkers.[16]

Not everyone needs to take a methylfolate supplement. Due to its ease of delivery into the cells, it is possible to overdose on this form more readily and cause hypohomocysteinemia.

Folinic acid, also known as 5-formyltetrahydrofolate (5-FTHF) or leucovorin, is a stable reduced form of folate that does not require enzymatic conversion in the body to be active. Folinic acid is readily absorbed and can be used directly in various metabolic pathways. This is another form that is often found in prenatal supplements. It is also found in food. There is limited research on this form, but it has been shown to function similarly to folic acid, where there is a more significant rise in serum folate levels after administration as compared to methylfolate but a reduced effect on biomarkers such as elevated homocysteine.[17] Folinic acid may be a better substitute for methylfolate in those without elevated homocysteine.

Supplementation with both vitamin B12 (cobalamin) and vitamin B6 (pyridoxine) has also been shown to lower homocysteine levels. Any nutritional supplemental regimen should be designed for the individual patient. If elevated homocysteine is detected, a complex nutritional regimen should be used. This would include nutrients that support both remethylation pathways and glutathione synthesis.

Additional Testing

complete blood count (CBC); comprehensive metabolic panel (CMP); vitamin B12 (cobalamin); serum folate; comprehensive thyroid profile II; thyroid peroxidase antibodies (TPOAb); thyroglobulin antibody (TgAb); c-reactive protein (CRP); functional genomic analysis

Causes of Low Homocysteine

See Vitamin B12 (Cobalamin) Section.

There is little research on hypohomocysteinemia and none related to pregnancy.

In one study, 41% of patients with idiopathic peripheral neuropathy were found to have low homocysteine levels.[18]

Inflammation/Oxidative Stress: The transsulfuration pathway that produces glutathione is one of the pathways in the breakdown of homocysteine. In cases of stress or inflammation overload, the conversion of glutathione from homocysteine in excess causes a decrease in homocysteine levels.[19] This may be seen in those with chronic inflammation associated with conditions such as inflammatory bowel disease (IBD), rheumatoid arthritis (RA), and systemic lupus erythematosus (SLE).

Other Possible Causes: low-protein diet, overdose of methyl vitamins, genetics

Treatment Strategies for Low Homocysteine

See Vitamin B12 (Cobalamin) Section.

Diet

If your patient has low homocysteine levels associated with inflammation and an increased need for glutathione, focus on dietary strategies that support both the methylation cycle and the synthesis of glutathione. Include foods rich in cysteine, an amino acid that is a precursor to glutathione. Examples include poultry, eggs, dairy products, legumes, and certain nuts (especially walnuts), as well as sulfur-rich vegetables like garlic, onions, and cruciferous vegetables (broccoli, Brussels sprouts, and cauliflower). Sulfur is a key component of glutathione.

Increase the intake of fruits and vegetables rich in antioxidants. These include berries, citrus fruits, tomatoes, and leafy greens. Antioxidants help protect cells from oxidative stress and can support overall health. Omega-3 fatty acids have anti-inflammatory properties and may contribute to the regulation of oxidative stress. Include sources such as fatty fish (salmon, mackerel), flaxseeds, and chia seeds. Reduce the intake of processed foods, sugary beverages, and refined carbohydrates, which may contribute to inflammation.

Lifestyle

Stress-reduction techniques, both for emotional stress as well as physical inflammation, are important for managing low homocysteine levels. Part of the treatment is identifying the triggers and either removing them or creating action plans for management. Sleep is important for regulating inflammation and stress levels, because that is when we detox and recover from cortisol needs throughout the day.

Supplements

N-acetyl cysteine (NAC) is commonly known for its role in supporting glutathione production and antioxidant activity. It may indirectly affect homocysteine levels. NAC helps replenish intracellular glutathione levels, which may modulate homocysteine metabolism and reduce the conversion of homocysteine to glutathione for antioxidant needs.

Additional Testing

antinuclear antibodies (ANA); complete blood count (CBC); comprehensive metabolic panel (CMP); c-reactive protein (CRP)

References

1. Walker M. C., Smith G. N., Perkins S. L., Keely E. J., Garner P. R. Changes in homocysteine levels during normal pregnancy. American Journal of Obstetrics and Gynecology. 1999;180(3):660–664. doi: 10.1016/S0002–9378(99)70269–3

2. Du Plessis JP, Nienaber-Rousseau C, Lammertyn L, Schutte AE, Pieters M, Kruger HS. The Relationship of Circulating Homocysteine with Fibrinogen, Blood Pressure, and Other Cardiovascular Measures in African Adolescents. J Pediatr. 2021;234:158–163.e2. doi:10.1016/j.jpeds.2021.03.034

3. Thakur P, Bhalerao A. High Homocysteine Levels During Pregnancy and Its Association With Placenta-Mediated Complications: A Scoping Review. Cureus. 2023;15(2):e35244. Published 2023 Feb 20. doi:10.7759/cureus.35244

4. Dai C, Fei Y, Li J, Shi Y, Yang X. A Novel Review of Homocysteine and Pregnancy Complications. Biomed Res Int. 2021;2021:6652231. Published 2021 May 6. doi:10.1155/2021/6652231

5. Chaudhry, S.H., Taljaard, M., MacFarlane, A.J. et al. The role of maternal homocysteine concentration in placenta-mediated complications: findings from the Ottawa and Kingston birth cohort. BMC Pregnancy Childbirth 19, 75 (2019). doi.org/10.1186/s12884–019-2219–5

6. Memon SI, Acharya NS. The Association Between Serum Homocysteine Levels and Placenta-Mediated Complications: A Narrative Review. Cureus. 2022;14(11):e31305. Published 2022 Nov 9. doi:10.7759/cureus.31305

7. Aishwarya S, Rajendiren S, Kattimani S, Dhiman P, Haritha S, Ananthanarayanan PH. Homocysteine and serotonin: association with postpartum depression. Asian J Psychiatr. 2013;6(6):473–477. doi:10.1016/j.ajp.2013.05.007

8. Xiaoyu Ding, Ying Wang, Jia Liu, Guang Wang, Impaired Sensitivity to Thyroid Hormones Is Associated With Elevated Homocysteine Levels in the Euthyroid Population, The Journal of Clinical Endocrinology & Metabolism, Volume 107, Issue 9, September 2022, Pages e3731–e3737. doi.org/10.1210/clinem/dgac371

9. Giovana Regina Weber Hoss, Soraia Poloni and Henk J Blom et al. Three Main Causes of Homocystinuria: CBS, cblC and MTHFR Deficiency. What do they Have in Common? Journal of Inborn Errors of Metabolism and Screening. 2019. Vol. 7. DOI: 10.1590/2326–4594-jiems-2019–0007

10. Chen TY, Winkelman JW, Mao WC, et al. Short Sleep Duration Is Associated With Increased Serum Homocysteine: Insights From a National Survey. J Clin Sleep Med. 2019;15(1):139–148. Published 2019 Jan 15. doi:10.5664/jcsm.7588

11. Ledda C, Cannizzaro E, Lovreglio P, et al. Exposure to Toxic Heavy Metals Can Influence Homocysteine Metabolism. Antioxidants (Basel). 2019;9(1):30. Published 2019 Dec 28. doi:10.3390/antiox9010030

12. Patanwala I, King MJ, Barrett DA, et al. Folic acid handling by the human gut: implications for food fortification and supplementation. Am J Clin Nutr. 2014;100(2):593–599. doi:10.3945/ajcn.113.080507

13. Pietrzik K, Bailey L, Shane B. Folic acid and L-5-methyltetrahydrofolate: comparison of clinical pharmacokinetics and pharmacodynamics. Clin Pharmacokinet. 2010;49(8):535–548. doi:10.2165/11532990–000000000-00000

14. Menezo Y, Elder K, Clement A, Clement P. Folic Acid, Folinic Acid, 5 Methyl TetraHydroFolate Supplementation for Mutations That Affect Epigenesis through the Folate and One-Carbon Cycles. Biomolecules. 2022;12(2):197. Published 2022 Jan 24. doi:10.3390/biom12020197

15. Sweeney MR, McPartlin J, Weir DG, et al. Evidence of unmetabolised folic acid in cord blood of newborn and serum of 4-day-old infants. Br J Nutr. 2005;94(5):727–730. doi:10.1079/BJN20051572

16. Obeid R, Holzgreve W, Pietrzik K. Is 5-methyltetrahydrofolate an alternative to folic acid for the prevention of neural tube defects? J Perinat Med. 2013;41(5):469–483. doi:10.1515/jpm-2012–0256

17. Elias E. Mazokopakis EE, Papadomanolaki MG, John A. Papadakis JA. The effects of folinic acid and l-methylfolate supplementation on serum total homocysteine levels in healthy adults. Clin. Nutr. ESPEN. 2023;58:14–20. doi.org/10.1016/j.clnesp.2023.09.002

18. Cullen CE, Carter GT, Weiss MD, Grant PA, Saperstein DS. Hypohomocysteinemia: a potentially treatable cause of peripheral neuropathology? Phys Med Rehabil Clin N Am. 2012;23:59–65. doi.org/10.1016/j.pmr.2011.11.001

19. Pizzorno J. Homocysteine: friend or foe? Integr Med (Encinitas). 2014;13:8–14

C-Reactive Protein (CRP)

The c-reactive protein (CRP), quantitative test measures the concentration of CRP in the blood.

CRP is primarily produced by the liver in response to certain signals from the immune system, particularly pro-inflammatory cytokines such as interleukin-6 (IL-6) and tumor necrosis factor-alpha (TNF-alpha). These cytokines are released by various cells, including macrophages and adipocytes, in response to tissue damage, infection, or inflammation.

CRP binds to certain substances released by damaged or inflamed cells, including phosphocholine residues on the surface of bacteria, damaged cell membranes, and nuclear material from dead cells. By binding to these substances, CRP helps to activate the complement system, enhance phagocytosis, and promote inflammation at the site of injury or infection. It is a key compound in the clearance of bacteria and dead cells.

There are two CRP tests: quantitative and high-sensitivity.

Quantitative CRP (qCRP)

The qCRP test measures CRP levels in the blood within a broader range. This test is often used to assess moderate to high levels of inflammation such as those seen in acute infections, autoimmune diseases, or inflammatory conditions like rheumatoid arthritis. It is less sensitive than the high-sensitivity CRP assay and may not detect low levels of CRP associated with lower-grade inflammation.

High-Sensitivity CRP (hs-CRP)

The hs-CRP assay is more sensitive than quantitative CRP tests and can measure CRP levels within a narrower range. This test is specifically designed to detect low levels of CRP associated with chronic low-grade inflammation. Hs-CRP testing is used as a marker of cardiovascular risk and is often included as part of cardiovascular risk assessment panels. It is more accurate in detecting subtle changes in CRP levels, even in the absence of clinically apparent inflammation.

Pregnancy

Pregnancy is a state of low-grade to moderate-grade inflammation. In response, c-reactive protein levels are increased in pregnancy. A significant increase is seen from 24 weeks through the first week of postpartum.[1] Some elevation is normal and protective in pregnancy.

Postpartum

CRP levels may initially remain elevated immediately after delivery due to the inflammatory response associated with childbirth, including uterine involution and tissue repair. Labor complications may increase CRP further. Women who birth via cesarean may have more prolonged elevations in their CRP values.

> The variability of CRP in pregnancy currently makes it an unreliable marker. Although it can be used to assess inflammation, it should not be used as a predictive biomarker at this time.

STANDARD LAB RANGE (QCRP): 0 – 10 mg/L*

Trimester	Standard Pregnancy Ranges	**Functional Pregnancy Ranges**
Preconception	0–10	**0–10**
First Trimester	Not Established	**0–10**
Second Trimester	0.4–20.3	**0.2–10**
Third Trimester	0.4–8.1	**0.2–10**
Postpartum	0.4–8.1	**0.2–10**

*Most research studies use quantitative measurements.

STANDARD LAB RANGE (HS-CRP): 0 – 3 mg/dL*

Trimester	Standard Pregnancy Ranges	**Functional Pregnancy Ranges**
Preconception	0–3	**0–3**
First Trimester	Not Established	**0–3**
Second Trimester	0–3	**0.2–3**
Third Trimester	0–3	**0.2–3**
Postpartum	0–3	**0.2–3**

*Most research studies use quantitative measurements.

Causes of Elevated C-Reactive Protein (CRP)

Elevated CRP has been associated with increased risks of preeclampsia, gestational diabetes, intrauterine infections, and preterm birth.

Elevated CRP levels have been found in preeclamptic women, with a median value of 8.8 and a range of 0.3 to 25.5.[2]

CRP >5.5 µg/mL increases the risk of spontaneous preterm labor.[3]

Infections: Bacterial, viral, fungal, or parasitic infections can lead to increased production of CRP. Examples include pneumonia, urinary tract infections, and sinusitis. Significant increases in CRP have been found in patients with COVID-19.[4]

Autoimmune Disease Inflammation: CRP is often used to assess autoimmune inflammation and tissue damage. Specifically, in conditions such as rheumatoid arthritis, systemic lupus erythematosus (SLE), and inflammatory bowel diseases (Crohn's disease, ulcerative colitis). These conditions are also associated with an inherent increased risk of pregnancy complications.

Tissue Injury/Trauma: Acute muscle injuries can be associated with an increase in CRP. In cases of acute tissue damage or injury, basophils will often be elevated.

Low DHEA/Estrogen: DHEA is inversely related to CRP. Interestingly, some studies have found higher CRP levels with both decreased DHEA and estrogen.[5]

Iron Overload/Hemochromatosis: Generally, iron overload alone will not raise CRP. If both ferritin and CRP are elevated, this is a sign of cellular damage and inflammation. If iron overload is present, further assessment of liver function is warranted.

Other Possible Causes: metabolic syndrome, liver disease, cardiovascular disease, asthma, vitamin D deficiency, excessive exercise, obesity, cancer

Treatment Strategies for Elevated C-Reactive Protein (CRP)

Diet

Flavonoids are a diverse group of polyphonic compounds found in fruits and vegetables. Certain ones—such as quercetin (found in onions, apples, and citrus); kaempferol (found in broccoli, kale, green tea, and beans); luteolin (found in parsley, celery, thyme, carrots, and olive oil); apigenin (found in parsley, celery, and oranges); and hesperidin and naringenin (found in citrus)—have been shown to help reduce CRP levels. Anthocyanins are antioxidants that give red, purple, or blue color to fruits and vegetables, and help to reduce mild inflammation and CRP levels. To increase diverse antioxidants that can help reduce CRP, make meals colorful.

Curcumin is the bioactive compound in turmeric. It has strong antioxidant and anti-inflammatory effects and has been shown to reduce cytokines and CRP. Caution should be used with curcumin supplements, but dietary intake should pose no increased risk of bleeding. Omega-3 fatty acids can reduce CRP and other inflammatory markers.[6]

Lifestyle

Adequate sleep is essential for overall health and well-being, including immune function and the regulation of inflammation. Poor sleep quality or insufficient sleep have been associated with an increase in inflammatory markers, including CRP. Chronic sleep deprivation or sleep disorders such as sleep apnea may cause increased inflammation. Sleep is crucial for cellular repair and detoxification. When we sleep, the glymphatic system becomes active, removing harmful substances.

Melatonin helps promote sleep and serves as an antioxidant. You can't change the oil in your car if the engine is running. One of melatonin's jobs is to turn off the cellular "engines" so that they can be cleaned out. Melatonin helps stimulate the production of other antioxidants such as glutathione. Adequate sleep is crucial for maintaining optimal glutathione levels.

If patients have issues with sleep and inflammation, help them identify ways to get adequate sleep. Both aerobic exercise and resistance training have been shown to lower CRP. However, excessive exercise or intense exercise without adequate recovery can increase inflammatory markers and CRP. Stress-management techniques can also be used to help reduce inflammation. Chronic stress can dysregulate the immune system and either cause or worsen inflammation. Psychological stressors such as relationship issues, work stress, financial worries, and trauma can elevate CRP over time. Increase stress-reduction techniques, including mindfulness, meditation, journaling, yoga, deep breathing, and spending time outdoors in nature.

Supplements

Omega-3 fatty acids, found in fish oils, have been shown to reduce inflammation and CRP levels, particularly in cardiovascular inflammation, specifically DHA.[7] Curcumin has been shown to reduce CRP levels by blunting the release of pro-inflammatory cytokines.[8] Some studies have linked curcumin use to negative changes in blastocyst development, implantation, and post-implantation embryo development. Use should be limited to late gestation and in cases of inflammation, and in very small doses, as it is also linked to increased bleeding risk. That being said, curcumin use has been shown to positively affect gestational diabetes mellitus (GDM), as well as preeclampsia in animal models. It has been found to be neuroprotective against environmental toxins.[9] The standard dosage for curcumin is 500 mg twice daily.

Glutathione is a powerful antioxidant that is produced by the body through the breakdown of homocysteine. Glutathione injection and IV therapy are becoming more popular and readily available. Although research is limited, especially in pregnancy, this may be an option for specific cases of inflammation. Thoroughly assess the patient to determine whether this is an option for their specific case.

N-acetyl cysteine (NAC) is the precursor to glutathione. Some studies have shown that NAC supplementation can reduce CRP. A 2023 meta-analysis found that those with positive COVID-19 who took NAC had significantly lower CRP and D-dimer levels than those who did not. This could be a potentially protective supplement for those who are pregnant and positive for COVID-19.[10]

Supplementing with vitamin D has been shown to reduce CRP in those with low vitamin D.[11]

Additional Testing
antinuclear antibodies (ANA); urinalysis; comprehensive metabolic panel (CMP); iron and TIBC; ferritin; sleep study

Causes of Low C-Reactive Protein (CRP)

Not considered pathogenic

Systemic Lupus Erythematosus (SLE): Interestingly, SLE patients tend to only have modest increases in CRP compared to other autoimmune diseases. The amount of change can vary based on the individual. CRP polymorphism rs1205 is a CRP-lowering polymorph that is overrepresented in SLE patients. In general, SLE patients have a decreased CRP reaction to elevating IL-6 levels. In these cases, CRP may be falsely decreased in correlation to the amount of inflammation present.[12]

Other Possible Causes: certain medications (aspirin, nonsteroidal anti-inflammatories/NSAIDs, steroids), hypothyroidism, vitamin B6 (pyridoxine) deficiency, zinc deficiency, vitamin D deficiency, copper deficiency

Treatment Strategies for Low C-Reactive Protein (CRP)

Not considered pathogenic

Additional Testing

antinuclear antibodies (ANA); comprehensive thyroid profile II; complete blood count (CBC); comprehensive metabolic panel (CMP); vitamin D, 25-hydroxy (25-hydroxycalciferol, 25OH-D)

References

1. Fink, N.R., Chawes, B., Bønnelykke, K. et al. Levels of Systemic Low-grade Inflammation in Pregnant Mothers and Their Offspring are Correlated. Sci Rep 9, 3043 (2019). doi.org/10.1038/s41598–019-39620–5

2. Ali Z, Bokhari FA, Zaki S, Zargham U, Tauseef A, Khakan S. Correlation of CRP levels in third trimester with fetal birth weight in preeclamptic and normotensive pregnant women. J Coll Physicians Surg Pak. 2015;25(2):111–114

3. Bullen BL, Jones NM, Holzman CB, et al. C-reactive protein and preterm delivery: clues from placental findings and maternal weight. Reprod Sci. 2013;20(6):715–722. doi:10.1177/1933719112466302

4. Ali N. Elevated level of C-reactive protein may be an early marker to predict risk for severity of COVID-19. J Med Virol. 2020;92(11):2409–2411. doi:10.1002/jmv.26097

5. Wander K, Brindle E, O'Connor KA. C-reactive protein across the menstrual cycle. Am J Phys Anthropol. 2008;136(2):138–146. doi:10.1002/ajpa.20785

6. Chun OK, Chung SJ, Claycombe KJ, Song WO. Serum C-reactive protein concentrations are inversely associated with dietary flavonoid intake in U.S. adults. J Nutr. 2008;138(4):753–760. doi:10.1093/jn/138.4.753

7. Khan SU, Lone AN, Khan MS, et al. Effect of omega-3 fatty acids on cardiovascular outcomes: A systematic review and meta-analysis. EClinicalMedicine. 2021;38:100997. Published 2021 Jul 8. doi:10.1016/j.eclinm.2021.100997

8. Gorabi AM, Abbasifard M, Imani D, et al. Effect of curcumin on C-reactive protein as a biomarker of systemic inflammation: An updated meta-analysis of randomized controlled trials. Phytother Res. 2022;36(1):85–97. doi:10.1002/ptr.7284

9. Filardi T, Varì R, Ferretti E, Zicari A, Morano S, Santangelo C. Curcumin: Could This Compound Be Useful in Pregnancy and Pregnancy-Related Complications? Nutrients. 2020;12(10):3179. Published 2020 Oct 17. doi:10.3390/nu12103179

10. Alam MS, Hasan MN, Maowa Z, Khatun F, Nazir KHMNH, Alam MZ. N-acetylcysteine reduces severity and mortality in COVID-19 patients: A systematic review and meta-analysis. J Adv Vet Anim Res. 2023;10(2):157–168. Published 2023 Jun 30. doi:10.5455/javar.2023.j665

11. Zhou A, Hyppönen E. Vitamin D deficiency and C-reactive protein: a bidirectional Mendelian randomization study. Int J Epidemiol. 2023;52(1):260–271. doi:10.1093/ije/dyac087

12. Enocsson H, Gullstrand B, Eloranta ML, et al. C-Reactive Protein Levels in Systemic Lupus Erythematosus Are Modulated by the Interferon Gene Signature and CRP Gene Polymorphism rs1205. Front Immunol. 2021;11:622326. Published 2021 Jan 28. doi:10.3389/fimmu.2020.622326

References

Antinuclear Antibodies (ANA)

The Antinuclear Antibodies (ANA) test looks for the presence of autoantibodies in the blood. It is a single analyte and is found in several other panels with differential ANA antibodies, such as the ANA Profile 12 (RDL); ANA by IFA, Reflex to 9-biomarker Profile; ANA by IFA, Reflex to 11-biomarker Profile; ANA 12 Profile, Do All (RDL); ANA 12 Plus Profile, Do All (RDL); and the ANA 12 Plus Profile (RDL).

Antinuclear antibodies attack the nucleus of cells. They can attack various components of the nucleus, including DNA, histones, nucleolar proteins, and nuclear antigens. The specific pattern in staining can provide insight into the type of attack. They are most associated with systemic lupus erythematosus (SLE) but can also be found in other autoimmune conditions. Here are the most commonly tested ANA antibodies.

Anti-Centromere B: These antibodies target the centromere proteins. These proteins play a role in the structure and function of the centromeres of chromosomes. Centromeres are specialized regions on chromosomes that serve as the primary site of stabilization in cellular division. They are important for mitosis and meiosis.

Anti-Chromatin: These antibodies attack the components of chromatin. Chromatin is a complex of DNA, histone proteins, and other proteins. It regulates gene expression, DNA replication, and DNA repair.

Anti-dsDNA (Double-Stranded DNA): These antibodies target double-stranded DNA, which is its typical structure.

Anti-Jo-I: These antibodies attack histidyl-tRNA synthetase. This enzyme regulates the translation of genetic material encoded in mRNA.

Anti-Ribosomal P (Anti-P): These antibodies attack ribosomal P proteins. This is a group of proteins associated with ribosomes and cellular organelles responsible for protein synthesis.

Anti-RNP: These antibodies attack ribonucleoproteins. Ribonucleoproteins are macromolecular complexes of RNA and proteins. They regulate gene expression and RNA processing.

Anti-Scl-70: These antibodies target DNA topoisomerase I. This is an enzyme that plays a role in regulating the structure and topology of DNA within cells.

Anti-Smith: These antibodies target the Smith antigen, which is part of the small nuclear ribonucleoproteins (snRNPs) involved in RNA processing.

Anti-SSA (Ro): These antibodies target the SSA antigen, which is found in the cell nucleus and cytoplasm. Ro is thought to play a role in RNA metabolism, stability, and cellular response to stress.

Anti-SSB (La): These antibodies target the SSB antigen, which is also found in the cell nucleus and cytoplasm. La protein binds to the 3' ends of newly synthesized RNA, helping in processing and stability.

ANA testing is reported as a titer (concentration). ANA titers are represented as a dilution factor in ratio to the highest dilution at which ANAs are still detectable. For example, 1:40 means the patient's serum was diluted 40 times before ANAs were still detected. The higher the titer, the more autoantibodies are present.

- **Borderline Titers:** 1:40
- **Low Titers:** 1:80
- **Intermediate Titers:** 1:160 or 1:320
- **High Titers:** 1:640 or higher

Positive ANA is often reflexed to a pattern if found positive as well. Pattern refers to the distinct staining that is observed when ANA testing is performed. These patterns provide valuable information about specific antigen targets.

- **Centromere:** In this pattern, the fluorescence stains the centromeric regions of chromosomes. It is associated with antibodies targeting centromere proteins.

- **Homogeneous:** In this pattern, the fluorescence is evenly distributed throughout the nucleus, causing a homogeneous or diffuse staining pattern. This pattern is most commonly associated with antibodies that target DNA and histones.

- **Nuclear Dot:** In this pattern, speckles are found within the nucleus in a pinpoint location. This occurs when antibodies attack specific nuclear antigens.

- **Nuclear Membrane:** In this pattern, the fluorescence is localized along the periphery of the nucleus, giving a rim-like or peripherally stained appearance.

- **Nucleolar:** This pattern involves staining the nucleoli, which are responsible for ribosome biogenesis. It is associated with antibodies that target nucleolar antigens.

- **Speckled:** In this pattern, the fluorescence appears in numerous speckles or dots within the nucleus. It is one of the more common ANA patterns and is associated with antibodies that target various nuclear antigens.

Pregnancy

ANA antibodies have been shown to be higher in pregnancy, even in normal pregnancies. Low titers are not associated with pregnancy complications. Higher ANA titers have been associated with pregnancy complications.

Postpartum

There is not enough data on how childbirth and postpartum affect ANA.

STANDARD LAB RANGE: <1:80

Trimester	Standard Pregnancy Ranges	**Functional Pregnancy Ranges**
Preconception	<1:80	**<1:80**
First Trimester	<1:80	**<1:80**
Second Trimester	<1:80	**<1:80**
Third Trimester	<1:80	**<1:80**
Postpartum	<1:80	**<1:80**

Causes of Elevated Antinuclear Antibodies (ANA)

ANA antibodies are not uncommon in women with unexplained recurrent miscarriages, suggesting a role for autoimmune disease in cases of unexplained pregnancy loss.[1]

Titers of >1:160 are highly associated with unexplained recurrent pregnancy loss, while titers of <1:80 are not.[2]

Elevated ANA antibodies are associated with decreased IVF transfer success.[3]

Medications: Several different medications have been known to cause elevated ANAs. This is called drug-induced lupus. It includes the following medications: hydralazine, procainamide, minocycline, sulfa drugs, penicillin, methyldopa, quinidine, and chlorpromazine.

Latent Viral Infections: During the initial infection, many viruses enter a state of latency, where they live in the host's cells without causing active replication. During the latency, the viral genome can integrate with the host's DNA, becoming a part of the host's genetic material. The most common viruses associated with this phenomenon are herpesviruses (such as Epstein-Barr, cytomegalovirus, human papillomavirus, and herpes simplex).

During times of stress, immunosuppression, or other triggers, the virus can reactivate and begin to replicate. This triggers an immune response. The immune system begins to attack the virus, but because it has integrated with the host's DNA, it mismarks the host's nuclear material, thus forming ANA antibodies. During both latent and active

Some studies have found that antinuclear antibodies occur more often in patients with preeclampsia, intrauterine growth retardation, fetal death, and placental abruption. Other studies, however, have not confirmed these results; therefore, there is not a clear connection.[4]

phases, the viral proteins may affect the immune system. Molecular mimicry is when the immune system, while attacking the virus, attacks similar proteins in the host's cells. The constant attack causes inflammation in the cells, which further increases immune responses in those tissues.

Environment Toxin Exposure: Common toxins can induce epigenetic changes in the body, bind to immune and endocrine receptors, reduce antioxidant reserves, promote immune barrier degradation, induce lymphocytic dysregulation, alter normal antigen presenting responses, bind to nucleic acids, and promote antinuclear autoimmunity.[5] This includes the following:

- Persistent organic pollutants: aldrin, chlordane, dichloro-diphenyl-trichloroethane (DDT), dieldrin, dioxins, endrin, furans, heptachlor, hexachlorobenzene, mirex, polychlorinated biphenyls, and tetrabromobisphenol A
- Toxic solvents: acetone, benzene, butanol, carbon tetrachloride, methanol, toluene, trichloroethylene, and xylene
- Heavy metals: arsenic, cadmium, lead, and mercury
- Endocrine disruptors: bisphenols, dioxins, perchlorates, phthalates, polybrominated diphenyl ethers, and polychlorinated biphenyls

These toxins can be found in contaminated water, food, air, soil, furniture, cosmetics, paints, glues, plastics, and canned food.

Glyphosate Exposure: Glyphosate use by farmers has been associated with both cancer and elevated ANAs.[6] It has now been established that glyphosate-based herbicides have endocrine-disrupting potential. There is a relationship between glyphosate exposure, immune-system dysfunction, and microbiome dysbiosis.[7]

UV Skin Damage: There has been a strong connection between ultraviolet radiation and sunlight and increased ANA antibodies going back decades.[8] UV light exposure can induce inflammation and damage skin cells; the corresponding release of cytokines increases apoptosis, damages cellular DNA, and increases the production of autoantigens. This increases immune-system activation, which causes the body to create autoantigens, thus increasing ANA antibodies. Sun exposure is known to flare certain autoimmune conditions.

Celiac Disease: False positive ANAs have been found in those with untreated celiac disease.

Vitamin D Deficiency: Vitamin D deficiency is very common in those with autoimmune disease. One study from Hungary found that 82% of those with SLE were low in vitamin D[9], and the severity of markers was inversely related to vitamin D levels.

Gut Dysbiosis: Emerging research[10] suggests that gut dysbiosis may be a driving factor in autoimmune disease development and progression. The gut microbiome plays a crucial role in immune function and maintaining immune-system homeostasis. Dysbiosis may compromise the intestinal barrier, leading to increased permeability and systemic inflammation, thereby activating the immune system. In addition, dysbiosis can promote molecular mimicry, where microbial proteins with similar structural components cause autoantibodies due to mistaken identity.

Other Possible Causes: stress, vitamin C deficiency, genetics

Treatment Strategies for Elevated Antinuclear Antibodies (ANA)

Diet

Diets high in processed and chemical-laden foods should be addressed, including fast food, sugary snacks, processed meats, packaged goods, and hydrogenated fats. Gluten-free diets have been shown to help reduce symptoms in those with non-celiac autoimmune disease.[11] A gluten-free trial can be done in these cases, with a minimum removal of three months.

There is limited research on the reduction of nightshades in autoimmune disease. Some studies do show benefits in those with autoimmune digestive disease. Some people with autoimmune disease notice more flares with nightshades. This family includes tomatoes, peppers, eggplants, and potatoes. Proper traditional preparations of these foods may be important, with the removal of skins and special cooking methods. Probiotics, fermented foods, and fiber-rich foods can help to rebalance the microbiome. Herbs and spices—particularly those that are high in antioxidants and phytochemicals such as turmeric, ginger, garlic, cinnamon, and rosemary—may help reduce autoimmune inflammation.

Supplements

Nutritional supplementation of vitamin D, vitamin C, vitamin B6 (pyridoxine), and omega-3 fish oils over the course of 12 weeks helps reduce inflammation associated with autoimmune disease. In various studies, 600 mg of N-acetyl cysteine (NAC) twice per day has shown promise of reducing symptoms of autoimmune disease over the course of three to six months.[12]

Additional Testing

vitamin D, 25-hydroxy (25-hydroxycalciferol, 25OH-D); c-reactive protein (CRP); comprehensive stool testing; leukocyte response testing; heavy metal testing; toxin testing; testing for latent viruses

Causes of Low Antinuclear Antibodies (ANA)

Not considered pathogenic

Treatment Strategies for Low Antinuclear Antibodies (ANA)

Not considered pathogenic

References

1. Molazadeh M, Karimzadeh H, Azizi MR. Prevalence and clinical significance of antinuclear antibodies in Iranian women with unexplained recurrent miscarriage. Iran J Reprod Med. 2014;12(3):221–226

2. Liu T, Guo X, Liao Y, Liu Y, Zhu Y, Chen X. Correlation Between the Presence of Antinuclear Antibodies and Recurrent Pregnancy Loss: A Mini Review. Front Endocrinol (Lausanne). 2022;13:873286. Published 2022 May 4. doi:10.3389/fendo.2022.873286

3. Ticconi C, Inversetti A, Logruosso E, et al. Antinuclear antibodies positivity in women in reproductive age: From infertility to adverse obstetrical outcomes: A meta-analysis. J Reprod Immunol. 2023;155:103794. doi:10.1016/j.jri.2022.103794

4. Afman IE, Cronjé HS, Joubert G, Badenhorst PN, Schoon MG. Antinuclear antibody testing in obstetric patients. S Afr Med J. 2003;93(12):932–937

5. Kharrazian D. Exposure to Environmental Toxins and Autoimmune Conditions. Integr Med (Encinitas). 2021;20(2):20–24

6. Parks CG, Santos ASE, Lerro CC, et al. Lifetime Pesticide Use and Antinuclear Antibodies in Male Farmers From the Agricultural Health Study. Front Immunol. 2019;10:1476. Published 2019 Jul 11. doi:10.3389/fimmu.2019.01476

7. Maddalon A, Galbiati V, Colosio C, Mandić-Rajčević S, Corsini E. Glyphosate-based herbicides: Evidence of immune-endocrine alteration. Toxicology. 2021;459:152851. doi:10.1016/j.tox.2021.152851

8. Veen JH, Lucas CJ. Induction of antinuclear antibodies by ultraviolet irradiation. Annals of the Rheumatic Diseases. 1970;29:556–558

9. Szodoray P, Tarr T, Bazso A, Poor G, Szegedi G, Kiss E. The immunopathological role of vitamin D in patients with SLE: data from a single centre registry in Hungary. Scand J Rheumatol. 2011;40(2):122–126

10. Mousa WK, Chehadeh F, Husband S. Microbial dysbiosis in the gut drives systemic autoimmune diseases. Front Immunol. 2022;13:906258. Published 2022 Oct 20. doi:10.3389/fimmu.2022.906258

11. Lerner A, Freire de Carvalho J, Kotrova A, Shoenfeld Y. Gluten-free diet can ameliorate the symptoms of non-celiac autoimmune diseases. Nutr Rev. 2022;80(3):525–543. doi:10.1093/nutrit/nuab039

12. Greco CM, Nakajima C, Manzi S. Updated review of complementary and alternative medicine treatments for systemic lupus erythematosus. Curr Rheumatol Rep. 2013;15(11):378. doi:10.1007/s11926–013-0378–3

APPENDIX A

Common Lab Panels

Complete Blood Count With Differential

White blood cell (WBC) count; red blood cell (RBC) count; hematocrit; hemoglobin; mean corpuscular volume (MCV); mean corpuscular hemoglobin (MCH); mean corpuscular hemoglobin concentration (MCHC); red cell distribution width (RDW); platelet count; percentage and absolute WBC differential counts; Immature granulocytes; nucleated RBC

Complete Blood Count Without Differential

White blood cell (WBC) count; red blood cell (RBC) count; hematocrit; hemoglobin; MCV; MCH; MCHC; RDW; platelet count

Iron and Total Iron-Binding Capacity (TIBC)

Iron, total; total iron-binding capacity (TIBC); unsaturated iron-binding capacity (UIBC); transferrin saturation

Ferritin, Iron and Total Iron-Binding Capacity

Iron, total; total iron-binding capacity (TIBC); unsaturated iron-binding capacity (UIBC); ferritin

Comprehensive Metabolic Panel

Glucose, serum; blood urea nitrogen (BUN); creatinine, serum; eGFR calculation; BUN/creatinine ratio; sodium, serum; potassium, serum; chloride, serum; carbon dioxide, total; calcium, serum; protein, total, serum; albumin, serum; globulin, total; albumin/globulin (A/G) ratio; bilirubin, total; alkaline phosphatase, serum; aspartate aminotransferase (AST/SGOT); alanine aminotransferase (ALT/SGPT)

Basic Metabolic Panel

Glucose, serum; blood urea nitrogen (BUN); creatinine, serum; eGFR calculation; BUN/ creatinine ratio; sodium, serum; potassium, serum; chloride, serum; carbon dioxide, total; calcium, serum

Thyroid Profile II, Comprehensive

Thyroid-stimulating hormone (TSH); thyroxine (T4); T3 uptake; free thyroxine index (FTI); triiodothyronine (T3)

Thyroid Profile with TSH

Thyroid-stimulating hormone (TSH); thyroxine (T4); T3 uptake; free thyroxine index (FTI)

APPENDIX B

Common Functional Lab Assessments

Comprehensive Stool Testing

Comprehensive stool testing is a diagnostic tool used to assess various aspects of gastrointestinal health and overall digestive function. Specific components will vary between laboratories, but some common elements include microbiome analysis, yeast and fungal analysis, parasitology, digestive enzyme activity and other digestive function markers, calprotectin and other inflammatory markers, secretory IgA, markers of intestinal permeability, and occasional markers of gluten intolerance.

Dried Urine Test for Comprehensive Hormones (DUTCH)

DUTCH is a commonly run test for the assessment of hormones and organic acids. It is used to assess overall, or a specific time of, hormone metabolism. It often includes levels of hormone metabolites, metabolite ratios, diurnal hormone patterns, sex hormone balance, adrenal function, and organic acids.

Nutrient Panels

Nutrient panels are used to evaluate the nutritional status, presence of nutritional deficiencies, and potential nutritional imbalances in an individual. These tests can include panels that assess micronutrient levels, amino acids, and fatty acid profiles. Occasionally, they will also include oxidative stress markers, inflammatory markers, and digestive function markers.

Food and Chemical Sensitivity Panels

The types and methods of analysis and results vary greatly among different labs. These panels are designed to identify immune-mediated reactions to specific foods or food components. They identify foods that may trigger adverse immune responses such as IgG-mediated immune reactions or other inflammatory responses. This includes panels that run the leukocyte response analysis (LRA) testing. These tests look for specific cellular responses in the immune system to selected antigens, unlike IgG testing, which looks for IgG levels in certain foods in the bloodstream. Leukocyte response testing tests the immune system against antigens and analyzes the immune-system response and release of inflammatory markers in reaction to select antigens.

Toxin Testing

Toxin testing can assess heavy metals, environmental toxins, or mycotoxin exposure. It helps identify the levels of chemicals in the blood, urine, or a hair sample.

Latent Virus Testing

Latent viruses remain dormant within a host cell after the initial infection. Testing for latent viruses can be challenging due to their inactive state. Antibody testing is the most common blood test used to identify past, present, and latent exposure. Some stool tests also provide latent virus testing.

Functional Genomic Analysis

Genetic testing focuses on understanding how genetic variations or mutations affect the function of genes and their biological pathways. Unlike traditional genetic testing, the primary goal is to identify variations in the DNA sequence that may affect nutrient needs or biochemical function. Some tests help identify underlying mechanisms of diseases or how specific mutations contribute to predispositions. Others help assess unique nutrient needs.

Oral Zinc Tolerance Test

Also known as the zinc tally test, oral zinc tolerance is a taste test used to assess the need for dietary or supplemental zinc.

APPENDIX C

Functional Reference Ranges for Serum Indices in Pregnancy

Analyte	Unit	Standard	Preconception	1st Trimester	2nd Trimester	3rd Trimester	Postpartum
WBC	× 10^9/L	4.5 – 11	5 – 8	6 – 11	6 – 11	9 – 15	5 – 11
Neutrophil AB	× 10^9/L	1.4 – 7	1.4 – 4.6	3.6 – 6	3.8 – 8	3.9 – 10	1.4 – 7
Neutrophil	%	30 – 70	40 – 60	60 – 80	60 – 80	60 – 80	40 – 60
Lymphocyte AB	× 10^9/L	0.7 – 3.1	1.4 – 4.6	1.1 – 2.9	0.9 – 2.9	1.1 – 2.9	1.4 – 4.6
Lymphocyte	%	20 – 40	20 – 40	12 – 20	12 – 20	12 – 20	20 – 40
Monocyte AB	× 10^9/L	0.1 – 0.9	0.1 – 0.7	0.1 – 1.1	0.2 – 1.1	0.3 – 1.4	0.3 – 1.4
Monocyte	%	2 – 10	2 – 8	2 – 9	2 – 9	2 – 9	2 – 8
Eosinophil AB	× 10^9/L	0.0 – 0.4	0.0 – 0.6	0.0 – 0.6	0.0 – 0.6	0.0 – 0.6	0.0 – 0.6
Eosinophil	%	0 – 7	0 – 3	0 – 3	0 – 3	0 – 3	0 – 3
Basophil AB	× 10^9/L	0.0 – 0.2	0.0 – 0.1	0.0 – 0.1	0.0 – 0.1	0.0 – 0.1	0.0 – 0.1
Basophil	%	0 – 3	0 – 1	0 – 1	0 – 1	0 – 1	0 – 1
Immature Granulocytes AB	× 10^9/L	0.0 – 0.1	0.0 – 0.05	0.003 – 0.09	0.007 – 0.247	0.018 – 0.456	0.018 – 0.456
Immature Granulocytes	%	0 – 1	0 – 1	0 – 1	0.1 – 2	0.2 – 3.8	0.2 – 3.8
Platelet Count	× 10^9/L	150 – 450	150 – 450	150 – 250	150 – 350	150 – 350	150 – 450
MPV	fL	6.4 – 11	6.4 – 11	7.7 – 10.1	7.7 – 10.3	8.2 – 10.4	6.4 – 11
Prothrombin Time	seconds	9.1 – 12	9.1 – 12	8.9 – 12.2	8.6 – 12.1	8.7 – 12.1	9.1 – 12
Activated PTT	seconds	24 – 33	24 – 33	24 – 33	24 – 33	24 – 33	24 – 33
Fibrinogen	mg/dL	193 – 507	200 – 500	300 – 500	300 – 500	300 – 500	200 – 500
RBC	× 10^6/µL	3.77 – 5.28	3.9 – 5.28	4.3 – 4.6	4 – 4.2	3.9 – 4.4	3.9 – 5.28
Hemoglobin	g/dL	11.5 – 15	13.2 – 14.5	11 – 14	10.5 – 14	11 – 14	11 – 15
Hematocrit	%	34 – 46.6	36 – 46.6	33 – 40	32 – 39	33 – 40	36 – 46.6
MCV	fL	79 – 97	80 – 95	80 – 95	85 – 97	85 – 99	80 – 99
MCH	pg	26.6 – 33	27 – 32	30 – 32	30 – 33	29 – 32	27 – 32
MCHC	g/dL	31 – 36	31 – 36	31 – 36	31 – 36	31 – 36	31 – 36
RDW	%	11 – 15	11 – 13	11 – 13	11 – 14	11 – 15	11 – 13
Reticulocytes	%	0.5 – 2	0.5 – 1.5	1 – 3	1 – 2	1 – 2	0.5 – 2
nRBC	%	0	0	<4	N/A	<13	0 – 1
Erythropoietin	mIU/mL	2.6 – 18.5	2.6 – 18.5	12 – 25	13 – 44	13 – 62	3 – 70
Serum Iron	µg/dL	27 – 159	50 – 170	50 – 170	50 – 170	50 – 170	50 – 170
TIBC	µg/dL	250 – 450	250 – 450	135 – 408	302 – 519	380 – 597	250 – 450
UIBC	µg/dL	131 – 425	131 – 425	131 – 425	131 – 425	131 – 425	131 – 425
Transferrin Saturation	%	15 – 50	15 – 45	20 – 45	20 – 45	20 – 45	15 – 45
Ferritin	ng/mL	15 – 150	30 – 150	30 – 80	30 – 80	15 – 80	15 – 80
Copper	µg/dL	63 – 121	90 – 140	150 – 305	190 – 330	222 – 380	90 – 140
Ceruloplasmin	mg/dL	19 – 39	19 – 39	30 – 49	40 – 53	43 – 78	19 – 39
Serum Glucose	mg/dL	70 – 99	80 – 95	70 – 85	75 – 90	75 – 90	80 – 95
Hemoglobin A1c	%	4 – 5.6	5 – 5.6	4 – 5.4	4 – 5.4	4 – 5.7	5 – 5.6
Sodium	mmol/L	135 – 145	135 – 142	130 – 140	130 – 140	130 – 140	135 – 142
Potassium	mmol/L	3.5 – 5.2	4 – 4.5	3.6 – 5	3.6 – 5	3.6 – 5	4 – 4.5
Chloride	mmol/L	96 – 106	100 – 106	101 – 109	101 – 109	97 – 109	96 – 106

Functional Reference Ranges for Serum Indices in Pregnancy

Carbon Dioxide	mmol/L	20 - 29	25 - 30	18 - 26	18 - 26	18 - 26	20 - 30
Anion Gap	mmol/L	8 - 16	8 - 16	10 - 20	10 - 18	10 - 18	8 - 16
Calcium	mg/dL	8.7 - 10. 2	9.4 - 10	8.8 - 10.6	8.2 - 9	8.2 - 9.7	8.2 - 10
BUN	mg/dL	6 - 24	10 - 15	7 - 9	3 - 9	3 - 9	10 - 24
Serum Creatinine	mg/dL	0.57 - 1	0.49 - 1	0.4 - 0.7	0.4 - 0.66	0.4 - 0.66	0.49 - 1
BUN/Creatinine	:1	9 - 23	10 - 15	10 - 20	10 - 20	10 - 20	10 - 20
eGFR	mL/min/1.73 m2	>60	>90	131 - 166	135 - 170	117 - 182	>90
Uric Acid	mg/dL	8 - 16	3 - 5	2 - 4.1	2.4 - 4.9	3.1 - 6.3	3 - 5
Protein	g/dL	6 - 8.5	6 - 8.5	6.2 - 7.6	5.7 - 6.9	5.6 - 6.7	6 - 8.5
Albumin	g/dL	3.9 - 5	4 - 4.8	3.1 - 5.1	3.3 - 4.5	3.3 - 4.5	3.9 - 5
Globulin	g/dL	1.5 - 4.5	2.4 - 2.7	2.5 - 4.5	2.5 - 4.5	2.5 - 4.5	2.4 - 2.7
A/G Ratio	:1	1.2 - 2.2	1.5 - 2	1 - 2	1 - 2	1 - 2	1.5 - 2
Bilirubin	mg/dL	0.0 - 1.2	0.0 - 1.9	0.1 - 0.4	0.1 - 0.8	0.1 - 1.1	0.1 - 1.9
ALP	IU/L	44 - 121	50 - 121	45 - 120	100 - 320	100 - 320	50 - 121
AST/ SGOT	IU/L	0 - 40	10 - 30	10 - 30	10 - 30	10 - 30	10 - 40
ALT/SGPT	IU/L	0 - 32	10 - 30	10 - 20	10 - 20	10 - 25	10 - 40
LDH	IU/L	121 - 224	140 - 210	120 - 200	120 - 200	150 - 400	140 - 210
GGT	IU/L	0 - 65	10 - 30	2 - 23	4 - 22	3 - 26	10 - 30
Bile Acids	µmol/L	0 - 10	0 - 10	0 - 4.9	0 - 9.1	0 - 11	0 - 11
TSH	uIU/L	0.45 - 4.5	0.5 - 3	0.1 - 2.5	0.2 - 3	0.3 - 2.5	0.5 - 3
Thyroxine, Total	µg/dl	5 - 12	6 - 12.5	7.5 - 18	7.5 - 18	7.5 - 18	6 - 12. 5
Thyroxine, Free	ng/dL	0.82 - 1.77	1 - 1.9	0.8 - 1.2	0.6 - 1	0.5 - 0.8	1 - 1.9
T3, Total	ng/dL	71 - 180	80 - 190	92 - 218	112 - 278	111 - 265	80 - 190
T3, Free	pg/mL	2 - 4.4	2 - 4.4	4.1 - 4.4	4 - 4.2	4 - 4.2	2 - 4.4
Reverse T3	ng/dL	9.2 - 24.1	9.2 - 24.1	34.8 - 83.4	18.2 - 74.7	20.1 - 84.5	9.2 - 24.1
T3 uptake	%	24 - 39	27 - 39	24 - 39	24 - 39	24 - 39	27 - 39
FTI	µg/dL	4.8 - 12.7	4.8 - 12.7	5 - 10.5	5 - 10.5	5 - 10.5	4.8 - 12.7
TPOAb	IU/mL	<34	<34	<34	<34	<34	<34
TgAb	IU/mL	<9	<9	<9	<9	<9	<9
TRAb	IU/mL	<1.75	<1.75	<1.75	<1.75	<1.75	<1.75
Iodine, Serum	µg/L	40 - 92	70 - 110	70 - 110	70 - 110	70 - 110	70 - 110
Iodine, Urine Spot	µg/L	28 - 544	150 - 250	150 - 250	150 - 250	150 - 250	150 - 250
Iodine, Urine 24hr	µg/24hr	100 - 466	150 - 460	150 - 460	150 - 460	150 - 460	150 - 460
Iodine:Creatinine	µg/g	29 - 536	150 - 250	150 - 250	150 - 250	150 - 250	150 - 250
Progesterone	ng/mL	0.1 - 12	0.3 - 15	15 - 35	30 - 95	90 - 175	0.1 - 0.9
Vitamin D, 25OH	ng/mL	30 - 100	40 - 100	40 - 80	40 - 80	40 - 80	40 - 100
Vitamin B12	pg/mL	232 - 1,245	400 - 1,245	280 - 800	280 - 800	280 - 800	400 - 1,245
Methylmalonic Acid, Plasma	µmol/L	0 - 378	0 - 370	0.5 - 275	0.75 - 275	0.75 - 275	0 - 370
Methylmalonic Acid, Urine	µmol/mmol creatinine	0.3 - 2.8	0.4 - 2.5	0.4 - 2.5	0.4 - 3.5	0.4 - 3.5	0.4 - 2.5
Homocysteine	µmol/mmol crt	0 - 14.5	5 - 12	4 - 7.3	3.5 - 5.3	4 - 7.3	5 - 12
C-Reactive Protein	mg/L	0 - 10	0 - 10	0 - 10	0.2 - 10	0.2 - 10	0.2 - 10
ANA	1:	<1:80	<1:80	<1:80	<1:80	<1:80	<1:80

Additional References

1. Eidenier H. *Balancing Body Chemistry with Nutrition.* 10th ed. Balancing Body Chemistry with Nutrition LLC, 2017

2. Abbassi-Ghanavati, Mina MD; Greer, Laura G. MD; Cunningham, F Gary MD. Pregnancy and Laboratory Studies: A Reference Table for Clinicians. Obstetrics & Gynecology 114(6):p 1326–1331, December 2009. | DOI: 10.1097/AOG.0b013e3181c2bde8

3. Gronowski AM ed. *Handbook of Clinical Laboratory Testing During Pregnancy.* Totowa , NJ: Humana Press , 2004: 402–403

4. Wallach, J. Interpretation of Diagnostic Tests, Eighth ed. Lippincott Williams & Wilkins, 2007

5. Fischbach FT, Dunning MB III, eds. *A Manual of Laboratory and Diagnostic Tests, 7th ed.* Philadelphia, Lippincott Williams and Wilkins, 2004

About the Author

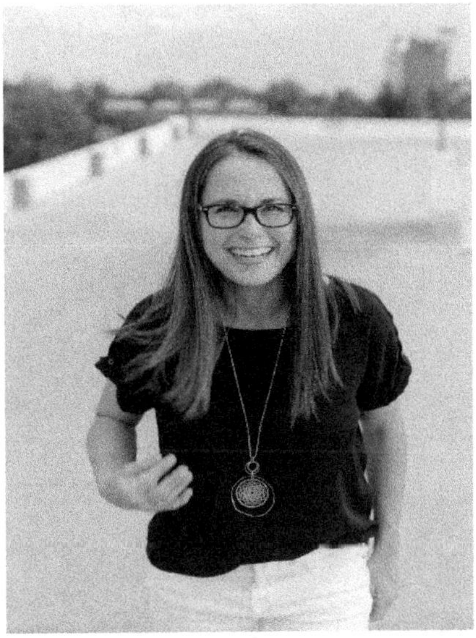

Sarah Thompson is a certified functional medicine practitioner, licensed acupuncturist, and doula. She began her career working alongside Western physicians, learning the value of collaboration in patient treatment success. She opened her private practice in 2012 with a passion for educating and empowering women to thrive throughout their childbearing years.

In 2021, she published her first book, *Functional Maternity: Using Functional Medicine and Nutrition to Improve Pregnancy and Childbirth Outcomes.*

Sarah currently runs a functional medicine clinic in Fort Collins, Colorado, lectures, and provides accredited continuing education courses for professionals.

Contact Information

Email: Hello@FunctionalMaternity.com
Instagram: @Functional.Maternity
Website: FunctionalMaternity.com

www.ingramcontent.com/pod-product-compliance
Lightning Source LLC
LaVergne TN
LVHW081942200926
848484LV00009B/2496